Food Beautiful

By Sarah King Feldman, BS
Forward by Dr. C. William Feldman, D.C.

Jenny + Demetri-
I love you so much.
You are so beautiful and enjoyable
to have as a beloved friend.
You are powerful beyond
measure. Live in Abundance.

For related titles and support materials, visit our online catalogue at www.foodbeautiful.com

Cover Design by Angelia Siverton

ISBN 1-4276-1273-0
First printing, December 2006

CIP data available from the Library of Congress

PRINTED IN THE UNITED STATES OF AMERICA

FORWARD

The Missing Link!? How do we live longer? Stay younger? Look more beautiful? Perform better? Every week in our wellness clinic we have people asking these questions and more. We all want to be full of energy, vitality, look great, and livelong! Doctors agree! "Everyone should read this book and apply the principles inside." Every doctor that has read this book has said that same thing!

This book covers a missing link in most of our lives and if applied will give you and your family amazing results. At the start this was an attempt by Sarah to fill one of the voids in our wellness clinic and it soon turned into a magnificent work. So many people were wondering what to eat, how to make it, where to buy it, and why they had not learned this before.

This is the only book of its kind! Everyone will enjoy this work from beginners to advanced it is an essential in every home in America! Sarah has brilliantly made this as a user-friendly book that can be used as a reference guide, instructional handbook, and I will not be surprised if it becomes a high school or college curriculum.

As a Doctor I have always searched for the best solution to a patient's problem. One of the major trends I saw as I was just starting practice was the rapidly increasing numbers of victims of disease and obesity. President Richard Nixon declared, "War on Cancer" when 1 out of 20 people were getting it, now the rumors are that 1 of 2 people will suffer from the ravaging effects of cancer. Heart Disease, Diabetes, Alzheimer's and about every other ailment is on a rapid rise and it is time for us to take control of our life and health and live life to our optimal potential. Most doctors and health professionals will agree that we are in a crisis and we need to go back to the basics!

There are a few principles that we can cling to that are the basics of life. We need clean air, pure water, nutrient rich food, proper neurological communication, a positive mental attitude, exercise and rest. They are so simple yet easily forgotten! The better the quality and balance of these principles the better the results in life you will have.

Food is such an amazing subject! I love food since many of my childhood memories, experiences with friends, and many travels have etched exquisite smells and tastes into my mind. To me taste and nutrition are very important and thanks to Sarah they can be found together. To most the conception is that "health" food is bland, filled with tofu, and unsatisfying. Well if that's what you think you are in for a Surprise! Just wait until you try some of the recipes in this book that are sure to become family favorites along with learning why your body craves certain foods and what you might be able to substitute for that junk food you might crave.

The best way to overcome disease and dis-ease is to stay healthy, fit and full of vitality. This book will get you and your family on that road and give you a great road map to follow! We were not born to be sick and tired, we were born to live and make a difference!

Oh one other thing. We all know too many people that are sick and dying too fast, we also know that the "things" that are good for us are not advertised very much since they don't make others a bunch of money! As a well-known comedian has said, "There ain't no money in a cure!" It is our social responsibility to help our fellow brothers and sisters our neighbors and friends. If you are like me you love to help others so as I read through this book I put the names of people I thought of on the borders so I could remember to tell them about this book and how it may help them or their family.

I cannot think of a better way to start turning this countries health around and it can start with us! When you find out how great the results you can achieve and how valuable this book can be if applied you will know that this information is far too valuable to not share! It is rare to find such a simple gift to share with someone that if applied can change their life and the lives of those around them in such a dramatic way! What if applying this book could give you just one more day on earth would it be worth it? Would your grandchildren or friends appreciate it? The possibilities are endless when you get rid of the roadblocks in your life that are holding you back. I still believe that if we all work together we can make this world a better place! Remember as Sarah says, "You were Born to be Beautiful!"

-Dr C. William Feldman DC
Founder, Feldman Wellness Centers
Founder & CEO, DoctorBeautiful.com

ACKNOWLEDGMENTS

This Book is dedicated to my husband and best friend, Dr. Will Feldman, who has believed in my mission and allowed me the means to accomplish it. Special Thanks to: Michael & Mary King; Dad, you never cease to amaze me with your knowledge and endless love!! Mom, you're desire to give never ceases. Michelle & Troy Warrick (Michelle, I will always look up to you!!), Alyssa King (you're so precious to me), Matt and Nicole King (you both have great strength and endurance!), Joe and Julie King (Joe, your blessings will always be cherished), Chuck and Marge Feldman (for being my second set of parents), Al & Carol Sparber ("one more question") and the McCain Family.

To my closest friends who have all inspired me; Dr. Tom Feldman, James and Mark Aleks, Stephanie Mullen (you're my sweetness), Chris & Hannah Knopping (we can live under any situation-in tents), Trent & Taylor Minshall (forever friends), Anna Graciela Medina, Alexandro & Faye, Chris Graham, Alan Kirk (my photo man), Angelia Sivertson (what a crush), Ashley & Manda Faherty, Biju (crazy Indian Chef), Britony Wilhelm (your prayers rock!), Elizabeth Reidel (best spiritual massage therapist ever!!), Cheri Stevenson, the entire King clan, Grandma Betty, Gram Lockwood, Jonathon & Brittony Keyser, Isaac Bunny, Junior, Angie & Luke Pucket (my second home), the Turano family, Shawn Crull, Emma Peters, Jenny Zehr, Isaac Slade (the best music ever), Joe Q, Travis Daniels, Michelle Staich, Kyle Kirby (next su-chef), Charlie Walk (you're too generous), Mike Flynn, Jason Ienner, Margo Plotkin, Marie King, Melody Braden, Allen & Nancy Gobel, Rico Cortez, Rosalinda Baca (Overcomer!), Silence & Nat Weeks, Joby Weeks (the Manna-man), Tom and Linda Phillips, Will Nuessle, and all my lovable clients. ALL have inspired me to be bold and give of myself without restraint.

It is my passion to help inform everyone who seeks to find truth, health, wealth, God and true joy in their lives. Most of all I give all the credit and glory to my heavenly Father, the Creator of the Universe, Who created this earth for our benefit.

May this book bring to you Abundant Health, Life, Love, Joy, and Prosperity Through the Creator of the Universe!!

CONTENTS

9 *Food Beautiful Recipes:*

1
Introduction

Dying to Be Told"

Your whole wheat and milk is killing you!! And you think your fortified, low-fat, high protein bars make you healthy? You already know you can't grow a plant in chocolate milk! So how do you grow? What you don't know is literally killing you.....As this was the case of my father in the winter of 96'. I was in my freshman year at C.U. Boulder, jamming along to tunes, studying for final exams week, daydreaming about stuffing my face with mom's homemade turkey and stuffing. It was about Thanksgiving time and my heart felt the excitement of going home. At this stage in my life nothing really worried me. I was fairly confidant that my life was going to be perfect!! No bumps, just a smooth road ahead. Well, I was in for the worst shock of my life. My Mom called me and cut right to the chase, "Sarah!" she said without letting me answer, "Your Dad has been diagnosed with stage three colon cancer!" I was speechless. I had no idea what cancer was. I knew cancer was bad, but I had no idea there were stages to this disease. There was no way my dad could be sick. He ran everyday, ate fruits and vegetables and loved God with all his heart. I said back to my mother, "He couldn't have cancer; he's done nothing to deserve it!" --- Exactly!!

He did nothing to prevent cancer, because no one ever educated him about prevention. We were taught that when you got sick you went to the doctor, he gave you some pills and in a couple of days you felt better. This time a pill wouldn't fix the damage. I was an emotional wreck for the next week-perfect timing for finals week. All I wanted was to be right beside my Dad. All my concentration was on worrying about what might happen to my Dad. My mom called me almost every hour to give me reports, which continued to fuel my fear and cause me more tears. My Father was told the only way to attempt recovery was by taking out one foot of his colon and then most likely start on chemotherapy. So, naively he plunged into what almost became his death sentence, in complete belief and trust that the doctors would fix everything. By the third dose of chemotherapy he was on his deathbed! My unbreakable father was broken; he lost 50 pounds in less than a month, looked like a Holocaust survivor, and needed help getting up and going to the bathroom. He began to realize that he wasn't dying from the cancer but was dying from the chemotherapy. Fortunately their method wasn't working! I say this because this is what brought him to find God's healing method.

He believed in the Divine power that God created within him, the innate wisdom, to heal himself. He chose to stop everything the doctor prescribed to him. He started to reeducate himself with books on Alternative healing and Medicine and hired a Naturopathic Doctor to begin educating and helping him. He threw himself into the search for truth and life, spending hours studying health books, researching on line and learning from experienced friends. He started on a 7-day Cleanse (very similar to the "Total Body Cleanse" as in this book), changed his diet to 80% raw / 20% cooked, proper food combining, took supplements and started to change his mindset. And within a 3-month period he was more vibrant and healthy than I had ever seen him look. He had loads of energy, was super fit, had radiant skin and most of all had a new passion and zest for the meaning of life. It was at this point I realized that food was a fundamental part in his healing process.

It is more than obvious that the western mindset and diet wouldn't prevent me or anyone else from getting cancer. Like my Dad's new passion for life, my new quest was to educate myself. With all his trial and error, I wanted to learn how to make healing foods taste amazing, yet still retain their healing properties. So I started learning what healing ingredients could replace the lesser quality ingredients in common foods. I was determined to learn why the body becomes sick and how God naturally heals it. I began daily investigations with hundreds of journal articles, diet plans, homeopathic books, integrative nutrition, and health magazines that started my journey. This opened my eyes to the lies we have been fed and are still being fed. I decided to stop living in ignorance, and made it my mission to seek out the truth and follow it.

This book is the culmination of all the research I've done in the field of "True Health". I pray this information reaches millions, so others won't have to go through what my Father went through (P.S. He has been cancer free since that time). What greater gift than to give life and get life.

May the words of my mouth, the foods I prepare bring healing to your body!

2

Food Beautiful Principles

FOOD BEAUTIFUL PRINCIPLES

"Did anyone ever tell you how beautiful you look when you're looking for what's beautiful in someone else?" -Anonymous

See, I have given you every herb that yields seed which is on the face of all the earth, and every tree whose fruit yields seed; to you it shall be for food   -Genesis 1:29

"Let your food be your medicine and your medicine your food."
                     - Father of Modern Medicine, Hippocrates.

You are an incredibly, sound and perfect being created in the likeness of God. You are perfect, beautiful, strong and full of abundant life. If you don't feel this way, than look deep into the principles and chapters of this book for answers that can reshape your outer and inner beauty. It is the rhythm of the right action creating momentum that gives power to your life! "Whatever a man sows, that he will also reap" Galatians 6:7. In the same fashion a Food Beautiful lifestyle requires effort to till the soil, plant the seeds, to nourish it so life may produce sweet aromatic fruit!! It is just the opposite that unhealthy life and actions produce rotten fruit that is sickly and unattractive. So as Hippocrates said, "Let your food be your medicine and your medicine your food." Honor this gift of life you've been given, create room for change and see the blessings you begin to manifest in your life.

Each of us sees the need for change all around us. Many of our friends and loved ones are laden with disease and Dis-Ease. Together we have a vision to empower millions of people to seek preventative health care methods and educational tools to reach physical and spiritual freedom. We cannot do this alone; we need your help!! We have found that those who share Food Beautiful Principles with others around them tend to manifest them in their own lives more abundantly. When we focus on blessing others, our lives naturally become more enriched physically, spiritually and monetarily. Start by planting seeds; give someone a book or teach them Food Beautiful Principles and watch the blessings unfold in your life and theirs. There are more than enough blessings to go around for all to give and receive in excess.

You already know that your life is worth more than diamonds and gold, and so are billions of others! Help us meet the challenge to get these truths out to millions of people around the world. We can not do it alone; we need your help and support. We envision sharing to the masses by use of the internet, radio, and television (and I believe Oprah would have an open heart to broadcast these truths) to reach and educate millions of amazing people. It is true that you were created in the image of God and you were born to be beautiful!! So, let us be a tree of life alongside living waters so we bear sweat aromatic fruit for others to taste and see!

"If you have a sound diet, of what use is a doctor? And, if you don't have a sound diet of what use is a doctor."   -Proverb in Ayurvedic Medical Tradition

"Beloved I pray that you may prosper in all things and be in health, just as your soul prospers."   3 John 2

Start by believing and applying one principle at a time and you will start manifesting the blessings the Creator of the Universe desired for you to receive. You deserve the best so don't let your negative self-talk get in the way. Allow this book to be an instrument to help empower your body and mind. This book is meant to empower you, giving you strategies and principles that will enable you to achieve greatness in your life.

Principle 1: Overcome the Mind

Principle 2: Cleanse the Body

Principle 3: Honor Your Food Source

Principle 4: Eat Volumes of

Fruits & Vegetables

Principle 5: Consume Healing Waters

Principle 6: Exercise with Purpose

Begin by adding one principle every 21 days and you will make lasting results. When you begin to apply ALL Food Beautiful Principles to your diet, you will see results within a couple of weeks. Remember if you ever fall of the Diet you are one meal away from getting back on track.

PRINCIPLE 1: OVERCOME THE MIND

Keep your thoughts positive because...Your beliefs become your thoughts. Your thoughts become your words. Your words become your actions. Your actions become your values. Your values become your destiny.

-Mahatma Gandhi

The foundations to a sound diet begin within your mind! What sets you apart from someone who is fit, youthful, vibrant and healthy? The difference is their mind believes they can have and deserve any goal they desire. Your mind is a powerful force that translates thoughts into their physical counterparts. It is your inner thoughts and beliefs coupled with outward action that bring you abundance or limitation. So if you believe yourself to be fat, ugly, poor, sick, worthless, then you will surely be just that. Begin today to allow your mind to let go of past failures, and start discovering the power of self suggestion that can harness the mind to believe whatever you so desire to be or have.

Begin by changing your inner thoughts and beliefs from what you don't want to what you want. And be specific!! For example "I will be a size 6 in 3 months because I love to eat a pound of vegetables and run 3 miles every day." It doesn't matter if you don't know the exact way in which you will achieve your goal, as that will come. Make your focus to believe your goal will be accomplished. Begin to activate the power of your mind to manifest these desires by visualizing, emotionalizing, believing and acting upon those goals. When you start to hear yourself say negative thoughts, stop yourself and correct those thoughts. If you are constantly entertaining negative thoughts, you will be, have and attract just that. Your life is the exact mirror of your inner self-talk. It may seem at first like a chore to monitor your thoughts, but soon you will start retraining your subconscious mind to believe you can achieve anything.

It takes active thinking, active organization and active action to attract what you want. Victor Frankel states, "Man's last great freedom of mankind is to choose your attitude under any given circumstances." So you must act now, don't delay, don't second-guess or doubt! When the opportunity, desire and impulse are there -- act upon it! Don't worry about how you will achieve your goal as you may not know exactly how to do it, but your willingness to align your thoughts with your desires and by the "Law of Attraction" you will naturally attract that goal. Martin Luther said, "Take the first step in faith; you don't have to see the whole staircase, just take the first step."

Principle Focus 1:

Start making a list of goals, what you want to receive and achieve this month, in 6 months and this year. Write these 5-10 goals down and put them where you can see them every day. Be very specific and clear about your desires, as this will help you pin down exactly what you want. Then set aside time every night, when there are no distractions, and allow your mind to nurture and manifest your desires. Spend this time visualizing and emotionalizing those goals and desires. Soon enough your body will manifest these thoughts into action, as long as you believe. Begin your sentences with words like; "I am..." "I act as if I..." or "I will be..." And soon enough your mind will start to believe, and you will start becoming what you have always known you could become. Now allow God to continue opening the power of your mind, building up in you the belief and promise of his blessings for you that will fulfill the desires of your heart and be manifested in your life.

PRINCIPLE 2: CLEANSE THE BODY

Detoxifying and Cleansing can be an uplifting experience, cleaning out areas of the body and mind that are stagnant and sick. Almost every religious and healing tradition recommends cleansing and fasting for physical and spiritual health. Cleansing is the way in which the body cleanses out, neutralizes or transforms toxins to be excreted out of the body. Our body produces toxins from and through normal metabolism of our food, air, water, stress, exercise and thoughts. These toxins can inflame cells and tissues, blocking normal healthy functions of the body. Toxicity occurs when we take in more than our body can utilize. Common toxicity symptoms include: backache, fatigue, headache, congestion, aching swollen joints, digestive problems, food allergies, seasonal allergies, sensitivity to the surrounding environment, and all types of diseases and illnesses. These toxins are what cause the body to hold onto weight, disease, stress, sickness, depression and unforgiveness. Many have never cleansed out the enormous amount of toxins sitting within their organs, tissues and cells.

Principle Focus 2:

If you want to let go of these issues, make it your goal to do a cleanse within the next 21 days. Choose one of the cleanses listed in the Cleanse and Detoxify Chapter. Please use caution if you currently have severe symptoms or known toxicity. Consult a healthcare provider first before starting any program. When you detoxify and cleanse you will experience greater health, vitality, energy, happiness, clarity and purpose in life. By cleansing you will naturally progress to begin eating a clean and healthy diet.

PRINCIPLE 3: HONOR YOUR FOOD SOURCE

Choose fresh organic whole foods to put into your temple. You were created divinely and need to honor what the earth created perfectly for you. Use foods that look closest to their original state. Man-made food is inferior for you! The less processed the more beautiful you will become. Use the Perfect Source shopping list in the Real Food Source Chapter to guide you into purchasing and making good food choices. God said, " See, I have given you every herb that yields seed which is on the face of all the earth, and every tree whose fruit yields seed; to you it shall be for food" Genesis 1:29.

Principle Focus 3:

Eat organic food as much as possible. Avoid eating fake-foods and unhealthy foods that are listed for you in The Real Food Source Chapter. Learn and add quality ingredients that replace the inferior food sources. Make your daily allowance of fake-foods or unhealthy foods at no more than 150 calories a day or 1,500 per week. Each week replace one unhealthy food item with one healthy food item.

PRINCIPLE 4: EAT VOLUMES OF FRUITS AND VEGETABLES

Eat foods dense in nutrients and in good combination! When you sit down to eat a meal, choose organic fruits and vegetables before any other food. Your appetite is controlled by high fiber nutrient-dense foods.

Listed in order are the foods highest in nutrients per calorie:

1- Raw Leafy Greens
2- Solid Green Vegetables
3- Non-green Vegetables
4- Beans and Legumes
5- Fresh Fruit
6- Grains
7- Nuts & Seeds

The more green foods you eat the more weight you will loose. You will require less food to be satisfied and find yourself being full much earlier in your meal (as long as you add the green leafy vegetables first). There is a favorable mix of all known essential nutrients found in a balanced whole-food diet. On the Food Beautiful Program you are not dieting, you are eating!! You don't need to count calories, just focus on consuming nutrient-dense foods before any other food.

As the principle does not focus on what to avoid, it is still important to have an understanding of what foods are low in nutrients comparatively to the top seven nutrient-dense foods. It is true that low-nutrient foods are not lacking in carbohydrate, fat and protein calories, they are lacking in vitamins, minerals and phytonutrients. These high calorie foods alone will not satisfy your body's hunger even though they fill you up. Just remember that any weight problem is not from the inability to control oneself, it's from malnourishment and deficiency. These foods will make you want more food, because you are not being nourished. Lack of nourishment from these foods will contribute to poor health, disease, obesity, fatigue etc. Some examples of low-nutrient foods are canned foods, bagels, chips, candy, pop, white rice, white flour, sugar, ice-cream, pasteurized dairy, red meat, chicken, turkey, fried foods, breads and pastries. (You can read more about these foods in the Fake Foods Section.) You already know these foods aren't good for you, and are extremely deficient in vitamins, minerals, essential fatty acids and amino acids. Fortunately there are healthier alternatives to low-nutrient foods which should still be eaten minimally, and, after nutrient-dense foods. Here are some foods that are healthier counterparts: organic meats, wild harvested and cold-water fish, sprouted grain breads, xylitol (sugar-substitute), organic dark chocolate (dairy free), brown rice crackers etc. Look at the options listed for you in the Perfect Source Shopping list.

Now take out a piece of paper; draw a line strait down the middle, dividing the paper in half. In the left column label it low-nutrient foods. In this column write down what low-nutrient foods you eat for breakfast, lunch, snack time and dinner. Then in the right column label this nutrient-dense foods I eat every day. Here you will take the foods listed above and write them next to the low-nutrient foods you will replace them with. Take your goals list, your food replacement list, and five motivating quotes from this book, copy them and tape this to your bathroom mirror, refrigerator, car stereo, computer, cupboards, closet door and at work. Read this every time you see it!! Then at night take 15 minutes to say these things, visualize yourself doing them, emotionalize the feeling of doing them, and you will start seeing amazing changes occur in your life. It is the action that produces the result!! Have these goals memorized so that if someone woke you up in the middle of the night, asking you, "What do you want most in life?" you would be able to say it without second-guessing.

Principle Focus 4:

The first foods into your mouth should be those highest in nutrient density. Make it a daily goal to consume 1 head of roman lettuce or spinach a day. Don't worry how you will do it just make it your goal and believe you can do it, and it will happen. Read your goals list every time you see it!! Then at night take 15 minutes to say these things, visualize you doing them and emotionalize them. Then keep low-nutrient foods to no more than 150 calories a day and you will see and feel the difference.

PRINCIPLE 5: CONSUME HEALING WATERS

Adequate hydration with improper water can cause your body to become a storehouse for sickness. The simple act of properly hydrating the body with water is extremely ineffective with the myriads of chemicals, hormones, viruses, and bacteria in it. However, using properly structured healing waters can greatly improve and rid the body of most disease.

Depending on what part of the country one resides, it is easy to find trace amounts of chlorination byproducts, organics, nitrates, pesticides, heavy metals, radioactive compounds, petrochemicals and parasites coming from the local municipal water supply. If you get your water from a private well, all of these contaminants except for the chlorination byproducts can be present. The toxins and free radicals in these waters are made significantly more toxic to humans by the addition of chlorine, a compound mandated by the public health department. The Environmental Protection Agency now reports that individuals who drink and bath in chlorinated surface waters (i.e., water from lakes, rivers and shallow wells) have a 50% greater likelihood of getting cancer in their lifetime. [1] [2] Even if you think you are safe because you drink bottled water, you may be surprised to learn that one can absorb up to 600% more contaminants in your body in a ten-minute shower than in all the water consumed in a day. [3] Chlorine gas had been banned from warfare long ago, but each morning we get up and shower in a hot steam bath of that same substance. Yet water is an essential element for our health and existence.

Water is the basic foundation for great health since that your body is over 70% water. Unfortunately not all water is created equal, and further more, the majority of people drink junk liquids that are caffeinated, carbonated and alcoholic causing the body to manifest life-threatening illnesses in bizarre ways. Improper hydration manifests itself into diseases like high blood pressure, high cholesterol, thyroid disorders, liver disease, constipation, autoimmune diseases, fibromyalgic pain, sleep disorders, joint aches, fatigue, hypertension, edema, acne, lupus, migraines, sinusitis, obesity, headaches, allergies, depression, anxiety, type 2 diabetes, Parkinson's disease, Alzheimer's, lymphoma, angina, heartburn, back pain, colitis, cancer and many more!!! So instead of hydrating with healing water, people take drugs that further dehydrate their body and exacerbate their illnesses.

What makes water good or bad for the body? There is a measuring scale called the "stability index" that indicates how stable water is in relation to the chemical and minerals in its environment. Water naturally seeks to have a zero index. If water has a positive stability index, it will release or precipitate minerals that are dissolved in it. A good example of how this occurs in water is when a water pipe develops deposits on the side leading to clogged pipes. A negative stability index has an aggressive action of dissolving minerals and metals from its environment. You see evidence of this when water corrodes or rusts the water pipes. Unfortunately distilled and reverse osmosis water has a negative stability index which can strip the body of calcium, magnesium, trace minerals etc. These types of water are good for short term use to detoxify the body but can cause long term health risks if used for more than a month at a time. The more mineral loss the greater the risk for osteoporosis, osteo-arthritis, hypothyroidism, coronary artery disease, high blood pressure etc.

So where can we find true healing water sources available for our consumption? Many health institutes, doctors, sports and fitness centers, and clinics around the world are now recommending a new Japanese filter system called Wellness Filter®. It has been shown to remove contaminants such as chlorination byproducts, MTBE chlorine, radioactive contaminants, pesticides, estrogens and many other toxic chemicals. The filter has multiple layers of purification and enhancement that add reduced ions producing a mild antioxidant effect, adding additional trace minerals that enhance cellular and biological function; has a natural resistance to the growth of harmful bacteria and fungi; increases the rate of hydration of the skin and tissue accelerating the rate of nutrient absorption into the bloodstream. Users have reported a noticeable increase of improved energy in all areas of health including improved digestion, natural elimination and weight loss.

In Japan many doctors routinely prescribe the water filter system to their patients to aid the body in fighting specific chronic conditions. The Chinese government conducted an international competition of water purification systems around the world and chose the Wellness Filter® as the number one in the world. And it became the first water filter system to be exhibited in the prestigious Smithsonian Institute.

By using natural purification processes in combination with advanced technology, the Wellness Filter® produces what many believe is the best drinking water on Earth right in your own home. The Wellness Filter® not only removes harmful contaminants but it also enhances the water through a patented process that creates a quality of water beyond the reach of conventional water filters. To order and get more information go to doctorbeautiful.com and place your order for a house system, sink system or shower unit today.

Principle Focus 5:

Start consuming and showering with healing water that hydrates, protects, nourishes and heals your body from illnesses. Drink a minimum of 2 liters of Wellness water a day which equals about a little less than 2 x 32 oz. drinking bottles worth of liquid. Keep carbonated alcoholic, sugar laden beverages to a minimum or omit them all together. Enjoy the healing benefits of showering daily in purified water as your skin is the largest organ that, on contact, absorbs almost every thing. As you already know, great products from Wellness Filters ® should replace your outdated purification and reverse osmosis house systems and shower units. "We must pay respect to water, and feel love and gratitude, and receive vibrations with a positive attitude. Then water changes, you change, and I change. Because both you and I are water." - Masaru Emoto author of New York Times best seller <u>The Hidden Messages in Water</u>.

[1] "Cancer Incidence and Trihalomethane Concentrations in the Public Drinking Water System", George L. Carlo. <u>American Journal of Public Health</u>, Vol. 74, No. 5, 1984, pp. 479-484.

[2] "Organic Chemical Contaminants in Drinking Water and Cancer", <u>American Journal of Epidemiology</u>, Vo. 110, 1979, p.420. [3] "Showers Pose a Risk to Health", Ian Anderson, New Scientist, 9/18/86 .

PRINCIPLE 6: EXERCISE WITH PURPOSE

Your body is designed to move and work at various intensity levels to produce strength, abundant health, joyfulness and success in life. We all know we need to exercise, but some of us still ignore the body's requirement for it. If you want an abundant life, you must give energy to get it! When you allow complacency into your life, this opens the door to slavery and you become a prisoner in your own body. Out of complacency come frustration, self-hatred, self-doubt, fear, stress, depression, disease, anger and sickness.

Does this sound like a life you want? On the flip side, with every negative thought there is a positive one. You can turn your complacency into action, with commitment. Physical action promotes self-love, self- belief, faith, joy, strength, passion, success and abundance. When you ignite action into your life, it makes you feel good and the more you do it, the more it makes you feel good and the more you do it... I think you get the idea! At any moment you can start a new life with a shift in your thoughts and action. You can either choose to move forward or sit back and watch your life pass you by. As I would say, "Don't let your past keep you from your future."

Your body was created to adapt to the stress and environment you place it under. When you participate in exercise, the forces you apply will cause you to get stronger, leaner and healthier. However, to reach the adaptation level, you must push through the uncomfortable stages. When you reach a peak and have become fully adapted, you will need to again increase the intensity and duration of your exercise to see further results, until you reach your desired health, beauty and weight. At this point you can maintain your workout schedule.

The key to exercising is to make sure you are doing it effectively. By doing so, you will ensure that all your hard work and time is not wasted and is having a positive effect on your body. To aid you in your efforts, there are three important variables to exercising:

- Length of time
- Frequency (times you workout per week)
- Intensity (workload)

Your exercise program should have a building stage of 6 weeks where you gradually increase workout time, frequency and intensity. Then follow this with the 7th week at half the workout intensity, time, and frequency. Then you will start the cycle all over again. Keep cycling the building periods every 6 weeks with the 7th week at half the time, frequency and intensity.

To better understand what intensity level you should reach you will need to understand the "talk test" measure. If you are able to talk without getting winded, you aren't working out hard enough. You will want to exercise hard enough so that you have a difficult time talking or carrying on a conversation with someone. Once you reach that level and you begin to feel it get too hard, you'll need to back off slightly. This is going to be your optimum training level. This means that walking will not work for everybody, unless you are walking up a strong incline, for periods of 30 minutes or more. You should have 2 workouts a week at the "talk test" level. Then you should have 2 workouts a week above the "talk test" level. For people exercising for 30 minutes and still having weight gain, you will need to increase the time to 60 minutes a day. If you are just starting to exercise you will gradually build up time and intensity over 6 weeks.

To more accurately measure your fitness level and intensity zone for workouts, you will need to know the following:

- Maximum Heart Rate (MHR) = 220 – Your Age.
- Fat-burning Zone (FUR) = 55 to 75% MHR
- Performance Enhancement Rate (PER) = 75 – 85% MHR

Maximum Heart Rate is the number of beats per minute your heart should not exceed during exercise. The safe zone for exercise is the Fat-burning Zone (FUR) = 55 to 75% MHR. Most people should shoot for 2 workouts a week in the 55% MHR Zone. While the higher intensity workouts should be at the 75% MHR Zone. For those who are experienced athletes, you can make your high intensity days at the Performance Enhancement Rate (PER) = 75 – 85% MHR.

<u>Example of how to calculate the Zone Heart Rates</u>
Age: 40
MHR: 220- 40 = 180 BPM (Beats Per Minute)
FUR: 55 – 75% of 180 = 99 – 135 BPM
PER: 75 – 85% of 180 = 135 – 153 BPM

For beginners or those who have not been working out, start out with 15 minutes of aerobic exercise 4 days a week. Each week you will add five minutes onto each workout until you have reached your desired time of 30 minutes or more of exercise. As a rule of thumb never dramatically bump up your exercise time, as this could lead to injury or lack of follow through. When you have completed the first 6 weeks of workouts, make the 7th week a back-off week as explained previously. At this point you can start adding intervals into your workout program. You can do this if you are running, walking, using the elliptical, doing aerobics, cycling or doing any other aerobic activity.

For the already active adult, begin adding interval workouts 2 times a week to your schedule of 4 or more workouts a week. Interval workouts are workouts that have a short period of high intensity followed by a recovery period of lower intensity. This produces a thermogenic response in the body to continue burning fat after you have worked out for about 6-8 hours. You can vary the length of your time by adding more or less time to your interval period of the workout. The more in shape you get the more time you will want for your interval time.

Beginner Level Intervals
5 min. easy warm up,
12 min. x (1 min. *above* "talk test" / 2 min. *at* "talk test" level)
5 min. cool down

Intermediate Level Intervals
7-10 minute easy warm up
20- 25 min. x (1 min. above "talk test" level / 1:30 min. at "talk test" level)
7-10 min. cool down

Advanced Level Intervals
10 min. warm up
25- 35 min. x (1 min. above "talk test: / 1 min. at "talk test" level)
10 min. cool down

Personalize Your Workout Routine:

1. Calculate MHR, FUR, and PER zones.
2. Pick an exercise.
3. Start the workout with 5-10 minutes of warm-up.
4. After the warm-up, increase the speed, tension or incline so you can reach desired zone.
5. End the workout with 5-10 minutes cool down.
6. Track your workouts by recording time, speed and intensity.

Principle Focus 6:

When you participate in exercise, the forces you apply will cause you to get stronger, leaner and healthier. The key to exercising is to make sure you are doing it effectively, with the proper length of time, frequency and intensity. Your exercise program should have a building stage of 6 weeks followed by a back-off period in the 7th week at half the time, frequency and intensity. Never go beyond your maximum heart rate zone. Use the Fat Burning Zones to tailor the intensity of your workouts. Beginners staying in the FUR zone and more experienced adult can use the PER zone for their higher intensity workouts. Create your own workout program using the information provided to you in this chapter.

3

Detoxify & Cleanse Your Body

Why Cleanse?

Since the early Biblical times, people have been abstaining from food, fasting and cleansing for many reasons including health, political ends and spiritual enlightenment. However, in our day and age the average person has no idea how to do a cleanse, let alone understand that most of their problems were created by their choices or lack of action. We can create healthy bodies and minds by eliminating the highly toxic foods and using the right foods. The better the mental and physical condition of a person, the higher the "vibration" of their cells become. Sick and dying cells do not vibrate with life; they do not move thus become magnets for disease, sickness and death. The person with a toxic free body and sound mind is the person unaffected by epidemics.

Cleansing is an excellent way of riding the body of toxins like pesticides, chemicals, parasites, artificial flavors, preservatives, artificial colors, rancid oils, and pollutants that are stored in various organs, cells and in fat tissue. Symptoms of toxic overload include digestive problems, joint pain, headaches, low energy, allergic reactions, asthma, allergies, anxiety, depression, mental confusion and disease. Cleansing is an opportunity for new beginnings, to recuperate, renew and regroup lost energy and health. For optimal health a cleanse is recommended once in the spring and once in the fall. If you have never done a cleanse before, this may be a challenge and uncomfortable for you. If you have been diagnosed with an illness and/or are taking drugs, cleansing should be done under the direct supervision of a health practitioner.

During the cleanse you may experience nausea, headaches, dizziness, extreme hunger and feverish-like chills. This is the body responding to major toxic overload. This may not happen to you but you should be aware when starting a cleanse.

Which cleanse is the best for your condition and how long should you do a cleanse? The Total Body Detox works on cleaning the liver, intestines, gallbladder and all the body's cells. This Detox can be done for up to seven days. The lemonade diet is meant to open the cells up to release toxins and allow weak organs and tissues to begin healing. The Parasite Detox is for those who know they have parasites in the blood, organs, colon and/or tissues. A doctor friend of mine that does dark field microscopy of the blood stated, "7 out of 10 people have parasites or fungus in their blood." I have laid out cleanses in this chapter for various conditions to get you jump started on your new life -- today!!

The length of the cleanse depends on your current condition and commitment level. The longer you cleanse the body the longer lasting and more effective the results will be. For first timers that have no life threatening conditions I suggest the Total Body Detox for 3 days. For those with serious health issues I suggest either the Lemonade Cleanse for a minimum of 10 days or the Total Detox for 7 days. As a rule of thumb when starting a cleanse of more than 3 days, you need to prepare your body for the process. Three days prior to doing the cleanse start by eating only fresh/raw vegetable, fruits, and seeds, abstaining from meats and heavy meals. During the cleanse use only distilled water as this helps reduce hunger pains; the molecules of purified, spring or tap water causes the body to search for food.

When completed with the fast, you need to allow yourself 2-3 days of transition to allow the colon to relearn how to digest whole foods. If you eat too soon, the body will experience digestion overload and will result in toxins being produced by any undigested food. The first day after the fast you should stick to juices (used during the cleanse) in the morning and afternoon, with clear organic soup broth and some protein powder (optional) in the evening. The second day after the fast you may have 1/2 a raw grapefruit or apple in the morning, followed by juices (same ones used during the cleanse) until mid afternoon. In the evening you may have lightly steamed veggies and clear organic soup broth. By the third day you may resume a diet of raw fruits, vegetables, and seeds. If you experience gas take two digestive enzymes with each meal. Remember your mind is a powerful tool; it can hinder or help you cleanse. So keep a positive attitude, read uplifting books, meditate, stretch, lie in the sun, take Epsom Salt baths and do moderate activity.

Where To Purchase the Ingredients:

Barley Life, Herbal Fiberblend and Just Carrots can be order through AIM Company. Call toll free 1-800-456-2462 and give them referral # 591683, so you can receive the discount member value. It is best if you purchase the Liquid Kyolic rather than capsules so you don't have to break down gelatin capsules during the cleanse. Other supplements and organic produce can be purchased from Whole Foods, Wild Oats, Vitamin Cottage, Trader Joes, on-line or your local health food store. Make sure to purchase only organic food products, as you do not need additional stress on the body from pesticides while you are cleansing.

TOTAL BODY CLEANSE

Warning: Seek the help of your health care provider before undergoing any cleanse. This cleanse is not advised for pregnant or lactating women and anyone with serious illness. This cleanse is done at your own risk. Those who have done cleanses before have reported having headaches, nausea, dizziness and fatigue. Occasionally the body is more toxic than it appears and can cause unforeseen problems. You may or may not experience these symptoms of cleansing, depending on your overall health. Proceed at your own risk!!!

You can do this cleanse for either 3 days or 7 days. The longer you do the cleanse the more lasting the results will be. This Cleanse helps to: rid the liver of toxic debris and excess bile, empty out the gallbladder of gallstones, clear out compacted fecal matter in the colon, clean out your cells, purify blood of bacteria, fungus, and viruses; and repair injured tissues (tendons, organs, muscles, etc.)

3-DAY CLEANSE

For the First Day it is recommended that you do 1 daily water enema (follow instructions below). If you do not have the time, follow all the instructions except for the enemas. Though the enemas are optional, they greatly improve the effectiveness of the detoxification process, helping to expel toxins much faster cleaning out the liver and gallbladder. Do the "water only" enema on day 1, and on the morning of the 2, 3 and 4th morning you will do 3 enemas (water, coffee and probiotic). Note: You may pass gall clots during day 2 and 3 of this part of the detoxification process. They are often the size of green peas, but can be much larger. They are usually dark green or bright chartreuse green in color. The 4th day you will start to resume a normal diet, and you do not need to take the Epsom salt before the enemas, only have the suggested amount of Barley Life before the enemas. Then on day 4 begin to follow the instructions at the beginning of chapter and in one of the following sections - Easing of the Detoxification.

SUPPLIES

2 Jars of Barley Life™ (by AIM)
1 Jar of Just Carrots™ (by AIM)
   (or carrots for juicing)
Bag of organic apples for juicing
   (or Organic Apple Juice)
1 Jar of Herbal Fiberblend™ (by AIM)

Liquid Kyolic™ or fresh garlic
4 organic grapefruit
5-6 organic lemons (optional)
Extra virgin olive oil
6 gallons of distilled water
Clove powder

UPON ARISING

DAY 1   Drink 1-2 TBS Barley Life with 6 oz water or 3 oz. freshly juiced wheat grass. (If your gallbladder has been removed do not proceed with the following use of olive oil). Wait 30 to 45 minutes then drink 2 tbsp. olive oil in 4 oz. freshly juiced or squeezed grapefruit or 8 oz. lemon juice. If possible, go back to bed and lay on your right side with your right knee to your chest for 20 minutes.

DAY 2-3   Drink an 8 oz glass of distilled water containing 1-2 tbsp of Epsom salts. 30 – 45 minutes later take 2 TBS Barley Life in 8 oz water or 3 oz fresh-juiced wheat grass. Follow with 2 or 3 enemas: distilled water, coffee or wheat grass and pro-biotic implant enema (see instructions below). It is highly recommended you do a minimum of 2 per day. If doing the coffee enema follow with a 3rd enema, the pro-biotic implant; use 2 caps of FloraFood™ from AIM or GI-Pro™ from Mannatech or Udo's Choice™).

DAY 4
Morning   Take 2 TBS Barley Life in 8 oz water or 3 oz freshly juiced wheat grass. Follow with 2 or 3 enemas: distilled water, coffee enema and pro-biotic implant enema (see instructions below). Must do all three!! Today you will start to resume eating some foods, make sure you follow the instructions for Easing of Detoxification provided for you in this chapter. Detoxification completed on the 4th morning.

START OF DAY

DAY 1-3   Mix and drink 2/3 cup fresh apple juice with 1/3 cup distilled water and 1 TBS Herbal Fiberblend. About 30 minutes later, begin drinking 5 cups apple juice (2/3 cup apple juice and 1/3 cup distilled water) until mid afternoon. Optional: add 1 lemon to the entire mix, and 10 drops of trace minerals 3 x day or a dash of Redmond's "RealSalt" sea salt 3 x day. Complete all 6 cups of apple juice before starting the carrot juice around mid afternoon.

MIDAFTERNOON

DAY 1-3   Carrot juice 5 x day (drink 7 oz of fresh carrot juice with 3 oz distilled water or 1 TBS of Just Carrots in 10 oz water.) Add to each 10 oz juice 1 tsp of Barley Life powder and 1 tsp of Liquid Kyolic garlic. Drink all five cups throughout the afternoon to early evening (up to 8pm). You can pre-mix the entire portion for the day.

LATE AFTERNOON

DAY 1-3   Drink one 8 oz glass of distilled water with 1-2 TBS of Epsom salts. You can have this between 4-6pm, BUT DO NOT SKIP THIS PART. It is crucial to the effectiveness of the cleanse.

PRIOR TO BED

DAY 1   Drink 1 TBS. Barley Life mixed with 4 oz of distilled water or 3 oz freshly juiced wheat grass.

DAY 2-3   In the evening of day 2 and 3, just prior to bed drink ½ cup of cold pressed extra virgin olive oil with ½ cup of fresh-juiced grapefruit or lemon juice. Add ¼ to ½ tsp of clove powder if you have a sensitive stomach (to prevent nausea). Immediately go to bed and lay on your right side with your right knee to the chest for 20 minutes.

7-DAY CLEANSE

For the First 5 Days it is recommended that you do 1 Daily water enema (follow instructions below). Enemas are optional, but this greatly improves the effectiveness of the cleanse, and helps to expel toxins much faster. Do the "water only" enema from days 1-5 and on days 6-7 and 8th morning do water enema, coffee enema and probiotic enema. Note that you may pass gall clots during days 6-8 of the detoxification process. They are often the size of green peas, but can be much larger. They are usually dark green or bright chartreuse green in color.

SUPPLIES

2-3 Jars of Barley Life™ (by AIM)
1 Jar of Just Carrots™ (by AIM)
  (or carrots for juicing)
2 Bags of organic apples for juicing
  (or Organic Apple Juice)
1 Jar of Herbal Fiberblend™ (by AIM)

Liquid Kyolic™ or fresh garlic
4 organic grapefruit
8-10 organic lemons (optional)
Extra virgin olive oil
12 gallons of distilled water
Clove powder

UPON ARISING

DAYS 1-5   Drink 1-2 TBS Barley Life with 6 oz water or 3 oz. freshly juiced wheat grass. (If your gallbladder has been removed do not proceed with the following use of olive oil). Wait 30 to 45 minutes then drink 2 tbsp. olive oil in 4 oz. freshly juiced or squeezed grapefruit or 8 oz. lemon juice. If possible, go back to bed and lay on your right side with your right knee to your chest for 20 minutes.

DAY 6-7   Drink an 8 oz glass of distilled water containing 1-2 tbsp of Epsom salts. 30 – 45 minutes later take 2 TBS Barley Life in 8 oz water or 3 oz fresh-juiced wheat grass. Follow with 2 or 3 enemas: distilled water water , coffee or wheat grass and pro-biotic implant enema (see instructions below). Must do a minimum of 2 per day. If doing the coffee enema follow with a 3rd enema –pro-biotic implant- (use 2 caps of FloraFood from AIM in enema).

DAY 8 **Morning**	Take 2 TBS Barley Life in 8 oz water or 3 oz fresh-juiced wheat grass. Follow with 3 enemas: distilled water enema, coffee enema and pro-biotic implant enema (see instructions below). YOU MUST DO ALL THREE. Today you will start to resume eating some foods, make sure you follow the instructions for Easing of Detoxification provided for you in this chapter. Detoxification is completed on the 8th morning.

START OF DAY

ALL DAYS   Mix and drink 2/3 cup fresh apple juice with 1/3 cup distilled water and 1 TBS Herbal Fiberblend. About 30 minutes later begin drinking 5 cups apple juice (2/3 cup apple juice and 1/3 cup distilled water) until mid afternoon. Optional: add 1 lemon to the entire mix, and 10 drops of trace minerals 3 x day or a dash of Redmond's "RealSalt" sea salt 3x a day. Complete all 6 cups of apple juice before starting the carrot juice around mid afternoon.

MIDAFTERNOON

ALL DAYS   Carrot Juice 5 x day (drink 7 oz of fresh carrot juice with 3 oz distilled water or 1 TBS of Just Carrots in 10 oz water.) Add to each juice 1 tsp of Barley Life powder and 1 tsp of Liquid Kyolic garlic. Drink all five cups throughout mid-afternoon to early evening (up to 8pm). You can pre-mix the entire portion for the day.

PRIOR TO BED

DAY 1-4   Drink 1 TBS. Barley Life mixed with 4 oz of distilled water or 3oz freshly juiced wheat grass.

DAY 5-7   In the evening just prior to bed drink ½ cup of cold pressed extra virgin olive oil with ½ cup of fresh-juiced grapefruit or lemon juice. Add ¼ to ½ tsp of clove powder if you have a sensitive stomach (to prevent nausea). Immediately go to bed and lay on your right side with your right knee to the chest for 20 minutes.

EASING OF DETOXIFICATION PROGRAMS
This starts on the morning of the last day of the cleanse!!!

UPON ARISING
Day 1-3   Have one 10 oz glass of apple juice with 1 TBS of Herbal Fiberblend, followed by a full glass of distilled water.

START OF DAY
Day 1   Drink 4 cups of (optional but recommended): Add 1 TBS Whey protein by Designer Protein or Goatien by Garden of Life to each glass of apple juice mix. You may eat 2 pieces of peeled fruits that are in season (grapefruit, apple, pear, 1 cup pineapple, or 1 cup papaya- no bananas!)

Day 2   You may eat 2-3 pieces of peeled fruits that are in season, followed by 2 cups of 10 oz fresh diluted apple juice (7 oz apple juice with 3 oz distilled water.)

Day 3   Resume a regular diet of fresh raw fruits, vegetable and legumes. Continue juicing fresh juices; choose from the juices section in the back of the book. Drink vegetable juices at a minimum of two 10 oz. glasses per day. Those battling serious chronic diseases should be drinking 104 oz of fresh carrot/vegetable/purified water juices. In order to maintain optimum health, it is important to maintain a diet that consists of 70% raw fruits and vegetables and 30% cooked foods. If you choose to eat meat it is recommended that you eat only game meat or organic meats and avoid milk products (except Kefir by Lifeway™), table salt, white flour, and white sugar and soft drinks. Do not eat poultry unless it is organic or scratch fed.

MIDAFTERNOON

Day 1 Drink carrot juice 3 x day (Drink 7 oz of fresh carrot juice with 3 oz distilled water or 1 TBS of Just Carrots in 10 oz water.) Add to each 10 oz. juice 1 TBS of Barley Life powder.

Day 2 Drink Carrot Juice 2 x day (Drink 7 oz of fresh carrot juice with 3 oz distilled water or 1 TBS of Just Carrots in 10 oz water.) Add to each 10 oz. juice 1 TBS of Barley Life powder.   Begin eating more grated raw vegetables.

LATE AFTERNOON

Day 1-2 2 cups organic vegetable broth or chicken with a 1 cup of cooked vegetables in the evening. On Day 2 you can have 2-3 cups organic butternut or broccoli soup (by Pacific or Imagine) with 1-2 cups of cooked vegetables in the evening.

ENEMA INSTRUCTIONS

Make sure to read and follow the instruction on the water/enema bags, which can be picked up at Wal-Mart, Walgreen's or local drug store. First clean the bowel with an enema bag of distilled water before doing 1 enema of wheat grass or coffee, or lemon, or hyssop tea. Note: an enema bag holds 2 quarts of fluid. Follow the distilled water enema with one of the following:

CHOOSE ONE TYPE OF ENEMA

1) Coffee & Probiotic Enema: Percolate or boil 4 – 6 tbsp of organic ground COFFEE per quart of distilled water for 15 minutes. Mix the coffee with 1 quart of distilled water. Warm the mixed coffee and distilled water to 98 degree F and pour into enema bag for use. Following the use of coffee enema is the PROBIOTIC Implant. It is recommended that if the coffee enema is used, that one additional enema be used

to implant PROBIOTIC back into the colon to establish health intestinal flora. Coffee kills the healthy intestinal flora in the colon. Add 2 capsules of probiotic with 2 quarts of warmed distilled (98 F) water to enema bag.

2) Wheat Grass Enema: Add the juice of 6 oz of wheat grass to 2 quarts of distilled water. Warm the distilled water to 98 degree F for use.

3) Lemon Juice Enema: Add juice of ½ lemon to 2 quarts of warmed distilled water. Bring to 98 degrees F and pour into enema bag for use.

4) Hyssop Tea Enema: Add 8 tsp of hyssop tea to a quart of water. Bring to a boil and allow steeping for 20 minutes. Combine the quart of tea with the one-quart of distilled water and bring to 98 degree F and pour into enema bag for use.

ENEMA PROCEDURE

Use and enema bag with a rectal tube or a Faultless brand fountain syringe. If you use a fountain syringe it is important to use the douche nozzle. The douche nozzle is long enough to extend beyond the nerve endings in the rectum. Lubricate the rectal tube or douche nozzle with KY jelly, or olive oil. DO NOT use Vaseline or any other petroleum product including mineral oil. These products will destroy the vitamins and minerals in the colon. Also have a small bucket of water containing a disinfectant solution available in which to place the nozzle following the enema procedure.

Enema Position:

Lie on a comfortable padded bathroom floor or slant board. Position the enema bag no higher than 20 inches above the hips when lying on the floor and even with the hips when using a slant board. Lie on your back and insert the lubricated tube or douche tip into the rectum. Release the clamp so as to allow the solution to enter slowly. When pressure builds, stop, lay on right side. You can place some olive oil on the stomach and massage the colon from right to left until more comfortable. When the pressure subsides, resume with the remainder of the enema. Never let the pressure get intolerable. Remove the nozzle and evacuate the solution if necessary. Remove the nozzle and place into the solution of disinfectant. When ready to resume the process begin the enema lying on the left side for 5-15 minutes while massaging the abdomen. Repeat this process again on the right side. Always try to massage following the line of the colon. Evacuate when necessary. For those using the coffee enema it is ideal to retain the coffee enema for 15 minutes before evacuating.

Congratulations!!! Now that you are done with the cleanse, take care to be cautious about the foods you choose to put into your body. This cleanse has cleared out thousand of little toxins that your body, mind and heart have accumulated over the years. It would be wise to use the rest of Food Beautiful Principles to create a temperate diet that increases the quality of your life. Use your willpower and good judgment to select and eat life giving foods, regardless of the ridicule or slander that friends or family may give to you.

LEMONADE CLEANSE

Warning: This cleanse is to be done at your own risk. Seek the help of your health care provider before undergoing. Those who have done cleanses before have reported having headaches, nausea, dizziness and fatigue. Occasionally the body is more toxic than it appears and can cause unforeseen problems. You may or may not experience these symptoms of cleansing, depending on your overall health.

Do this cleanse for 3-10 days as this cleanse is meant to open up the toxins within your cells and allow weak organs and tissues to begin healing. This cleanse should be done before undertaking any new lifestyle/diet change.

INGREDIENTS
Per 10 oz. of distilled water add:

2 TBS freshly squeezed lemon or lime juice (1/2 Lemon)

2 TBS grade B maple syrup (Grade B has more minerals to help replace those lost during the cleanse)

1 Container of Redmond "RealSalt"

1/10 tsp of cayenne pepper - 40,000 BTU is the highest heat content recommended for this cleanse and you may if desired increase the amount to 1/8 tsp. Cayenne has been noted to increase circulation and kill blood born pathogens.

DIRECTIONS FOR CLEANSE:

Premixes the entire days worth of ingredients anywhere from 6-12 glasses per day, but never vary the amount of lemon juice per glass. Feel free to drink whenever you want and have any extra purified/distilled water if so desired. To maintain sufficient elimination you may add the following internal Salt Water Bath. Prepare a full quart of lukewarm water and add 2 teaspoons of sea salt (Redmond "RealSalt" brand is the best). Do not use iodized salt; it will not work the same!!! The salt water has the same specific gravity as the blood, so the kidneys do not pick up the water and the blood cannot pick up the salt (thus no water retention). Drink the entire quart first thing in the morning on an empty stomach, before any juice. Do this every morning during your cleanse.

Note: Do not take supplements on this cleanse, allow your body to rest from any supplements or herbs. A good indication the cleanse is near completion is when the formerly fuzzy coated tongue becomes clear and pink looking again. If you are on prescription drugs consult your physician before starting on any cleanse.

HOW TO BREAK THE DIET:

Day One - drink several 8 oz. glasses of fresh squeezed/juiced orange or grapefruit juice as desired in the morning this prepares the body for assimilation of regular food. Dilute the juice with 1/3 distilled water. For example you have a 12 oz. cup fill 8 oz with juice and 4 oz with water.

Day Two - drink fresh orange or grapefruit fruit juice all throughout morning. By early afternoon start drinking diluted carrot spinach juice. Have 3, 12 oz (diluted 1/3 water) glasses until evening. At this time you may have Clear Vegetable broth with ¾ cup of steamed veggies.

Day Three – drink orange/grapefruit juice in the morning followed with raw fruit for lunch (no bananas). At night you can have a fresh fruit or vegetable salad with only lemon juice and 2 TBS olive oil. Do not over eat!! After day three you are ready to eat a normal healthy diet.

THE CANDIDA CLEANSE

If you have Candida it is best to follow this type of cleansing diet after you do the Total Body Cleanse. This Candida cleanse is for the individual who suffers from an overgrowth of Candida Albicans. You can get Candida from: taking antibiotics, eating sugar, having parasites, fungus or bacteria in your blood, or drinking high volumes of coffee. Candida acts like a fungus that stays inside your blood feeding on the foods you eat. Candida has been linked to conditions such as arthritis, cancers, chronic fatigue syndrome, constipation, anxiety, hypoglycemia, food allergies, and environmental allergies, to name a few. It may also be noted that my doctor friend claims that 7 out of 10 people have visible signs of Candida in their blood when looked at under a dark field microscope.

Below is a list of foods you should avoid for 6-9 months, as Candida is extremely hard to get out of the blood. The less of these foods you eat the faster you can rid your body of the Candida. Eat only the following foods recommended during this time as listed below

FOODS TO AVOID DURING CLEANSE

Avoid Sugars and Sugar Containing Foods:
Brown, granulated and powdered sugar as well as other sugars such as dextrose, fructose, galactose, glucose, glycogen, lactose (milk sugar), maltose, mannitol, monosaccharides, polysaccharides, sorbitol, sucrose, barley malt, honey, maple syrup, molasses, maple sugar, date sugar, turbinado sugar. Whenever possible, avoid artificial sweeteners such as NutraSweet (aspartame). Read all labels of packaged foods to make sure there are no hidden sugars.

Avoid Yeast
Brewers yeast, baker's yeast, vitamins, minerals (unless labeled "yeast free" and sugar free), and yeast-leavened bakery products: breads, crackers and pastries.

Avoid Fruit Juices
canned, bottled or frozen. Freshly prepared juices as tolerated (after initial three months).

Avoid Coffee and Tea
Regular coffee, instant coffee, decaffeinated coffee and teas. Recommended herbal tea - Traditional Medicinal™ caffeine-free teas. Green tea is permissible to have.

Avoid Caffeine
or anything that contains caffeine (including chocolate).

Avoid Dairy Products and Dairy-containing products:
Milk contains lactose, a simple carbohydrate which feeds the yeast, and should be avoided at least until you improve. Many people are allergic to milk. Some can tolerate plain yogurt, which is free of fruit, sugar or other sweeteners, preservatives, additives, and unsalted butter.

Avoid Black Pepper
Black pepper is hard to digest, so it is not recommended. In contrast, however, cayenne (red) pepper seems to promote digestion.

Avoid Edible Fungi:
All types of mushrooms, morels, and truffles.

Avoid Smoked & Processed Meats:
Smoked fish, pickled and smoked meats, including sausages, hot dogs, corned beef, pastrami, and ham.

Avoid Condiments, Sauces, and Vinegar-Containing Foods:
Mustard, ketchup, Worcestershire, Accent, steak Sauce, BBQ sauce, pickles, green olives, sauerkraut, horseradish, tamari, mayonnaise.

Avoid Dried & Candied fruits:
Raisins, apricots, dates, prunes, figs and pineapple.

Avoid Leftovers:
Mold grows in leftover food unless it is properly refrigerated. Freezing is best.

FOODS YOU CAN EAT FREELY

VEGETABLES

Artichoke
Asparagus
Beet
Broccoli
Brussel Sprouts
Cabbage
Carrots
Cauliflower
Celery
Chard
Cucumber

Eggplant
Garlic
Green bean
Collards Kale
Leek
Lettuce, all types
Mustard
Okra
Onion
Parsley
Parsnip
Peas, all types

Peppers, all types
Potatoes, red skinned
Pumpkin
Radish
Rutabaga
Spinach
Tomato
Turnips
Tofu
Yam

FISH

Cod
Crab
Halibut
Orange Roughy
Salmon
Trout
Tuna

WHOLE GRAINS

Barley
Kamut
Millet
Oats
Rye
Spelt

Wild Rice
Amaranth
Buckwheat
Quinoa
Brown Rice
Teff

NUTS

EAT RAW:
Almond
Brazil
Filbert
Macadamia
Pecan
Pine nut
Walnut

FRUIT

Avoid all fruit for 3 months and then reintroduce fruits 1 at a time. Eat all fruit alone on an empty stomach!!

Apple - Apricot - Tomato
Banana - Grapefruit - Mango
Nectarine - Orange - Papaya
Peach - Pear - Pineapple

MEATS

Antelope
Beef
Buffalo
Lamb
Veal
Venison
Other red meat

POULTRY

Chicken
Cornish Hen
Duck
Goose
Game birds
Turkey

SEEDS

Pumpkin
Sesame
Sunflower
Poppy seeds
Hemp seeds
Flaxseed

BEANS

Black   Lima
Pinto   Aduki
Navy   Mung
Kidney
Garbanzo
Soybean

BUTTERS

Raw Almond
Raw Sesame
Raw Sunflower
Raw Cashew

FATS

Organic Butter
Coconut Oil
Olive Oil
Sunflower Oil
Sesame Oil
Walnut Oil

BEVERAGES

Wellness Water
Sparkling Water
Lemon or Lime Herbal Tea
Pau D'Arco Tea
Green Tea
Herbal Teas

EGGS

Goose
Pheasant
Turkey
Chicken

DAIRY

Organic Butter
Yogurt, plain and unsweetened only!!
Kefir (by Lifeway)

4

<u>Food Combining</u>

GET SKINNY BY FOOD COMBINING

Proper food combining is not a new fad or a passing craze. Its earliest roots are found in ancient Greece and its usage in the U.S. is seen beginning approximately 155 years ago. In the U.S. food combination principles find their roots in the health care philosophy of Natural Hygiene. Natural Hygiene is based on natural body cycles and proper food combination. Natural Hygienists believe there are three cycles through which the body operates during a 24-hour period. If these cycles are ignored then confusion is created in the body's systems and breakdown in system function is observed.

BODY CYCLES:

4:00 A.M. to 12:00 P.M. = **Elimination** (Body wastes and food debris)
fruits Only during   this cycle.

12:00 P.M. to 8:00 P.M. = **Appropriation.** (Eating and digestion)
fruits, vegetables, proteins and starches in proper
combinations are eaten during this cycle.

8:00 P.M. to 4:00 A.M. = **Assimilation** (Absorption and usage)
Avoid eating during this cycle.

Everyone at one time or another has eaten a late night meal and the following morning been extremely fatigued. The reason for this fatigue: is that during this night time cycle (8:00 P.M. to - 4:00 A.M.) the body is supposed to be absorbing nutrients and repairing the system from daily wear and tear. If you eat during this time period the digestion process robs the energy needed to absorb and heal. The digestion process is a very energy intensive mechanism and does not leave much room for rest and healing while it is occurring. Therefore, following an improperly eaten evening meal, you will wake up the next morning feeling as if you had not received enough rest.

Since digestion requires so much energy to accomplish, it is logical that we should want it to occur as efficiently and in the least amount of time as possible. This is where proper food combining is extremely beneficial. 1f foods are improperly combined, digestion can take up to eight hours to complete. If food is properly combined this process will only take approximately 3 hours. This means that with properly combined foods we can save a lot of our body's energy for the things we need to do every day (work, play, healing, detoxifying, etc.). By properly combining your foods you may feel much more energetic, mentally acute, emotionally stable, and able to handle stress more appropriately. If you have a hard time controlling your food cravings, maybe it is time to do some spiritual cleansing and ask God to give you self-control and patience. I will lightly touch on the benefits of spiritual cleansing later in the book, and will hopefully be writing my next book on this subject.

RULES FOR PROPER FOOD COMBINING:

1) Protein and vegetables combine perfectly! Do not mix starches with proteins!!!

2) Starches and vegetables combine perfectly! Do not mix starches with protein!!!

3) Fruit must be eaten alone; it is best to start the day with fruit and not to eat it between meals. Apples are an exception (see next page). Do not mix or eat any melon with other fruits.

4) "First meat then wheat"-When eating throughout the day, have your meat at lunch and starches at dinner, as the protein is digested in the lower end of the stomach while the starch is digested in the upper part of the stomach. Mind you, I do not promote the usage of wheat; I just like the catchy title.

5) Do not eat fats and proteins together - in a meal unless you are having a salad or significant amount of fresh vegetables. The fat has a distinct inhibiting influence on secretion of gastric juices that are required for protein digestion.

6) "Sugar and protein no good"- Do not mix sugars with protein! The sugars inhibit the gastric juices needed to digest protein. Sugars need to be digested in the intestines, so they end up fermenting in the stomach. Take sugars alone or with vegetables only, as then they are not held up in the stomach.

7) Dairy, which is counted as a fat should be eaten alone or with fresh raw vegetables. For example, it would be okay if you had goat cheese on a salad with beans-- this would digest well.

8) A rule of thumb, if you have an abundance of vegetables, you can usually get away with having fat, a little bit of sugar, and meat in one meal. Obviously, do not eat a Snickers bar with your meal, as this is too much sugar (and a very bad food combination) to be digested. So for example, you can have vegetables with raspberry vinaigrette (which has sugar in it,) with some fish and flax seed oil on top.

9) A starchy meal- more than one kind of starch at a meal can lead to overeating which leads to bacterial activity. Be sure to drink your water 15-20 minutes before meals as water with a starchy meal weakens the action of the saliva on the starch. Chew your starches very well (30-50 chews) before swallowing.

ILL EFFECTS OF IMPROPER FOOD COMBINING:

1) Excess energy expenditure; leads to fatigue.

2) Enzyme depletion; leads to aging and disease.

3) Increased tissue toxins and inability to rid the body of toxins.

4) Putrification of foods in intestines; which leads to increased gas, bloating and poor elimination from the bowel. Putrification will rob you of the vital nutrients to create healthy life giving cells, free of disease and Illness.

5) When starches, sugars, and protein undergo fermentation, they are broken down into unusable substances like carbon dioxide and acetic acid, which act like poisonous gases in the body.

All these factors combined may lead to impaired body function and ill health. So remember, foods that rot do not supply the body with many vitamins. To derive sustenance from foods they must be properly digested. Anything that reduces the digestive power favors bacterial activity, such as overeating, eating right before a work out, eating when cold or hot, eating when feverish, eating when in pain, eating when not hungry, eating when worried/anxious/fearful/angry...all lead to bacterial activity. Try to spend 10-20 minutes defusing any unfavorable emotions or thoughts before a meal. I suggest relaxing to classical music, easy listening music, and do deep breathing combined with stretching. Take the time to now learn the basic rules of food combining and you will feel and see the difference.

Exceptions to the Rules of Proper Food Combining:

1) You can have fats and proteins in a meal only if you have an abundance of green, uncooked vegetables.

2) You can have an apple with any meal or at any time of the day as it has a neutral effect on the stomach, and it helps to satiate hunger, balance blood sugar, and reduce fermentation in the colon and small intestines.

3) Salad dressings that have sugars in them (maple, cane sugar, molasses etc.) are fine on salads, as the green vegetables help to carry them through to the intestines.

4) You can have celery or lettuce with any fruit, or after any meal.

5) Eggs combine well with other proteins, fats, or dairy but not with starches.

6) Acid fruits with nuts- acid fruits like grapefruit, lemons, and tangerines mix well with nuts, as the acids of the stomach do not delay the digestion of nuts. For example, a good combination breakfast meal would be- a grapefruit, orange, apple, pineapple, nuts and some avocado. However I would again suggest having this at the beginning of the day. Some people may still find this to be a bad combination and should avoid having nuts with acid fruit.

7) Even though tomatoes are a fruit they can be added with vegetable salads and meat.

PROPER FOOD COMBINING EXAMPLES
What to eat & at what times!

- **Upon arising**----Daily starter: 2 pieces of fruit.

- **20 min.-1 hour later**------Breakfast: handful of nuts (raw pumpkin, almonds, etc.), 2 slices Ezekiel bread with apple sauce.

- **Mid morning** -----Between breakfast and lunch you can have some green tea with rice milk and stevia, great mid morning pick me up.

- **12--2 p.m. Lunch:** Veggie juice followed 30 minutes later with a large salad with protein of choice.

- **3-4 p.m. Snack:** One of the following with raw nuts: apple, baby carrots or celery sticks.   1 cup kefir or a healthy food bar with some raw nuts. Most health food bars do not follow the food combining rules, but since these are eaten only once a day, it is a good alternative for busy people. Some good bars: Lara Bar™, Organic Food Bar™, Bobo's Oatmeal bars™, and any other bar with few ingredients that is raw or minimally processed. Note that 10-12 raw almonds have been used to help balance blood sugar. To make them even more absorbable soak the raw nuts in water overnight and the next morning drain out water and store in the fridge!

- **6-7 Dinner:** Light meal cooked with vegetables and a starch food of choice. Do not eat later than 8:00 p.m.

Other Guidelines & Suggestions

1) Most of the recipes in the back follow the food combining rules. If you have a serious disease or illness, it is in your best interest to follow the food combining chart 100% of the time.

2) Juice combination: ½ cucumber, 3 celery sticks, 3 leaves of kale, ½ apple, 2 carrots, 1/4 purple cabbage, handful parsley, 1 clove garlic. Add ginger, turmeric, and/or cayenne for extra nutrition. More juicing tips and recipes are in the back of the book.

3) Foods that are adulterated (refined) are to be avoided, eat foods that look most like how it came out of the earth, and if it didn't come out of the earth, don't eat it. The occasional splurge on junk food can be done one time a week, and this does not give you the freedom to overeat. Pray that God will give you self-control and patience!!

4) When eating out remember you can ask for substitutions. For example, replace rice with veggies when eating a protein, ask for salad dressing on the side, ask for an open-faced sandwich, ask for extra veggies, and bring your own healthy dressings. These are only a few of many suggestions when eating out.

FOOD COMBINING CHART

PROTEIN

Beans	Meat
Fish	Legumes
Nuts	Seeds
Eggs	Cheese
Milk	All Dairy

VEGETABLES

Broccoli	Zucchini
Lettuce	Yellow Squash
Spinach	Bell Peppers
Cabbage	Eggplant
Beet	Asparagus
Turnip	Sprouts
Parsley	Green Beans
Carrot	Cauliflower
Onions	Sweet Peas

STARCHES

Bread	Potatoes
Grains	Squash
Corn	Artichoke
Cereal	Chips
Pasta	

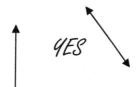 *YES*

 YES

NO

DO NOT COMBINE FOODS LISTED ABOVE WITH FOODS LISTED BELOW
For exception to the rule read pages above

Always eat melons alone!

ACID FRUITS

Pineapple	Kiwi
Lemon	Orange
Grapefruit	Lime
Tomato	
Pomegranate	

MELONS

Honey Dew
Cantaloupe
Watermelon

SWEET FRUITS

Banana	Cherry
Raisins	Dates
Mango	Figs
Persimmon	
Dried Fruits	

 YES

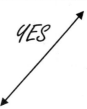 *YES*

SUB-ACID FRUITS

Strawberry	Pear	Blueberry
Plum	Grape	Nectarine
Peach	Apple	

5

Why Buy Organic?

TOP REASON TO BUY ORGANIC

#1 Dangers of GMO (Genetically Modified Organism) Food

GMO's are plants that have been inserted with another gene from various sources to increase the color, growth, and look of the product. Once a gene is inserted into an organism, it can cause unanticipated side effects. Mutations and side effects can cause GMO foods to contain toxins, allergens, and lower nutritional value. There is no way to control the effects that these have on people.

The Dangers of GMO foods:

1- They damage the ecosystem; harm wild life and natural habitats.

2- GMO's can transfer their new characteristic to other organisms, making that organism unable to reverse back to its original state.

3- Increased pollution in food and water supplies; GMO's increase resistant bacteria resulting in the need for tripling herbicide amounts on crops.

4- Unpredictable and permanent changes in the action and nature of our food; the new GMO can give rise to novel proteins in our food with unknown results for our health.

5- Deletion of beneficial properties to foods.

6- Decreased effectiveness of antibiotics.

7- Cause allergic reactions.

8- Cause livestock to become sick and suffer because they are being fed these GMO Foods.

#3 Soil Erosion, Depleted Soil; Resulting in Low-nutrient Foods
The Soil Conservation Service estimated that more than 3 billion tons of topsoil is eroded from United States croplands each year. Soil is the foundation of the food chain in organic farming. They rotate the crop and allow the soil to rest so more vitamins and minerals can be absorbed into the food. But, in most conventional farming, the soil is used more as a medium for holding plants in a vertical position so they can be chemically fertilized, resulting in 50-

75% fewer nutrients than organic produce, that are loaded with pesticides that reduce the nutrient value even further. The commercial soil has little nutrient left in it and as a result American people are suffering.

#4 Protect Your Water Quality Water makes up 70% of your body mass and covers 75% of the planet. Despite its importance, the Environmental Protection Agency (EPA) estimated pesticides – most cancer causing -- contaminate the ground water in 38 states, polluting the primary source of drinking water for more than half the country's population, resulting in unknown diseases and illnesses than ever before recorded. Another emerging issue is prescription drugs and the hormones being leached into the water supply. The hormone is too small to be filtered out. There is only one filter system we've found that takes the hormones out. It is a Japanese made technology called Wellness Water System. Their number is (352)-333-0480 and email is www.wellnessfilter.com

#5 Buy Organic Food, You'll Save Energy & Money American farms have changed drastically in the last three generations, from family-based small businesses dependent on human energy to large-scale factory farms highly dependent on fossil fuels. Modern farming uses more petroleum than any other single industry, consuming 12 percent of the county's total energy supply. More energy is now used to produce fertilizers than to till, cultivate and harvest all the crops in the Unites States. Organic farming is still mainly based on labor-intensive practices such as weeding by hand and using green manures and crop covers rather than synthetic fertilizers to build up soil. Organic produce also tends to travel fewer miles from field to table.

#6 Keep Chemicals Out of Your Body and Off Your Fork! Pesticides, herbicides, and fungicides are all poisons designed to kill living organisms and can be harmful to humans both in and out of the body. Many pesticides approved for use by the EPA were registered long before extensive research linking these chemicals to cancer and other diseases had been established. The EPA considers that 60% of all herbicides, 90% of all fungicides and 30% of all insecticides are cancer causing. A 1987 National Academy of

Sciences report estimated that pesticides might cause an extra 1.4 million cancer cases among Americans over their lifetimes. In addition to cancer, pesticides are linked to birth defects, nerve damage and genetic mutations.

The National Cancer Institute did a study and found that farmers exposed to herbicides had a six times greater risk than non-farmers of contracting cancer. In California, reported pesticide poisonings among farm workers have raised an average of 14 % a year since 1973 and doubled between 1975 and 1985. Field workers suffer the highest risk of occupational illnesses in the state of Colorado. The average child receives four times more exposure than an adult to at least eight widely used cancer-causing pesticides in food. The food choices you make now will impact you and the health of others. Total estimates of 1 million people are poisoned annually by pesticides and are experiencing the effects of choosing non-organic products.

#7 You'll Help Small Farmers And Support a True Economy

Most organic farms are small independently owned and operated family farms of less than 100 acres, although more and more large farms are making the conversion to organic practices. It is estimated that the United States has lost more than 655,000 family farms in the past decade. Although organic foods might seem more expensive than conventional foods, conventional food prices do not reflect hidden costs born by taxpayers, including nearly $74 billion on federal subsidies in 1988. Other hidden costs include pesticide regulation and testing, hazardous waste disposal, clean-up and environmental damage. Author Gary Null says, "If you add in the real environment and social costs of irrigation to a head of lettuce, its price can range between $2 and $3".

#8 Buying Organic-You're Food Will Taste Better

There's a good reason Sarah and other chefs around the world use organic foods in their recipes -- they taste better! Organic farming starts with the nourishment of the soil, which eventually leads to the nourishment of the plant and, ultimately, our palates. Organic foods have much higher amounts of vitamins, minerals and phytonutrients than any conventional product has. So choose organic foods when shopping and you will see and feel the difference!!

6

Healing Properties of Foods

HEALING PROPERTIES OF FRUIT

APPLE:

Moistens dryness in the lungs, protects the lungs from cigarette smoke, benefits low blood sugar conditions, and stimulate appetite. Remedies indigestion, due in part to the presence of malic and tartic acid which inhibits the growth of fermented food and disease-producing bacteria in digestive tract. Contains pectin, which removes cholesterol, toxic metals (such as lead and mercury) and the residues of radiation. Apples and their juice are cleansing for the liver and gallbladder which help to soften gallstones.

APRICOT:

Moistens lungs, used for thirst and asthma. Because of its high copper and cobalt content, it is commonly used for those suffering from anemia and constipation.

AVOCADO:

Builds the blood, harmonizes the liver, lubricates the lungs, and intestines. A natural source of lecithin, a brain food containing more than 80% of its calories from easily digested fat, primarily in the form of polyunsaturated oils. Rich in copper and potassium, which aids in red blood cell formation. A nutritious protein source often recommended for nursing mothers.

BANANA:

Helps with constipation and ulcers *if eaten ripened*. Bananas eaten *before completely ripened* will halt diarrhea, colitis, and hemorrhoids. Detoxifies the body, and is useful in helping to overcome drug addictions (especially alcoholism). Rich in potassium and easy to digest, bananas are great for helping those with hypertension and high blood pressure.

CANTELOPE:

Helps to clean out the liver by stimulating bile flow (when eaten on an empty stomach). Helpful for those with depression; eat the seeds while eating the fruit. You can save the seeds and eat later, as it is not necessary to eat all at once.

CHERRY:

A well-known remedy for gout, arthritis, and rheumatism. Helps overcome numbness in the limbs and paralysis as a result of rheumatism. Rich in iron, makes them useful for treating anemia.

FIG:

One of the most alkalinizing foods. Balances acidic conditions from highly refined foods and meats, helps with dysentery, hemorrhoids, has a detoxifying action, cleanses the intestines, helps iron absorption. Used to clear up skin boils and discharge, and is high in mucin which has a soothing laxative affect.

GRAPE:

Has natural tannins in the dark varieties that act as natural antioxidants.
Contains carotanoids, which prevent oxidation of fats that lead to hardening of the arteries. A blood tonic, known to build and purify the blood and improve the cleansing function of the glands. Benefits the liver and kidneys and thus strengthens their corresponding tissues-the bones and sinews. Positively affects those with arthritis, rheumatism, edema and urinary difficulty.

GRAPEFRUIT:

Helps with poor digestion, belching, increases appetite during pregnancy, helps overcome alcohol intoxication, allergies, hay fever, strep throat, candida overgrowth, giardia, athlete's foot, parasites, flu, staph infections, nail fungi, dandruff, yeast infections, sinus problems, and ear infections. Grapefruit peel regulates digestive energy, resolves mucus conditions of the lungs and can treat lung congestion and coughs. Bioflavonoids and vitamin C in the peel strengthen the gums, the arteries, and circulation in general. To extract properties of the peel, place fresh grapefruit peel in simmering water for 20 min. The CITRUS SEED EXTRACT is extremely beneficial as it is a natural antibiotic, antifungal, and antibacterial. It inhibits many types of microbes; parasites (protozoa, amoebas, bacteria, viruses) and 30 types of fungus, including candida yeast-like fungi.

LEMON & LIME:

A natural astringent, antiseptic, anti-microbial that promotes weight loss, cleanses the blood, treats high blood pressure, poor circulating blood and weak blood vessels, destroys putrefactive bacteria in the intestines and mouth, is mucus resolving for dysentery, colds, flu, hacking cough, and parasite infestation. Benefits the liver encouraging the formation of bile, improving absorption of minerals.

MULBERRY:

Builds blood, moistens the lungs and gastrointestinal tract, strengthens liver and kidneys, used to treats vertigo, paralysis, stomach ulcers, diabetes, dry cough, ringing in ears, poor joint mobility. Is also beneficial for blood deficiencies such as anemia, prematurely gray hair, irritability, insomnia, and constipations from fluid dryness.

ORANGE:

A general tonic for weak digestion, poor appetite, inflammation, high acidic diseases, arthritis, high fevers. The peel has stimulating, digestive, and mucus resolving properties similar to grapefruit peel.

PAPAYA:

Tonifies the stomach, acts as a digestive aid, alleviates coughing, used for dysentery, indigestion, mucus excesses, and pain from rheumatism. Under ripe papaya has high amounts of papain that is good for digesting protein and breaking down deposits on the teeth. Has a vermicidical action capable of destroying most intestinal worms (follow the parasite cleanse in the cleanse detoxify section). Contains carpain, an anti-tumor activity compound.

PEACH:

Moistens the lungs, used for dry cough, and helps to lower high blood pressure. An astringent and tends to limit perspiration while tightening tissues. Can be used as a remedy in facial creams. The kernel inside strengthens blood circulation, is used in anti-tumor formulas and for those with uterine fibroids. Peach leaf taken as a tea destroys worms.

PEAR:

Used for diabetes, loss of voice, coughing, gallbladder inflammation and obstruction.

PERSIMMON:

Used to moisten the lungs, reduce phlegm, sooth mucus lining of digestive tract, halts gastrointestinal inflammations, canker sores and chronic bronchitis. Unripe persimmon has high amounts of tannic acid, which is desirable for treating these conditions; diarrhea, dysentery, vomiting blood, and coughing up mucus.

PINEAPPLE:

Helps to relieve summer heat in the body by quenching thirst. Helps individuals overcome sunstroke, indigestion, anorexia, diarrhea, and edema. Contains enzyme bromelin, which increases digestive ability, has anti-inflammatory action, and destroys worms in the colon/intestines. Large amounts of bromelain found in ripe pineapples help those with severe disc inflammations. Note: Do not us pineapple for those with peptic ulcers or skin discharges.

PLUM:

Used for liver disease and diabetes; cirrhosis of the liver, hardened or expanded liver conditions, dehydration, and poor assimilation of carbohydrates. The Umeboshi salt plum treats indigestion, diarrhea, removes worms, and stops dysentery.

POMEGRANATE:

Destroys worms in intestinal tract, strengthens gums, soothes ulcers of the mouth and throat. Loaded with vitamin C and Iron.

RASPBERRY & BLACKBERRY:

Raspberry enriches and cleanses the blood of toxins, regulates menstrual cycle (raspberry leaf tea), controls urinary function, anemia, as well as excessive urination (especially at night). Raspberry leaf strengthens uterus, balances excessive menstrual flow, and restrains bleeding in general. Blackberry is similar in effects to the raspberry.

STRAWBERRY:

Improves appetite, moistens the lungs and body fluids; used for thirst, sore throat, and hoarseness. Eating before meals helps with poor digestion accompanied by abdominal pain and swelling. Helps to relieve urinary difficulties, painful urination and inability to urinate. Rich in silicon and vitamin C, it is useful for arterial and all connective tissue repair. One of the first fruits to appear in spring, it is helpful for cleansing the body. Those who are allergic to strawberries, for the most part, are those who buy and eat the unripened and non-organic berries.

WATERMELON:

Very cooling, great for quenching thirst in the summer, loaded with electrolytes so great for an after workout snack or juice. Great for those with urinary difficulty, edema, canker sores, depression, kidney and urinary tract inflammations. The seed of the watermelon contains cucurbocitrin, a nutrient that dilates capillaries, lowering cholesterol. The rind is useful for high blood pressure, diabetes, and calcium needs.

HEALING PROPERTIES OF LEGUMES

ADUKI BEAN:

Aids adrenals and kidneys, detoxifies the body, reduces swelling, diuretic. Beneficial for conditions such as jaundice, diarrhea, edema, boils, and promotes weight loss. For prolonged menstruation, daily chew well 5 raw aduki beans until menses stops.

BLACK BEAN:

Benefits kidneys and reproductive function. Used for low back pain, knee pain, infertility, and involuntary seminal emission.

BLACK SOYBEANS:

Improves blood circulation and water metabolism; diuretic, removes toxins from the body, used to treat rheumatism and kidney disease.

FAVA BEAN:

Diuretic, strengthens the spleen and pancreas. Used to treat edema and swelling.

GARBONZO BEAN:

Beneficial to pancreas, stomach and heart.

KIDNEY BEAN:

Diuretic, used in treating edema and swelling.

LENTIL:

Beneficial to heart and circulation and stimulates the adrenal system.

LIMA BEANS:

Highly alkalinizing, benefits lung and liver. Neutralizes acidic conditions such as those that arise from excessive meat and refined food consumption. Best for most Americans.

MUNG BEAN:

helps to heal + repair

Detoxifies the body, benefits liver and gallbladder, diuretic, reduces swelling in lower legs. Used as a cure for food poisoning (drink liquid from mung soup), dysentery (cook with garlic), diarrhea, painful urination, mumps, burns, lead and pesticide poisoning, boils, heat stroke, conjunctivitis, and edema (especially in the lower extremities), beneficial for treating high blood pressure, acidosis, gastro-intestinal ulcers, skin outbreaks, thirst, and restlessness.

PEAS:

Harmonizes digestion and reduces the effect of an overworked, excessive liver on the stomach spleen and pancreas. Reduces vomiting, belching, hiccups and coughing. Mildly laxative, also used for spasms, edema, constipation and skin eruptions such as carbuncles and boils.

SOYBEAN:

Used occasionally in small amounts --- improves almost all organs, cleanses blood vessels and heart by improving circulation, promotes clear vision, diuretic, lowers fever, eliminates toxins form the body, boosts milk secretion in nursing mother, a remedy for dizziness, and childhood malnutrition. Good for toxemia during pregnancy, food poisoning, and is a natural source of lecithin (good for the brain). Easily digested by young children! However, well-cooked soybeans can inhibit the digestive enzyme, trypsin, making then hard to digest. It is best to use the fermented types of soy; tempeh, tofu, and miso. If used too much, soybeans can cause anemia, amenorea, osteoporosis, weakened kidney and adrenal function, hypothyroidism and mineral deficiencies.

STRING BEAN:

Used for diabetes, frequent urination and thirst.

Herbal Combinations for better digestion and taste of Legumes:
- Mint, garlic --- garbanzo, lentil
- Coriander, cumin, ginger --- lentil, mung, black, aduki
- Dill, Basil --- lentil, garbanzo, split pea
- Sage, thyme, oregano --- black pinto, lentil, kidney
- Fennel or cumin --- pinto, kidney
- Seaweeds (Kombu or kelp) add while cooking to make legumes more digestible and tasty.

HEALING PROPERTIES OF GRAINS

AMARANTH:

Used to help fulfill protein and calcium requirements. Benefits the lungs, high in protein, fiber, amino acids, Vitamin C, and calcium.

BARLEY:

Cooling nature, strengthens the spleen-pancreas, regulates the stomach, builds blood, benefits gallbladder and nerves; very easily digested, alleviates painful and difficult urination; quells fever, helps reduce tumors, swelling, and edema.

BROWN RICE:

Soothes the stomach; expels toxins; hypoallergenic; concentrated in B vitamins therefore beneficial for the nervous system and helps relieve mental depression. A handful of raw brown rice thoroughly chewed, as the only food in the morning, helps to expel worms.

BUCKWHEAT:

Cleanses and strengthens intestines and improves appetite. Helpful for dysentery, chronic diarrhea, strengthens capillaries and blood vessels, reduces blood pressure, increases circulation to the hands and feet.

CORN: Improves appetite, helps regulate digestion, notifies the kidneys.

> Corn silk: is highly diuretic and can be used as a tea infusion for urinary difficulty, high blood pressure, edema, kidney stones, and gallstones.

KAMUT:

Called the "Ancient Wheat", which is great for those sensitive to today's wheat and glutenous products, high in protein and in vital nutrients.

MILLET:

A natural diuretic, strengthens kidneys, benefits stomach and spleen-pancreas, alkalizing, sweetens breath by retarding bacterial growth, helps prevent miscarriage, anti-fungal (best grain for those with candida). Helps those w/ diarrhea (roast millet before cooking), indigestion, diabetes, and soothes morning sickness (eat millet soup).

OATS:

Restores nervous and reproductive systems, removes cholesterol from the digestive tract and arteries. Rich in silicon which helps renew the bones and connective tissue. Nourishing for young children which helps to develop their nervous system. Cooked oatmeal once cooled has been used to sooth burns of the skin (make a paste with water and oats and apply to affected area).

QUINOA:

High in protein, a good source of iron, B vitamins, vitamin E, and has more calcium than milk. Tonifies the kidneys and the pericardium functions.

RYE:

Increases endurance; aids muscle formation; cleanses and renews arteries; aids fingernail, hair and bone formation.

SPELT:

Benefits the spleen and pancreas, benefits the frail and deficient person. Often used for treating diarrhea, constipation, poor digestion, colitis, and other intestinal disorders.

WHEAT:

Encourages growth, weight gain, and fat formation- good for children and frail people. Should be eaten in small amounts, if at all, for obese individuals and those with growths or tumors. Wheat can provoke allergic reactions as the flour becomes rancid from oxidation within 2 weeks. Wheat flour should be used right after grinding, otherwise, it needs to be kept in an airtight container, refrigerated, and used within two weeks.

"TEA FOR HEALING"

"Tea for Healing" is known in Eastern Medicine as Congee Tea. This tea is a thin porridge of rice with other grains, beans, vegetables or herbs. To make the tea, measure out 6 cups of water, one handful of brown rice, then place in a crock-pot or covered pot with your ingredient of choice (listed below). What is the right measurement for the tea? For beans use one handful, for vegetables use 4 cups, for herbs and seeds use 2-5 TBS. Cook the congee tea four to six hours on warm at the lowest temperature possible. It is better to use more water than not enough. It should end up being a porridge type drink; you may strain it or drink it all together. It is best to drink 3 cups of congee tea a day for chronic conditions. You can use other ingredients in the tea that are listed in the Healing properties of foods section.

Aduki Bean: A natural diuretic, curative for swelling, edema and gout.

Carrot: Digestive aid, eliminates flatulence.

Celery: Cooling in summer, benefits large intestine.

Chestnut: Strengthens kidneys, knees and loin; useful in treating anal hemorrhages.

Fennel: Harmonizes the stomach, expels gas, heals hernias.

Ginger: Used for digestive weakness: diarrhea, anorexia, vomiting, and indigestion.

Mung Bean: Reduces fevers, a food for summer heat, relieves thirst

Mustard: Expels phlegm, clears stomach congestion

Purslane: Detoxifies body,, recommended for rheumatism and swellings

Sweet Brown Rice: Used for diarrhea, vomiting, and indigestion.

Sesame Seed: Lubricates intestines, helps those with rheumatism.

Rye: Helpful for easing migraine headaches.

Taro Root: Nutritious, aids stomach, builds blood and good for those who are anemic.

HEALING PROPERTIES OF NUTS AND SEEDS

The best way to eat seeds or nuts is to soak them overnight in water to initiate there sprouting process. This makes the protein and fats more digestible. Drain the water and dry them, eat them raw or lightly roasted. Store hulled seeds in dark glass bottles in cold places. Do not store in plastic, as the oil rich food combines with plastic to form plasticides.

ALMOND:

Relieves stagnant energy in the lungs, alleviates cough and lubricates the intestines. Used for lung conditions including coughing and asthma. For lung conditions use almond milk (brand: Almond Breeze unsweetened vanilla flavor). Almond is the only nut to alkalinize the blood.

BLACK SESAME SEED:

Strengthens the liver and kidneys, lubricates the intestines, strengthens heart, liver, kidney, spleen-pancreas and lungs. Used to relieve rheumatism, constipation, dry cough, blurry vision, ringing in ears, blood in urine, low back pain, weak knees, stiff joints, nervous spasm, headaches, insufficient mother's milk, dizziness and numbness.

CHIA SEED:

Next to flax, this seed is the highest source of omega-3 fatty acids.

COCONUT:

Used for weakness, fungal infections, emaciation, nosebleed and childhood malnutrition. Coconut milk is helpful in treating edema resulting from heart weakness and diabetes. There are many claims that coconut oil helps those with an under active thyroid.

FLAX SEED:

A natural and mild laxative, mucilaginous, relieves pain and inflammation, rich source of omega-3 fatty acids, and pulls out excess estrogen in the blood.

PEANUTS:

Buy only organic as they have a carcinogenic fungus that grows inside the nut and are heavily sprayed with chemicals and synthetic fertilizers. Should be avoided by overweight individuals, cancerous persons, and yeast infected individuals. Used to increase the milk supply of the nursing mother, stops bleeding including hemophilia and blood in urine and helps to lowers blood pressure (drink tea of shells).

PINE NUTS:

Mildly laxative, helpful for dizziness, dry cough, spitting up blood and constipation.

PISTACHIO:

Influences the liver and the kidney, purifies the blood, lubricates the intestines, used for constipation. Is an important tonic for the whole body when eaten raw.

PUMPKIN & SQUASH SEEDS:

Influences the colon and spleen-pancreas, diuretic, vermifuge (expels worms and very effective on tape worms and round worms). Beneficial for those with motion sickness, nausea, impotency, and swollen prostate. Is a great source of zinc and omega-3 fatty acids.

SUNFLOWER SEED:

Influences the spleen-pancreas, acts as an energy tonic, lubricates the intestines, beneficial for constipation, and hastens the eruption of measles. These seeds go rancid quickly because of their high polyunsaturated fatty acid content. It is best to shell them before eating.

WALNUT:

Walnuts reduce inflammation and alleviate pain, due to high content of omega-3 oils. They moisten the lungs and intestines, help relieve coughing and wheezing, nourish the kidney-adrenals-brain, and enrich sperm. Beneficial for those with involuntary emission, impotency, painful back and knees, and constipation in elderly. May harbor parasites so it is best to roast them lightly.

HEALING PROPERTIES OF VEGETABLES

ASPARAGUS:

Contains diuretic asparagine, which helps to eliminate water through the kidneys. Beneficial for those with kidney problems, but should not be used when there is inflammation. Helps cleanse out cholesterol from the arteries and is useful for those with hypertension and arteriosclerosis.

BEET:

Strengthens the heart, improves circulation, purifies the blood, benefits the liver, helpful for those with anemia, moistens the intestines and promotes menstruation. For hormone regulation during menopause, use in conjunction carrot and chlorophyll rich foods (greens) to impart hormone balance. Helps those with liver stagnancy and liver ailments, as well as constipation, nervousness, and congestion of the vascular system. Rich in silicon, which increase the body's ability to absorb calcium.

BROCCOLI:

A natural diuretic, brightens the eyes, used for eye inflammation and nearsightedness. Contains high amounts of pantothenic acid and vitamin A, aids weight loss, helps to alleviate rough skin, cold sores, and other forms of herpes. Has more vitamin C than citrus and is high in natural sulfur, iron, and B vitamins, which build the immune system, and ability to fight of infections. Lightly cooked, broccoli will retain its rich chlorophyll content, which counteract gas formation resulting from its sulfur content, allowing you to absorb the iron.

CABBAGE:

Green and purple cabbage moisten the intestines, benefit the stomach, improve digestion, and beautify the skin. Is also beneficial for those with constipation, the common cold, whooping cough (cabbage soup or tea), chronic cold feet, mental depression, and irritability. Also helps to rid the digestive system of worms (taken with garlic makes it more effective against parasites), and purifies the blood. Contains vitamin U, an ulcer remedy for either stomach or duodenal ulcers (drink 1 ½ cups of freshly made cabbage juice 2-3 times a day between meals for at least 2 weeks). Cabbage is a good source of iodine and Vitamin C. Studies indicate that cruciferous vegetables (cabbage, broccoli, and brussel sprouts) inhibit cancerous growth in the large intestine.

CARROTS:

Benefit the lungs, strengthen the spleen and pancreas, improve liver function, dissolve accumulations such as stones and tumors, help with indigestion, skin lesions, heartburn and eliminates putrefactive bacteria in the intestines that cause poor assimilation. Also used for diarrhea, chronic dysentery, and destroys roundworm and pinworms in the intestines. Alkaline-forming and clear acidic blood conditions including acne, tonsillitis, rheumatism. Protective against cancer, night blindness, ear infections, earaches, and deafness. The large amount of beta-carotene/vitamin benefits the skin, lungs, digestive tract, and urinary tract infections. Ease whooping cough and coughing in general. Contain large amounts of silicon, thereby strengthening connective tissues and increasing ability to absorb and metabolize calcium.

CELERY:

Improves digestion, purifies the blood, helps to control appetite, promotes sweating, helps to clear digestive fermentation, rheumatism, arthritis, gout, and nerve inflammation. Useful for burning urine, blood in urine, acne, and canker sores. A natural diuretic, high in potassium, celery juice combined with lemon juice is a remedy for the common cold, headaches, and a great workout recovery drink. Very high in silicon that helps to renew joints, bones, arteries and all connective tissues. Though a vegetable, celery combines well with fruit!

CUCUMBER:

A natural diuretic that helps alleviate edema from the lower legs, cleanses the blood, counteracts toxins, and lifts depression. Helpful for those with inflammatory conditions, such as sore throat, acne, stomach inflammation, conjunctivitis, and discharge. A tonic for the heart, spleen-pancreas, stomach, and the large intestines. Quenches thirst, moistens lungs, purifies the skin and acts as a digestive aid. High in erepsis, a digestive aid, that breaks down protein and cleanses the intestines enabling the body to destroy worms (especially tapeworms). Applied to the skin, beautifies complexion and relieves hot, inflamed, swollen, dry eyes.

JERUSALEM ARTICHOKE:

Helps to relieve asthmatic conditions, cleanses the liver, eases constipation, and stimulates insulin production. Contains inulin, which reduces insulin need, thereby highly beneficial for diabetics.

KALE:

Eases lung congestion, benefits the stomach, and good for anemic/weak persons. Abundant in sulfur and can be used to help those with stomach and duodenal ulcers (make fresh juices of kale and other veggies). An exceptional source of chlorophyll, amino acids, calcium, iron, and vitamin A, which can meet most of your daily nutrient requirements.

KOHLRABI:

Helps to increase circulation, eliminates blood coagulations, helps with indigestion, and blood sugar imbalances. Used for hypoglycemics and diabetics, relieves painful urination, stops bleeding in the colon, reduces swelling of scrotum, and alleviates effects of intoxication from drugs and alcohol.

LETTUCE:

Dries up damp conditions in the body such as edema and digestive ferments and yeasts. Helpful in fighting hemorrhoids, acts as a natural diuretic, and alleviates scant urine and blood in urine. Is the highest source of silicon of common vegetables (silicon allows the body to metabolize and absorb calcium effectively). Used for increasing mothers milk production. Helps to relax the nerves without impairing digestion. Not to be used if eye disease exist.

MUSHROOM:

Decreases fat level in blood, helps rid excess mucus in lungs, has antibiotic properties, can aid in fighting contagious hepatitis, increases white blood cell count, has anti-tumor activity, can help stop post surgery cancer metastasis, and promotes appetite.

SHIITAKE MUSHROOM:

Natural source of interferon, a protein which appears to induce an immune response against cancer and viral diseases. Used to help the body fight stomach and cervix cancers. Decreases both fat and cholesterol in the blood and helps discharge the excess residues of accumulated animal protein.

MUSTARD GREENS:

Influences the lungs, tonifies the intestines, clears chest congestion, improves energy circulation, and reduces white copious mucus associated with lung infections. A remedy for colds and coughs (heat up mustard greens in a tea and drink). Note: Not for those with inflamed eye disease or hemorrhoids.

EGGPLANT:

Reduces swelling, clears stagnant blood dissolving congealed blood and accumulations such as tumors specifically congealed blood in uterus and helps reduce excess bleeding. Not good for pregnant mothers as it can cause miscarriages. Used for conditions such as bleeding hemorrhoids, blood in urine, dysentery, diarrhea and canker sores (apply charred eggplant powder). A rich source of bioflavonoids which renew arteries, prevent strokes, and aid in calcium absorption. Influences liver and uterus and is particularly helpful for resolving repressed emotions and their harmful effects on these organs.

POTATO:

Contains abundance of sugar, potassium, and minerals. Neutralizes body acids which help relieve arthritis and rheumatism.

TOMATO:

Relieves thirst, tonifies the stomach, cleanses the liver, purifies the blood, detoxifies the body, encourages digestion and diminished appetite, alleviates indigestion, food retention, anorexia, and constipation. Relieves high blood pressure, red eyes and headache. Alkalinizing, reducing acidic blood from rheumatism and gout. Large amounts of tomato weaken everyone, and should be avoided by those with arthritis.

ONIONS:

Resolve stagnant blood, reducing clotting. Expels coldness, lowers blood pressure, lowers cholesterol, cleanses the arteries and retards growth of viruses, yeasts, ferments, and other pathogenic organisms. The richest food in sulfur, helps purify the body, remove heavy metals, parasites, and facilitates protein/amino acid metabolism. Eastern tradition believes if eaten too often, they can foster excessive emotional desires.

CHIVES:

Influences repair in the kidneys, liver, and stomach. Increases circulation (specifically for bruises, swellings and other joint injuries). Strengthens the kidneys and sexual capacity making them beneficial for those with leukorrhea, urinary incontinence, spermatorrhea, and pain from arthritis. Note: Avoid when eye diseases and skin eruptions are present.

GARLIC:

Promotes circulation and sweating, eliminates toxins from the body (including poisonous metals such as lead), removes abdominal obstructions, inhibits the common cold virus as well as viruses, amoebae, and other microorganisms. Eliminates worms, unfavorable bacteria, and yeast (candida albican). Used for tuberculosis, asthma, hay fever, dysentery, Lymes disease, anthrax infection, warts, abscesses and hepatitis. Good for colds, sore throats, and sinus headaches (hold a clove of garlic in mouth for at least 15 minutes, and then consume it). To ward off mosquitoes, eat garlic at least once a day. For athlete's foot, sprinkle garlic powder on wet feet and let dry—socks may be worn. A drop of garlic in the ear canal once a day helps clear ear infections.

LEEK:

Leeks can be used by those with dysphagia (difficulty swallowing), bleeding, and diarrhea.

SCALLION:

Used in cases of both chest and heart pain. Promotes urination and sweating, relieves edema, diarrhea, abdominal swelling/pain, and arthritis. Note: Avoid if you have yellow mucus, fever, and great thirst.

PARSLEY:

Improves digestion, detoxifies body from meat or fish poisoning, ripens measles to hasten recovery, strengthens optic and brain nerves, strengthens adrenals, promotes urination, good for treating obesity, and mucus in bladder. Contains loads of vitamin C, vitamin A, chlorophyll, calcium, natural sodium, magnesium, and iron. Note: Parsley should not be used by nursing mothers, as it dries up milk production.

PARSNIP:

Benefits spleen-pancreas and stomach, helps clear liver and gall bladder obstructions, promotes perspiration, lubricates intestines, acts as an analgesic, and a source of concentrated silicon. Used in soups or teas for cough, cold, shortness of breath, headaches, dizziness, rheumatism, and arthritis. Note: Avoid parsnip leaves, as they are poisonous.

PUMPKIN:

Relieves dysentery, eczema, edema, helps regulate blood sugar imbalances, benefits the pancreas—used for diabetes and hypoglycemia. Promotes discharge of mucus from lungs, bronchi, and throat, and if used regularly helps benefit bronchial asthma. Cooked pumpkin destroys intestinal worms, but not as effective as the seeds.

RADISH:

Moistens the lungs, cuts mucus, detoxifies the body, clears sinuses, hoarseness, phlegm, and sore throats. Helps cleanse the gallbladder, relieves indigestion and abdominal swelling. The toxin purging property of radish makes it useful for detoxifying old residues in the body during healthy diet upgrades.

SPINACH:

Builds the blood, stops bleeding, is a natural laxative and diuretic, builds red blood cells for those with anemia, quenches thirst, and cleanses blood of toxins that cause skin disease. Can assist in riding the body of constipation, and urinary difficulty Its sulfur content relieves herpes irritations. Good for night blindness.

SQUASH:

Helpful for stomach and spleen-pancreas, reduces inflammations and burns (fresh squash juice applied to relieve burn), improves circulation, and alleviates pain. Summer squashes and zucchini help overcome summer heat, water retention/ edema, and difficulty urinating. Eat steamed summer quash or zucchini with its skin and seeds to destroy worms in the colon.

SWEET POTATO & YAM:

Strengthens spleen-pancreas, increases quantity of milk in lactating women, removes toxins from the body, aids kidneys, treats thinness and diarrhea. Rich in Vitamin A - helpful for night blindness. Spirulina and organic animal liver added to sweet potato soups some to makes a highly effective night-blindness formula.

TURNIP:

Improves circulation, detoxifyies, builds blood, resolves mucus conditions, relieves coughing, clears food stagnancies, and improves appetite. Generally helpful for indigestion, hoarseness, diabetes, and jaundice. Best to use it in its raw form.

WATERCRESS:

Influences lungs, stomach, bladder, and kidneys. Is a diuretic, purifies blood, removes stagnant blood, helps reduce cancerous growths, benefits night vision, and clears facial blemishes. Is a rich source of vitamin A, chlorophyll, sulfur, and calcium. Helps to dry up and eliminate yellow phlegm from flu and colds.

HEALING PROPERTIES OF HERBS & SPICES

ANISE- relaxes nerves, a variety of basil.

DILL- helps eliminate flatulence and digestive disturbances, anticancer and antimicrobial effects, promotes liver detoxification.

SAGE- antispasmodic (calms nerves and muscles),high estrogen content, antioxidant, hypoglycemic, uterine stimulant, suppresses perspiration, heals mucus membranes.

GINGER- calms upset stomach, increases circulation to lower extremities

FENNEL- digestive, aids bean digestion, anti-inflammatory, circulatory stimulant, stimulates milk flow in nursing mothers, encourage mental alertness.

CUMIN- high in iron, digestive aid, anti-cancerous, anti-tumor, aids liver detoxification.

CELERY SEED- reduces fluid retention and arthritic conditions. Aids urinary and kidney function.

CORIANDER- bean digestive, antidiabetic plant, anti-inflammatory properties, antimicrobial, has anxiety lowering action and cholesterol lowering effects.

CARDAMOM- digestive stimulant, stimulates mind and heart, used in pregnancy for morning sickness and help combat miscarriage, carminative.

CLOVES- stops nausea, digestive aid, helpful for reproductive organs and kidneys, used to

reduce gum irritation and inflammation.

CINNAMON- balances blood sugar, antibacterial, antifungal, antiviral, improves circulation.

CAYENNE PEPPER – increases circulation, antifungal, and antibacterial.

CHILI PEPPER- antibacterial and digestive.

WHITE PEPPER- digestive aid, soothes the stomach.

LICORICE- antispasmodic, antitussive (stops coughing), relieves constipation and gastric ulcers, anti-allergenic, avoid if you have high blood pressure.

SPEARMINT- cooling for excess heat.

PEPPERMINT- cools body from over heating, digestive aid, reduces flatulence, a diaphoretic, reduces nausea. DO NOT use on children under four.

PAPRIKA- improves blood circulation, reduces indigestion, aids stomach ulcers, aids heartburn, and helps combat colds and sinus infections.

LEMON BALM- improves circulation, headache relief, anti-depressant, digestive stimulant, antibacterial, antiviral, anxiety, headache relief.

MARJORAM– antimicrobial, kills amoebas, inhibits growth of bacteria, antioxidant

ORANGE OIL- helps stop diarrhea

TARRAGON- antifungal, antimicrobial, antioxidant, benefits diabetics, reduces desire to overeat and aids weight loss.

TUMERIC- soothes joints, antioxidant, aids injury recovery, improves flexibility, reduces cholesterol levels, improves skin, reduces pain.

THYME- digestive, clears phlegm and combats chest infections, antimicrobial, antispasmodic, antibiotic, wound healer.

GARLIC- antifungal, antibacterial, antiviral, reduces cholesterol.

ONION – cleanses the blood, antibacterial, antiviral.

CHIVES- reduces edema in lower legs, part of onion family.

ROSEMARY- brings oxygen directly to the brain, digestive, carminative, relieves headache/migraine, and indigestion, used to darken graying hair, anti-dandruff.

OREGANO- antifungal, antibacterial, antiviral.

NUTMEG- improves appetite, provides migraine relief, helpful with nausea, reduces abdominal bloating, indigestion, colic, anti-inflammatory.

BASIL- antidepressant, antiseptic, adrenal stimulant, digestive, anti-parasitic, combats fever and headaches.

BLACK PEPPER- stops diarrhea, antibacterial, circulatory stimulant, (the only time I suggest its use), avoid if you have fungal or candida infections.

SEA SALT- (by Redmond) Natural mineral and a good source of iodine.

7

<u>Deadly Foods</u>

DEADLY FOODS TO AVOID

Always read the labels on the side for listed ingredients. If the product contains anything listed below, it is not healthy for you, and is robbing your body of life and health. The more of these ingredients included the more harm it does to your body. Don't just look at calorie amounts from fat, sugar, carbohydrates and protein as they only tell you part of the story. You need to look at the full story and read the ingredients! Use wisdom when shopping as flashy products can makes claims like "fat-free, low-sodium, sugar-free, high-protein, all natural," but are far from being healthy for you. Take your time while shopping; be smart when choosing products and you will start to see the difference.

OILS & FATS TO AVOID

Hydrogenated Oils	Rapeseed Oil	Margarine
Vegetables Oil	Animal Lard	Soy Butters
Corn Oil	Peanut Oil	Partially-Hydrogenated Oil
Canola Oil	Non-organic Butter	

PRESERVATIVES TO AVOID

Salt & refined Sea Salt	Sulfur Dioxide	Distilled Vinegar
Chloride	Artificial Flavors	White Vinegar
BHT	Natural Flavors	Potassium Sorbate
Artificial Colors	MSG	Hydrolyzed Yeast
Ferrous Fumerate	Spices	

SUGARS TO AVOID

Corn Syrup	Refined Honey	Sweet & Low
White Sugar	Fructose	Aspartame
Brown Sugar	Glucose	High Fructose Corn Syrup
Sucralose	Refined Can Sugar	

OTHER FOODS TO AVOID

The items followed with a * are okay to use if they are organic. There are also healthy replacements for most of these foods under the Fabulous Food Replacements List.

Highly Refined Foods	Graham Crackers	Buttermilk*
Soy Protein Isolate	Packaged Frosting	Sour Cream*
Bleached Wheat Flour	Sugar Cereals	Cornmeal*
Unbleached Wheat Flour	Puddings	Enriched Flour
Catsup/Ketchup	Corn*	Enriched Products
Milk in cartons	Peanuts	Mayonnaise
Soy Milk*	Wheat Gluten	Pasteurized Cheese
Processed Meats, Deli Meat*	Vital Wheat Gluten	Peanut Butter
Butter*		

BEVERAGES TO AVOID

The items followed with a * are okay to use if they are organic.

Decaf Coffee	Carbonated Beverages	Hard Liquor
Tap Water	Energy Drinks	Soy Milk*
Most Alcohols	Fruit Juices (with sugar)*	Black Tea
Soda/Pop	Pasteurized Milk	

FABULOUS FOOD REPLACEMENTS

The foods listed on the left are Unhealthy Foods, which can easily be replaced with the items listed on the right that are Healthy Replacements, as the replacements mimic the taste and use of the unhealthy foods.

UNHEALTHY FOODS

Sugar.............................

White Flour............................
Pasta....................................

Canola Oil, Vegetable Oil...............

Cheese..................................
Peanut Butter............................
Bacon & Sausages.......................

Yogurt...................................

Milk......................................
Sour Cream.............................
Salted & Roasted Nuts...................
White Rice...............................
Fat called for in recipes.................

Black Pepper............................
Salt ....

HEALTHY REPLACEMENTS

Succanat, Agave Nectar, Pure Maple Syrup, or Stevia
Whole Spelt, Rice, Barley, or Oat Flour
Ezekiel Sprouted grain pasta, Spelt or Brown Rice Pasta
Sunflower and Sesame Oil, Walnut, Olive and Coconut Oil, Flax Seed Oil, Organic Butter
Raw Cheese, Almond or Rice Cheese
Raw Almond and Sesame butter
Pork Free Turkey or Chicken sausage/bacon (Welshire Farms, Applegate Farms)
Kefir (by Lifeway) made from unpasteurized cows milk
Almond, Rice or Soy Milk
Toffuti Sour Cream or Rice Sour Cream
Raw Nuts
Brown Rice, Spelt or Barley
Applesauce, mashed bananas, ground flax seed, ground zucchini.
Cracked White or Red Pepper
Sea Salt that has natural discoloring –Redmond's Real Salt™

UNHEALTHY FOODS	HEALTHY REPLACEMENTS
Ketchup.....................................	Fruit Sweetened Ketchup
Vinegar.....................................	Apple Cider Vinegar or Lemon Juice
Soy Sauce.................................	Bragg's Liquid Aminos
Mayonnaise..............................	Vegenaise (by Follow Your Heart)
Tomato Soup.............................	Fresh tomatoes pureed in blender, with almond milk, oregano, stevia, sea salt, thyme, basil and olive oil- warm up and serve.
Chips...	Organic selections made with sunflower, olive, safflower oil.
Cheese Dip................................	Recipe in back No Cheese-Cheese Sauce & Dip.
Canned Foods............................	Fresh or frozen raw vegetables or fruits.
Dried Fruits with Sulfur..............	Unsulfured dried fruits
Meat and Deli Meats..................	Raw nuts, seeds, beans, sprouts and organic meats.
Café Latte, Coffee...................... & Black Tea	Green Tea with Almond milk, stevia, ginger, cinnamon, cardamom and nutmeg
Pop and Canned Juices..............	Water, Fresh Juices (Knudson) Lemon in water or Watermelon.
Gelatin......................................	Agar-Agar (tasteless, colorless seaweed).
Refried Beans...........................	Cooked Organic Pinto or Black beans that you mash up adding little Olive oil.

"KILL YOUR CRAVINGS" REPLACEMENTS

Now that you have started eating life-giving foods, you may occasionally experience cravings for processed, "low nutrient foods". Below are suggested replacements for those unhealthy low nutrient foods. The column on the left is unhealthy food cravings, which can be replaced by the list of foods to the right. These foods have the vitamins and minerals your body is searching for yet not getting. The items marked with a * can be found in the recipe section in the back of the book.

When You Crave This: Choose This:

Apple Pie-----------------------→*Charosset or Raw Apple Pie

Burritos ------------------------→ Ezekiel Tortilla with lightly stir-fried grated veggies, Toffuti sour cream, and 505 green chili sauce.

White Bread ---------------------→Toasted Ezekiel Bread, Spelt Bread

Candy Bar -----------------------→ Raw Cashews and dried Papaya

Candy --------------------------→ Dried Fruit or *Breakfast Roll

Chocolate ----------------------→ Dairy free Chocolate or Carob Chips

Cheese -------------------------→*Dairy Free Cheese Sauce, Almond Cheese

Chip Dip -----------------------→* Hummus with Organic Chips

Dessert ------------------------→*Oatmeal cookies, Dried Fruits

Drugs and Alcohol---------------→*Green Machine Juice

Fried Foods --------------------→* Salmon Pineapple Stir-Fry or Roasted Baby Vegetables.

When You Crave This:	Choose This:
Hamburger	→ Organic Buffalo Burger on sprouted grain bun or * Lentil Loaf with Barbecue sauce.
Ice Cream or Milk Shake	→ Fruit Smoothie made with Almond milk, 1 banana, 1 cup frozen berries, ½ avocado, 2 dashes of stevia (by SweetLeaf)
Milk	→ Almond or Rice Milk
Pancakes	→ *Oatmeal/Kamut/Spelt Pancakes *Grande Puffed Pie
Pastries & Breakfast Cereals	→ *Multi-Grain Breakfast Recipe *Sarah's Puffed Pie *Spelt Breakfast Cake
Pizza	→ * California Spelt Crust Pizza
Pudding & Jello	→ Rice milk pudding/tapioca, tofu pudding
Pop or Juices	→ Fresh fruit or vegetable juices
Salad Dressings	→ *All varieties in the salad dressing section
Thai Food	→ Steamed Veggies with *Thai Red Curry Sauce or * Green Curry Sauce

8

Food Beautiful

Shopping List

FOOD BEAUTIFUL SHOPPING LIST

We recommend that all foods be organic if possible. Foods marked with a * are heavily sprayed with pesticides if purchased conventionally (meaning non-organic). Health food stores like Wild Oats, Whole Foods, Vitamin Cottage, and Sunflower Market carry a variety of these foods, however, organic foods are becoming more readily available in your local grocery store (sometimes a bit pricier). If you do most of the shopping you will find that Vitamin Cottage or your local health food store has more reasonable prices than the larger chain Health food stores. You will want to check out all the stores and compare their selection, quality, and price to one another. And be careful at markets that mix organic with conventional!! In the lists that follow, parenthesis indicate the best brands found thus far-though not an exhaustive list.

GRAINS, FLOURS & BREADS

While you are out shopping keep in mind to buy organic grains, which are higher in nutritional value and have no pesticides and herbicides on them. When you get home store these grains in your refrigerator or freezer so they do not spoil. Some grains you should avoid are the non-organic wheat, corn and their flour forms. Non-organic wheat flour spoils within two weeks of milling, making it very toxic for you. Sprouted grain is the best form of bread to eat as it has three times more nutritional value than flour breads and is much easier to digest. Alvarado St. Bakery and Food for Life are some companies that make excellent sprouted grain breads, bagels, tortillas and pasta.

___ Amaranth Grain/Flour	___ Brown Rice	___ Sprouted Bread
___ Oat Groats	___ Brown Rice Flour	(Food for Life)
___ Rolled Oats	___ Sweet Brown Rice	___ Tapoica
___ Spelt Flour	___ Rye Grain	Flour/Grain
___ Spelt Grain	___ Rye Flour	___ Mannabread
___ Kamut -rolled	___ Coconut Flour	___ Spelt
___ Tritical Flakes	___ Almond Flour	

FRUITS & FRUIT JUICES

Some of the fruits below can also be purchased frozen by Stahlbush or Cascadian Farms. For Fruit Juices, always dilute 1/3 with purified water, and choose the brands from either Knudson, Santa Cruz, or Lakewood Organics.

____ Apples
____ Apricot *
____ Banana
____ Kiwi
____ Figs
____ Prunes
____ Date
____ Raisins *
____ Lime

____ Nectarine
____ Melons
____ Mango
____ Pineapple
____ Papaya
____ Grapefruit
____ Lemon
____ Avocado * (by Hass)
____ Grapes- seeded

____ Strawberries *
____ Blueberry
____ Pear
____ Peach *
____ Black Berry
____ Raspberry
____ Cranberry
____ Tangerine
____ Tomato- all varieties *

VEGETABLES

I highly encourage you to purchase these and all foods organic as many of the conventional vegetables are genetically modified. Those marked with a * are definitely genetically modified unless they are organic.

____ Alfalfa Sprouts
____ Artichoke
____ Asparagus
____ Baby Corn *
____ Bamboo Shoots
____ Beets
____ Beet Greens
____ Bell Peppers- all colors
____ Broccoli *

____ Eggplant
____ Endive
____ Escarole
____ Garlic
____ Ginger
____ Horseradish
____ Jicama
____ Kale- all varieties
____ Lettuce- all varieties

____ Radish
____ Rutabaga
____ Shallots
____ Sorrel
____ Spinach
____ Sprouts
____ Squashes- All Varieties
____ Sugar Snap Peas

_____ Cabbage- all colors
_____ Carrots
_____ Cauliflower
_____ Celery
_____ Chicory
_____ Chili Pepper
_____ Chives
_____ Collard Greens
_____ Cucumber *
_____ Dandelion Greens

_____ Leeks
_____ Mushrooms
    (Portabello, Shitakii)
_____ Mustard Greens
_____ Onion- all kinds
_____ Okra
_____ Parsley- all varieties
_____ Parsnips
_____ Potatoes (red) *
_____ Pumpkin

_____ Swiss Chard
_____ Taro Root
_____ Turnip
_____ Water chestnuts
_____ Watercress
_____ Yellow Squash
_____ Zucchini

UNPASTUERIZED DAIRY & NON-DAIRY

Try to avoid items that are enriched with vitamins, as these products contain synthetic vitamins which deplete your body of nutrients. I do not recommend using Canola Oil regularly, however some of the cheese alternatives have canola oil in them. Try to keep canola based oil products to a minimum and use the healthier recommended oils listed under Fantastic Food Replacements.

_____ Rice Milk- vanilla or plain
    (Rice Dream)
_____ Organic Yogurt
    (Brown Cow, Alto, Horizons)
_____ Organic Raw Cheese
    (Organic Valley, Alta Denta)
_____ Chocolate Chips
    (Tropical Source, Sunspire)
_____ Carob Chips
    (Sunspire, Chatfields)

_____ Oat Milk (Pacific)
_____ Multi Grain Milk (Pacific)
_____ Almond Milk
    (Blue Diamond Natural)
_____ Organic Butter
    (Alto, Horizons)
_____ Rice Cheese (by Aromatic)
_____ Almond Cheese
    (by Aromatic)
_____ Kefir –(Lifeway Organic)

HEALTHY OILS

Choose cold pressed organic oils as they are not heated up to extract the oil, preserving the nutrients and healing properties of the oil.

____ Olive Oil -extra virgin (Olio Beato, Omega Nutrition)
____ Coconut Oil (Omega Nutrition, Garden of Life)
____ Walnut Oil (Spectrum)
____ Flax Seed Oil- (Barleans Organics)
____ Hempseed Oil (Manitoba Harvest)
____ Sesame Oil (Flora, Spectrum)
____ Sunflower Oil (Spectrum)
____ Organic Butter (Horizons, Organic Valley)

RED MEAT, POULTRY, FISH & OTHER PROTEIN SOURCES

____ Free Range Deli Turkey (Deisel, Applegate Farm)
____ Free Range Deli Chicken (Deisel, Applegate Farm)
____ Free Range Buffalo (Order; Custer County Bison (719)-783-2530)
____ Venison & Elk Meat
____ Free Range Beef
____ Organic Lamb
____ Tofu– (Denver Tofu)
____ Silken Tofu (Nori)
____ Tempe- fermented soy beans.
____ Eggs -Organic Free Range/Roaming (Nest Fresh, Chino Valley)
____ Tofu Pups
____ Fish without dye, not farm raised, wild harvested, Alaskan or fresh water.
____Salmon ____ Halibut ____Yellow Perch ____Trout ____Tuna
____ Mackerel ___ Herring ___ Bass ___ Cod ___ Haddock

NUTS & SEEDS

It is best to keep all nuts and seeds refrigerated as they can go rancid (spoil) quickly if unshelled. I do not recommend roasted nuts or seeds (with exception to pumpkin seed) as this causes them to lose their vitamin E (which protects the other vitamins and minerals in the nut/seed) and denatures the quality of the natural oils within them.

___Almonds –raw

___ Coconut Meal

___ Coconut Flakes- without sugar

___ Brazil Nuts- raw

___ Peanuts- raw

___ Cashews- raw

___ Chestnuts- seasonal

___ Pecans-raw

___ Hazelnuts- raw

___ Walnuts-raw

___ Pumpkin Seeds- roasted or raw

___ Black Sesame Seeds- raw

___ Sesame Seeds- raw & unhulled

___ Sunflower Seeds - raw

___ Poppy Seeds - raw

___ Flax Seed- raw or ground

BEANS & LEGUMES

Beans can be found dried in bulk or canned by Eden, Westbrae Organics, or by Natural Value. You can sprout beans to increase their mineral, amino-acid, and enzymatic composition.

___ Aduki & Sprouts

___ Adzuki

___ Black Beans

___ Bean Sprouts

___ Garbanzo Beans /Chickpeas

___ Kidney Beans

___ Black Eyed Peas & Sprouts

___ Navy Beans

___ Organic Refried Beans

___ Green Lentils

___ Red Lentils

___ Yellow Lentils

___ Lima Beans

___ Mung Beans & Sprouts

___ Peas- frozen (by Stahlbush)

NOODLES, CHIPS, PASTA & PACKAGED FOODS

____ Brown Rice Noodles (Thai Kitchen, Tinkyada)

____ Kamut Noodles (Cleopatra's Noodles, Eden Organics)

____ Spelt Pasta & Noodles (by VitaSpelt)

____ Sprouted noodles and pastas (Food For Life)

____ Bean Noodles

____ Rice Cakes (by Lunberg)

____ Rice Crackers (Hol-Grain, Edward & Sons, San-J)

____ Blue & Red Corn Chips (by Kettle, Guiltless Gourmet)

____ Potato Chips (Kettle, Terra-Red Bliss) made with Olive Oil

____ Cheeto Replacement – Tings (by Robert's American Gourmet)

____ Cookies- (Enjoy Life, Small Planet Foods)

____ Flax Crackers – by Foods Alive (order at Foodbeautiful.com)

____ Amaranth Crackers- (Nu World Foods)

____ Healthy Bars (by Organic Food Bar, Lara Bars, BubbleBar's)

____ Chocolate Bars (Dagoba, Endangered Species, Newman's Organics)

CONDIMENTS

It seems as though more products are adding canola oil, which is a hybrid seed that has high amounts of Omega 6's, which, in excess, can cause physical problems. It is not recommended that you use canola oil regularly; it can cause cholesterol and plaque build up in your arteries, and cause arthritic type symptoms.

____ Ranch Dressing (by Tammy's Second Chance Ranch)

____ Applesauce (Solana Gold, Santa Cruz) from organic apples

____ Mustard – made with Apple Cider vinegar (Annie's Natural)

____ Apple Cider Vinegar (Bragg's)

____ Liquid Aminos (by Bragg's) -soy sauce alternative

____ Almond Butter-raw (Maranatha)

____ Tahini- raw (by Maranatha) sesame butter

____ Brewer's Yeast (by Lewis Labs, KAL)

____ Lemon Juice (by Lakewood Organic, Santa Cruiz)

____ Jams- fruit sweetened (by St Daflour, Crofters, Fiordifrutta)

____ Honey – Raw (Ambrosia, Really Raw Honey, Clark's Raw Honey)

____ Maple Syrup (by Shady Maple)

____ Succanat – 100% Raw Cane Sugar- not refined!

____ Date Sugar

____ Black Strap Molasses-unsulphured (by Plantations)

____ Stevia (by Now, Sweet Leaf) powdered or liquid

____ Sour Cream (Toffuti Sour Cream)

____ Rice Sour Cream (by Rice)

____ Mayonnaise Replacement- Vegenaise (by Follow your Heart)

____ Salsa (505 Organics, Emerald Valley Kitchen – Fresh & Organic)

____ Ketchup (by Muir Glen Organics) Fruit juice sweetened

____ Green Chili- Pork free (505 Organics)

____ Red Chile Sauce (505 Organics)

____ Coconut Milk (Natures Forest)

____ Xylitol- (by The Ultimate Sweetener)- birch sugar

TEA

Green tea is the pure un-roasted leaf filled with antioxidants and minerals. Black Tea's are roasted leaves with very little antioxidants, to many tannins, and cause flair ups for those dealing with candida or fungus issues.

Green Tea	Herbal Teas	Other Teas
Celestial Seasoning	Milk Thistle	Yogi Teas
St. Daflour	Dandelion	Celestial Seasoning Teas
Lotus Island	Chamomile	Alvita Teas

SPICES & HERBS

If you have had your spices for more than a year, replace them with fresh herbs. You can store spices in the freezer to preserve their effectiveness, freshness, and taste, otherwise, use your cupboard spices within a year from purchasing. Simply Organic, Frontier, Spice Island and The Spice Hunter are the best brand names to purchase from. Feel Free to purchase spices that are premixed for Mexican, Thai, Italian... dishes. Make sure that none of your spices have ingredients such as salt, MSG, spices, natural flavors in them as these are neurotoxins, that stimulate your hypothalamus (taste center of your brain) to crave more food. Always remember that any vegetable meal can transform from boring to fabulous by adding more spices, stevia, or fruit juice.

____ Anise	____ Cloves	____ Paprika
____ Dill	____ Cinnamon	____ Lemon Balm
____ Sage	____ Cayenne Pepper	____ Marjoram
____ Ginger	____ Chili Pepper	____ Orange Oil
	____ Lemon Peel	____ Tarragon
____ Fennel	____ White Pepper	____ Turmeric
____ Cumin	____ Licorice	
____ Celery Seed	____ Spearmint	____ Sea Salt (by Redmond)
____ Coriander	____ Peppermint	
____ Cardamom		

NUTRITIONAL SUPPLEMENTS

These are a list of the supplements I recommend and use myself, as they are the highest quality around, free of toxins and pollutants. You can order most of these products on my web site FoodBeautiful.com and DoctorBeautiful.com
on my web site www.foodbeautiful.com and www.doctorbeautiful.com Otherwise you can order the AIM products by calling 1-800-456-2462 and give them referral # 591683, so you can order the products at cost. Mannatech products can be requested for purchase via email Sarah@foodbeautiful.com for associate enrollment. These are many of the supplements we suggest to our clients. There are products listed on our websites that are not on this list.

____ Ambrotose- 8 essential glyconutrients (Mannatech)
____ Ambrotose AO - antioxidant (Mannatech)
____ Plus- endocrine system balancer (Mannatech)
____ EFA's –Omega 3's (Nutri-West, Carlson's)
____ Cod Liver Oil – Omega 3's and vitamin D (Carlson's)
____ Multivitamin - Food based (Mannatech, Megafood, Innate)
____ Probiotic (AIM, Mannatech. Nutri-West)
____ Digestive Enzymes (AIM, Mannatech, ReNew Life Formulas)
____ Amino Acids (Nutri-West)
____ Calcium (Nutri-West, Bone-up, Innate, Green Herb)
____ GenaSlim (Country-Life) weight management supplement
____ Liquid Iron- food derived source (Floridix)
____ Barley Life (AIM)
____ Just Carrots (AIM)
____ Herbal Fiber Blend (AIM)
____ Oil of Oregano & Olive Leaf Extract (GAIA)

Resource Guide for Purchasing Organic Foods

REJUVENATE FOODS
Telephone: (800) 805-7957
Web site: www.rejuvinate.com
They offer the highest-quality raw
fermented and cultured vegetables.

ORGANIC PASTURES DAIRY
Telephone: (559) 846-9732
Web site: www.organicpastures.com
They produce raw dairy products
that are from certified organic
pasture-grazed cows.

WHITE EGRET FARM
Telephone: (512) 267-7408
www.whiteegretfarm.com
They sell raw organic goat dairy
products; raw cheeses, milk and
yogurt. Free range turkey, goat
and beef.

EAT WILD
Web site: www.eatwild.com
Go to suppliers page and you can
find out how to purchase organic
foods of all varieties.

RAISED RIGHT
College Hill Poultry
220 North Center St.
Fredericksburg, PA 17026
Web site: wwwraisedright.com
Certified organic, free-range poultry

REAL FOODS MARKET
743 West 1200 North, Suite 200
Springville, UT 84663
Telephone: (886) 284-7325
www.realfoodsmarket.com
Organic grass-feed beef and wild
salmon. Raw dairy products; butter,
yogurt, kefir and cheese.

BRISTOL BAY

Telephone: (207) 223-4353
Wed site:
www.bristolbaywildsalmon.com
Wild sockeye salmon

FREY VINEYARDS

1400 Tomki Rd
Redwood Valley, CA 95470
Telephone: (800) 760-3739Web site:
www.freywine.com
Certified organic, biodynamic, and
sulfite-free wines

ORGANIC VALLEY

507 W. Main St.
LaFarge, WI 54639
Telephone: (608) 625-2602
Wed Site: www.organicvalley.com
Certified organic high omega-3 eggs.

ARROWHEAD MILLS

Telephone: (800) 749-0730
Web site: www.arrowheadmills.com
Packaged and bulk organic grains
and flour.

ORGANIC WINE WORKS

Web site: www.organicwineworks.com
This site sells the finest certified organic
wines from around the world.

THE RAW WORLD

P.O. Box 16156
West Palm Beach, FL 33416
Telephone: (866) RAW DIET
Web site: www.therawworld.com
Supplier of raw foods, snacks, live
food supplements, juicers, blenders,
and many other excellent products.

GLASER ORGANICS

19100 SW 137th Ave
Miami, FL 33012
Telephone: (305) 238-7747
Web site:
www.glaserorganicfarm.com
Supplies a variety of organic raw nuts,
seeds, and butters.

9

Food Beautiful Recipes

Breakfast

Date-Pecan Squares

Ingredients

1 cup dates
½ cup pecans
1 tsp. Vanilla extract
1 cup organic raisins
2 cups unsweetened shredded coconut

Directions

In a food processor, using the "S" blade, grind pecans into a fine meal; add pitted dates and raisins, process until dough like consistency is reached. By hand, work in ½ cup of the coconut. Sprinkle ¾ cup coconut in a pan, place date pecan mixture on top and spread to cover bottom payer. Top with remaining coconut. Cover and place in refrigerator. When chilled cut into squares and serve.

Date Coconut logs

Ingredients

2 cups organic dates- pitted
1 cup unsweetened, shredded coconut
½ cup apple juice

Directions

In a food processor using the "S" blade or blender grind date and juice until dough like consistency is reached. Wet hands and shape into logs, and roll them in coconut until they are covered.

Orange Poppy Seed Muffins

Ingredients

1 cup oat or spelt flour
2 tsp baking powder
4 TBS Xylitol or Succanat
1/4 tsp salt
1 tsp vanilla

¼ cup poppy seeds
2 tsp orange oil
1/2 cup water
2 TBS walnut oil

Directions

Preheat oven to 400 degrees. Oil spray (with sunflower or olive oil by Spectrum) 6 muffin pans. Sift dry ingredients into a bowl. Add cold water and mix until smooth then stir in oil. Pour into muffin cups that have been sprayed. Bake for 25 minutes. Makes 6 to 8 muffins.

Carob Muffins

Ingredients

1/3 cup pecan nuts
1/2 cup coarsely chopped pecans
1 cup boiling water
2 tsp baking powder
1/4 cup walnut oil
3/4 tsp ground cinnamon

1/4 cup honey
1/4 tsp baking soda
1 cup spelt flour
2 eggs
1/3 cup carob powder
1 tsp pure vanilla extract

Directions

Grind 1/3-cup pecans to a fine powder in a blender, add water and blend for 30 seconds, add oil and honey, blend again. Allow to cool to lukewarm. Combine flour, carob, chopped pecans, baking powder, cinnamon and baking soda in a large bowl. Mix well. When the liquid mixture has cooled to lukewarm, blend in the eggs and vanilla. Pour liquid mixture into the flour bowl. Mix until all ingredients are blended well together. Bake in muffin cases at 350 F for 25 minutes.

Breakfast of Champions

Ingredients

1-2 cups of cooked brown rice &
    sweet brown rice or spelt

Juice of 1 lemon or lime

1 TBS Agave Nectar
    (honey replacement)

1-2 tsp. Flax Oil

1-2 tsp Bragg's Liquid Aminos®
    (soy sauce replacement)

½-1 Avocado sliced and/or sunflower seeds

2 TBS Almond slivers

1 firm Tomato

1 tsp of Spice Hunter's® Garlic
    Herb Bread Seasoning

Directions

Warm the rice up if you have time! Slice the avocado and tomato into chunks. Mix in the oil, Liquid Aminos, lemon juice, agave nectar and sprinkle seasoning over the top.

Cashew Butter Roll

Ingredients

20 Dates

½ cup Raisins

½ cup Cashew Butter

¼ cup chopped cashews

¼ cup sesame seeds

Directions

Pit the dates and blend raisins, dates and cashew butter together in a food processor or champion juicer with the screen plugged. Take out and place in bowl, stir in chopped cashews. Then take small amounts and roll it over the sesame seeds so the roll is coated. Serves 4. Prep time 10 min.

Grande' Puffed Pancake

Ingredients

1 ¼ cup spelt flour
1 ¼ cup oat milk or rice milk
5 organic eggs
¼ tsp sea salt

1 tsp of cinnamon
¼ tsp Nutmeg
1 tsp Vanilla Extract
¼ stick Organic Butter
   or 4 TBS coconut oil

Directions

Preheat Oven to 425F. Beat the eggs until slightly stiff. Add the milk and vanilla mix to the eggs and stir until well combined. Then in a separate bowl mix all dry ingredients (spices, sea salt and flour) together. Slowly stir in the eggs to dry mix. Mix together completely until there are no lumps. Melt in oven ¼ stick of butter or 4 TBS Coconut oil in a 4-quart baking dish (casserole dish). Remove pan from oven stir butter around the pan until it is evenly spread. Then pour mixture directly in the center, place in oven for 12-15 min. It will come out puffy. Serve with maple syrup, applesauce, or jam. Serves 4.

Fruit Verdé

Ingredients

25 fresh green grapes
2-3 small-medium green kiwi

1 pear
2 TBS pineapple concentrate

Directions

Wash and cut grapes in half. Peel kiwi and chop in fairly small chunks. Chop pear into fairly small chunks as well. Place all fruit in bowl and pour pineapple concentrate over evenly. Serves 2.

Multi-Grain Cereal

NOTE: This is recommended as a cereal replacement.
It's packed with nutrients & loaded with flavor!

Ingredients

½ c. Oat Groats
½ c. Sweet Brown Rice
½ c. Spelt
3 ½ c. Water
1/8 tsp of cinnamon

Dash of nutmeg
¼ tsp. Sea salt
¼ cup Almond flakes
2 dashes Stevia
1 cup Rice Milk or Almond Milk

Directions

Bring water to a boil, add grains, turn to low, let simmer for 45 minutes. Strain out water and add cinnamon, nutmeg, sea salt, almond flakes and stevia. Serve hot or cold with Almond milk.

Berry Packed Smoothie

Ingredients

1 c. Berries of choice
½ c. Kefir (by Lifeway)
1 tsp. black strap molasses
1 dropper full of Stevia

½ c. Almond milk or papaya juice
½ banana
1 cup of ice

Directions

Place all ingredients into blender and mix until creamy.

Walnut Raisin Breakfast Cake

Note: You will need to purchase the arrowroot powder at a health food store. Arrowroot is a natural healthy thickener for recipes.

Ingredients

1 2/3 cups water

1/2 cup raisins

1/2 pound pitted dates, chopped.

1/3 walnut oil

2 tsp lemon juice

1 cup spelt flour

1 cup arrowroot powder

1 tsp baking soda

1 tsp ground cinnamon

1/2 cup chopped walnuts

Directions

Combine water, raisins and dates in a 3 quart saucepan. Boil for 10 minutes, then set aside to cool. Stir in the oil and lemon juice into a medium bowl, sift the flour, arrowroot, baking soda and cinnamon. Stir the flour mixture into the saucepan, mix well, stir in the walnuts. Spread batter into an oiled 8" or 9" square baking pan. Bake at 400 F for 20 minutes, or until the top is firm when touched.

Brain & Joint Food

Note: Kefir is cultured un-pasteurized cow's milk and tastes like plain yogurt.
This drink adds in repair of all tissues (tendons, bones, and joints), increases vascular growth, clears plaque out of the arteries, highly absorbable form of calcium. Aids brain function, muscular growth, and fat metabolism.

Ingredients

½ cup Plain Kefir

1 TBS Cod Liver Oil –plain flavor
(by Carlson's®)

2-3 dashes of Stevia (by Sweet Leaf)

1 tsp carob powder

2 dashes cinnamon

2 dashes nutmeg

2 dashes ginger

Directions

Place all ingredients into a cup and mix until emulsified together.

Granola Gone Nuts

Ingredients

In a large bowl mix together:

4 or 5 cups rolled oats

¾ cup wheat germ

½ cup bran or bran flakes
   (optional)

½ cup sesame seeds

¾ cup fresh or dried coconut

¾ cup raw sunflower seeds

½ cup almonds, slivered

½ cup walnuts, chopped

¾ cup flax seeds

In a separate bowl mix together:

3/4 cup raw unfiltered honey

2 tsp. Vanilla

1/3 cup fresh apple juice

Directions

Pour wet ingredients over dry ingredients a little at a time, stirring to distribute evenly. Preheat oven to 300 F. Line a 9 x 13 inch cooking pan with a thin layer of soy lecithin then pour mixture onto pan. Bake for one hour, stirring every 15 minutes. After removing from the oven add dried fruit, cool to room temperature and store in airtight container.

A Berry Delicious Tart

Note: Agar- Agar, a tasteless seaweed that is used as a gelatin replacement.

Ingredients

2 cups fresh strawberries

2 cups fresh blueberries

½ cup apple juice

2 ripe bananas

2 ripe nectarines

1 ½ TBS. Agar-agar

½ cup shredded coconut

1 ¾ cup applesauce

Directions

Mix ½ cup apple juice with Agar-Agar and heat gently until dissolved, stirring constantly. Set aside to cool. Wash, hull and slice strawberries, wash blueberries, peel and slice nectarines. Set these items aside. In blender combine 2 ripe bananas and 1 3/4 cup applesauce, and blend until smooth. Combine with Agar-agar and apple juice mixture, add coconut, and pour over fruit. Mix gently. Pour into round pan or decorative ring and chill until it sets.

Mediterranean Fruit Salad

Ingredients

1 banana

4 dates

¼ cup organic apple juice

¼ cup organic raisins

½ avocado

Directions

Soak the raisins in the apple juice for 30 min. Peel and slice the bananas, peel and dice the avocado and cut dates into small pieces. Combine everything into a bowl and eat.

Oatmeal Pancakes

Note: Succanat or Xylitol is a healthy sugar substitute

Ingredients

3/4 cup ground oat (flour)
1/4 tsp baking soda
1 1/2 cups purified water
1/2 cup ground oats
1 TBS Succanat or Xylitol
1 tsp baking powder
½ tsp sea salt

Beaten together:

3 TBS Walnut or Grape seed Oil
2 TBS purified water
1 tsp baking powder

Directions

Combine oats, baking soda and 1 1/2 cups water; let stand for 5 minutes, so mixture rises. Combine ground oats, date sugar, 1 tsp baking powder and salt. Add to this beaten together oil, water and baking powder and beat well. Pour 1/4 cup batter for each pancake onto a hot greased griddle. Bake to a golden brown, turning once. Makes 10 pancakes.

Sweet Fruits Salad

Ingredients

8 dates
2 apples
¾ cup Organic Raisins

3 ripe bananas
2 ripe pears
½ cup organic apple juice

Directions

Peel apples pears and bananas. Cut all fruit into small pieces, add raisins, pour apple juice over fruit, cover and refrigerate. Serve cold. Coconut flakes may be added if desired.

Jewish Charosset

A traditional food used in Passover. It also makes a great morning breakfast meal eaten with toasted Ezekiel 4:19 bread.

Ingredients

3 apples, cored and grated
1 cup Walnut Pieces
¾ cup sliced apricots
1 TBS grated lemon rind
1 ½ tsp ground cinnamon

1 tsp nutmeg
3 tsp lemon juice
½ cup honey
½ cup raisins
4 TBS sweet red wine or
        pineapple juice

Directions

Cut the apples in half, remove their core and grate. Chop the dried fruit into bite size pieces. Place all ingredients into a large mixing bowl and mix together. Cover and chill

Citrus Salad Delight

Ingredients

2 oranges
½ pineapple
2 tangerines

1 grapefruit
1 pint strawberries
½ cup blueberries

Directions

Peel and segment oranges, tangerines, grapefruit and cut into smaller pieces. Cut pineapple into cubes, slice strawberries and put all ingredients into a bowl. If additional juice is needed, juice two oranges and pour over before serving.

Raisin Victor Salad

Ingredients

1 apple

1 peach

2 bananas

¼ cup of raisins

3 cups of red grapes

Directions

Wash grapes and cut in half, peel and dice apple and peach into ½ inch chunks, cut banana into quarters and slice. Combine all fruits together and serve.

Soups & Salads

Mozzarella Basil Rolls
& Creamy Tomato Soup

Note: Pick up 1 box of Organic Creamy Tomato Basil Soup (by Imagine). This is a dairy free soup mix. This recipe is okay for those dealing with fungal or Candida related issues when you use the rice or soy mozzarella cheese.

Ingredients:

1-2 large eggplant
3 tbs. Olive oil
8 oz. raw mozzarella cheese
or mozzarella rice cheese

2 tomatoes
8 large fresh basil leaves
Annie's Balsamic Olive Oil
  Vinaigrette

Directions

Preheat oven to 400F. Cut the eggplant into 8 lengthwise slices, sprinkle salt onto both sides to draw out bitter flavor. Leave on for 20 minutes, then rinse off and pat dry. Oil a large flat baking sheet, place on the eggplant and drizzle over with the Vinaigrette Dressing. Cook in oven for 8-10 minutes. Meanwhile cut the tomato into ½ inch half moon slices, and cut the cheese into ¼ inch lengthwise slices. Pull the Eggplant out of oven. Place in order on top the cheese slices, tomato and basil leaf then fold eggplant over the filling. Turn your oven to broil and cook for 3-4 min. or until cheese melts. Take out of oven and serve warm, with Tomato soup.

Lemony Lentil Soup

Ingredients

1 cup green or brown lentils
1 carton (32oz) veggie broth
2 cups water
1 medium yellow onion,
  chopped very fine
1 tsp oregano
1 cup cooked sweet brown rice
2 bay leaves

2 TBS Olive Oil
1/2 tsp fresh ground white pepper
1 tsp pre-packaged curry powder
1 tsp sea salt (less or more to taste)
4 TBS honey or agave nectar
2 lemons and their peel
  (puréed in food processor)

Directions

Rinse lentils in strainer, until water runs through clear, place into a soup pot along with the veggie broth and 2 cups water. Bring to a boil, lower heat to medium high, and simmer (steady bubbling, but not boiling). Add bay leaves, oregano, pepper, curry powder, then cover and let cook for 25 minutes. While the lentils are cooking, chop onion very fine and sauté in 2 TBS olive oil until the onions are soft (about 5-6 minutes). When the soup has cooked for 25 minutes, add the sautéed onion, cooked rice, and honey. Continue cooking covered for another 20 minutes. Finally add the white pepper and puréed lemons, stir until evenly combined. Remove bay leaf and serve. Enjoy with spelt or rye crackers.

Black Nile Salad

Ingredients

1/2 cup quinoa
1 cup sweet corn
2 scallions chopped
1/2 cup finely chopped tomatoes
1/2 cup celery thinly sliced
1/2 cup chopped green peppers
1 can black beans, drained and rinsed

Dressing Ingredients

3-4 TBS Olive Oil
2 TBS Lemon juice or Balsamic vinegar
1 TBS Apple cider
2 clove garlic minced
1 tsp sea salt
3 dashes stevia powder
1 tsp chili powder
1 tsp ground white pepper
2 TBS both fresh cilantro and parsley

Directions

Soak ½ cup quinoa for five minutes then drain. Cook either in 1 cup vegetable stock or water for 15 minutes. In the last five minutes put in the corn if using frozen. After it is done cooking drain and allow to cool. Mix the dressing and then add the remaining ingredients together in a bowl and mix well. This salad is best served cold. Feel free to add a couple of jalapeno peppers before serving or a couple of dashes of cayenne if you like it hot. Serves: 4-6.

Cabbage Peanut Salad

Ingredients

2 cups red cabbage
2 cups green cabbage (finely chopped or shredded)
3/4 cup ground raw peanuts or roasted cashews if you are allergic to peanuts (you can use more or less as you like.)

1 tsp sea salt and pepper to taste
1 TBS lime or lemon juice
4 TBS Honey or Agave Nectar
2 TBS red Chili Oil
1/4 cup finely chopped cilantro leaves

Directions

In a saucepan heat up honey and oil. Then in a large bowl toss in all the ingredients, mix well and serve. You can serve immediately or chilled if you prefer.

Greek Salad

Ingredients

1 carrot, finely diced or grated

2 cucumbers, finely diced

2 onions, finely chopped

3 green chilies, finely chopped

1 tomato, finely diced

½ cup Coriander leaves, chopped

3 mint leaves-minced

2 tsp fresh chopped ginger

4 TBS. Agave nectar

4 lettuce leaves, finely cut

½ cup cabbage, finely sliced

Juice of 1 lemon

1 tsp sea salt or to taste

1 cup Greek Dressing (by Annie's®)

Directions

Mix all the grated and chopped items together with sea salt and lemon. Add Greek dressing (by Frontier Culinary Spices or Annie's) and mix together and serve chilled or as is. Serves 3

Marinated Cucumber Salad

Ingredients

2 medium cucumbers

1 TBS sea salt

½ cup date sugar or honey
    or 1/8 tsp powdered stevia

1/2 cup brown rice vinegar

1 TBS apple juice

3 TBS fresh dill, chopped

4 dashes ground white pepper

Directions

Slice cucumbers thinly and place them in a colander, sprinkling with salt between each layer. Set the colander over a bowl large enough to catch the water and let drain for 1 hour. Thoroughly rinse the cucumber slices under cold running water to remove excess salt. Pat dry with paper towels and set aside. Gently heat the sugar or honey with brown rice vinegar and apple juice in a sauce pain until the sugar/ honey dissolves. Remove from heat and let cool. Place cucumbers into a bowl, pour the vinegar mixture over them and let marinate for 2 hour. Drain the cucumber and sprinkle with dill and pepper. Chill until ready to serve.

Rainbow Salad

Ingredients

1 cup red cabbage, grated

½ a beet, grated

2 carrots, grated

1 zucchini, grated

1 cup jicama, grated

1 cup fresh green peas

1 cup sprouts of choice

1 apple, grated

1 cup pumpkin seeds

1 cup Tahini Mint Dressing
in sauces section

Directions

Grate all the vegetables and toss in a large salad bowl with salad dressing.

Hot and Sour Chinese Salad

Ingredients

2 cups snow peas or early peas,
   Slightly cooked
4 cups rice noodles, cooked
   and drained and cut into
   2-inch length strips

Dressing Ingredients

1 green onion, chopped

1 TBS Umeboshi Paste

2-3 tsp mustard

Juice of 2 lemons

Pinch of stevia

1 TBS Oil

Directions:

Combine the peas with the noodles. Blend ingredients for the dressing together. Add dressing to noodle mixture. Mix lightly and serve before noodles become mushy.

Simply Sprouts

Ingredients:
Simple Sprouted Salad
2 cups alfalfa sprouts
2 cups mung sprouts
1 cup sunflower sprouts

Directions
Arrange an outside ring of alfalfa sprouts on a plate. Next make a ring of mung sprouts. Place sunflower sprouts in center. Serve with your favorite salad dressing.

Rutabaga-Parsley Salad

Ingredients
1 cup boiling water with
1 tsp sea salt
½ bunch of parsley
1-2 large rutabaga or turnips

2 TBS Vegenaise (mayo)
¼ cup sauerkraut
A pinch of stevia
½-1 tsp sea salt

Directions
Plunge the parsley into salted boiling water for 3 minutes. Remove and chop finely. Cut rutabagas into round slices and cook in the parsley water (without the parsley). Mix the sauerkraut, stevia, salt, and mayonnaise together. Arrange the rutabaga over the bed of parsley and pour the dressing over top. Serve with protein of choice!

Pineapple Broccoli Salad

Ingredients

2 bunches of fresh broccoli

1/2 red onion

½ cup sunflower seeds

1 cup grated carrots

2 cups Pineapple

1 cup Vegenaise (Mayo replacement)

3 TBS Xylitol or Succanat

2 TBS apple cider vinegar

2 dashes of cayenne pepper

1 tsp sea salt or to taste

Directions

Cut broccoli, red onion, pineapple (cubed) into bit size pieces, and mix all ingredients into a bowl and let stand several hours in refrigerator. Recipe can be adjusted to one's taste by adding more cayenne or sea salt. Serves: 6-8 Preparation time: 10 minutes

Lunch & Dinner:

Meat, Vegetarian & Side Dishes

Salmon Pineapple Stir-Fry

Ingredients

1 cup baby corn, halved
1 orange bell pepper, thinly sliced lengthwise
1 green bell pepper, thinly sliced lengthwise
1 red onion, sliced
2 TBS sesame/sunflower oil
1 lb. salmon fillet, skin removed
½ cup bean sprouts
2 TBS paprika
2 dashes powdered stevia (by Sweet Leaf)
8 oz. of freshly ripened pineapple, cubed
2 TBS fruit sweetened Ketchup
3 TBS soy sauce or Bragg's Liquid Aminos®
2 TBS white wine
1 tsp cornstarch or 1/8 tsp xanthan gum

Directions

Heat the oil in a large wok or pan. Add the onion, bell peppers, and baby corn to pan and stir-fry for 5 min. Rinse the salmon fillet under cold water and pat dry with paper towels. Cut the salmon into thin strips and place in large bowl. Sprinkle heavily with paprika and toss until well coated. Add the salmon to the wok/pan, together with the pineapple, stir-fry 3-4 min. further until fish is tender. Add the bean sprouts to the pan and toss well. Mix together the Ketchup, soy sauce, wine, stevia and cornstarch. Add the mixture to the wok and cook until the juice thickens. Transfer to warm serving plate and eat immediately. Serves 4.

Red Curry Delight

Sauce Ingredients

2 garlic cloves, minced
2 roasted red bell peppers chopped
1 TBS Ginger root, chopped or pressed
2 TBS fresh mint, roughly chopped
¼ onion, chopped
¾ cup lime juice
1 tsp ground cumin

2-3 pinches ground cloves
cayenne pepper, to taste
¾ tsp. paprika
14 oz. Coconut milk
2 TBS Red Curry
    (from "Thai Kitchen")
½ cup honey or Succanat
    (is 100% raw cane sugar)

Other Ingredients

4 cups cooked brown rice
1 head broccoli, chop into bit size pieces
1 zucchini- cut half moon shape, ¼ inch thick
2 carrots – chopped ¼ inch thick
½ head of green cabbage, chop into 6 pieces
1 can of baby corn

Directions

In a food processor or blender mix well the garlic, roasted bell peppers, ginger, mint, onion, lime juice, cayenne, cumin, cloves, paprika. Set aside. In a large saucepan simmer coconut milk then add the red curry sauce with blended herbs, and honey for 5 min. Cook the brown rice. Chop the vegetables and steam until lightly cooked, make sure they are still crunchy. You can also serve with organic chicken! Serves 3-4.

Green Curry Halibut

Note: You can make this a curry soup dilute with 3/4 cup water during cooking

Sauce Ingredients

4 garlic cloves, minced
2-3 mild chilies, chopped
1 TBS Ginger root, pressed
2 dashes cayenne pepper
1 tsp ground cumin
2-3 pinches ground cloves
1 pinch cinnamon
¼ onion, chopped

½ cup lemon juice
14 oz. Coconut milk
1-2 TBS Green curry from
   Thai Kitchen®
½ cup honey
1 TBS fish sauce (optional)
1 tsp of sea salt

Other Ingredients

2 steaks Halibut or Cod, cooked
3 TBS Olive Oil
1 head broccoli

1 zucchini
2 carrots
½ head of green cabbage
1 can of baby corn

Directions

In a food processor or blender mix well the garlic, ginger, chilies, onion, lemon juice, cayenne, cumin, cloves, and cinnamon. Set aside. In a large saucepan simmer coconut milk then add the green curry sauce with blended herbs and honey, stir occasionally for 5 min. Slice fish into 1" square pieces. Pour 3 TBS Olive Oil on top and season with 1 tsp. sea salt cook on stove until it flakes apart (about 8-10 min). While fish is cooking, chop broccoli, slice carrots and zucchini into ¼ inch thick half moon pieces, chop cabbage into large chunks and steam until lightly cooked. Then in a large flat serving dish place in the fish baby corn, steamed vegetables, pour the sauce over top or place in a bowl and dip food into it. Serves 3-4.

Miso Sweet Potato Casserole

Note: Miso is a fermented brown rice or soy paste that is traditionally used in Japanese style meals and soups. Aduki beans are known for their weight loss and cleansing properties. You can pick these products up at the health food store.

Ingredients

16 oz can Aduki beans

1 medium carrot

1 cup Sliced green beans

1 medium red onion

2 sweet potatoes/yam cubed

4 TBS succanat or Xylitol

4 TBS Olive Oil or Organic Butter

1/2 cup frozen peas

1/2 cup rolled oats

2 tsp paprika

1 tsp dried thyme

1 TBS. miso

3 TBS Bragg's Aminos®
   (soy sauce replacement)

¾ cup water

¾ cup soy milk

Directions

In a 2-3 quart casserole dish dissolve miso with ¼ cup boiling water. Add Aduki beans, stir in rolled oats, paprika, thyme, and Liquid Aminos. Chop vegetables and dice onion, place into medium sized pan and add to casserole dish. Cover with 1/2 cup water, 3/4 cup soy milk and drizzle over 4 TBS Olive Oil. Cook at 300 F for 1 hour 35 minutes. Stir a couple of times during cook time to make sure it is not drying out. Add additional oil or soymilk if needed. It may need thickening before serving, you can add 1-2 TBS of ground flax seed, or ¼ tsp Xanthan Gum. Serves 2.

Veggie Tortilla Wraps

Ingredients

1 cup zucchini, grated
1 cup carrots, grated
½-1 cup finely chopped broccoli
1 tomato, finely chopped
1 tsp sea salt
1 tsp onion powder
1 tsp basil
1 tsp garlic powder
2 tsp paprika
2 dashes cayenne (optional)

2 dashes ground white pepper
½ tsp sage
2 TBS Olive Oil
½ cup black beans or
   organic refried beans
5 oz pepper jack rice cheese, sliced
½ cup 505 Chili sauce
Toffuti™ sour cream
2 sprouted grain tortilla's
   (Food for Life™)

Directions

Place the zucchini, carrots and broccoli in a medium size bowl, mix in the herbs and sea salt. Then place a frying pan with 2 TBS olive oil on medium heat until oil is warmed up. Pour in the vegetables, stir and cook for 5 minutes. Meanwhile place the sliced cheese, beans and tomato in the middle of the tortillas. Remove the vegetables from heat place into the tortilla wraps and fold over. Place back into the pan over medium high heat for 2 minutes each side. You may want to place a plate on top of the tortilla's to keep them from opening up. Top with the chili sauce and sour cream to your liking.

African Pineapple Cashew Moussaka

Ingredients

1 cup Onions, Chopped

2 Garlic Cloves, Minced or Pressed

1 1/2 TBS Coconut Oil or Olive Oil

4 cups Kale, Sliced

2 cups Pineapple (Fresh is best)

1/2 cup Cashew Butter
    (or raw Peanut Butter)

1 TBS Tabasco or Hot Pepper Sauce

3 TBS Honey

1/2 cup Cilantro, Chopped

2 tsp. Sea salt

½ tsp. Mint

Directions

In a covered saucepan, sauté the onions and garlic in the oil for about 10 minutes, stirring frequently, until the onions are lightly browned. While the onions sauté, wash the kale and remove the stems. Stack the leaves on a cutting surface and slice crosswise into 1-inch-thick slices. Add the pineapple and its juice to the onions and bring to a simmer. Stir in the kale, cover, and simmer for about 5 minutes, stirring a couple of times, until just tender. Mix in the peanut butter, hot pepper sauce, sea salt, mint, cilantro, and honey simmer for 5 minutes. Serve warm and enjoy with toasted Ezekiel bread.

Tofu & Cauliflower Explosion

Note: You can substitute the tofu with ½ lb. shredded Organic chicken

Ingredients

1/2 head cauliflower, cut into florets

1/2 lb. extra firm tofu, pressed
and drained, cubed

4 cloves garlic, crushed

1 can chickpeas/garbanzo beans

2 diced tomatoes or 1 can diced
tomatoes

1/2 onion, quartered and sliced

1/8 cup sliced jalapeno peppers

2-3 tsp curry powder

1 tsp cumin

2 TBS toasted Sesame oil

1 tsp sea salt

½ tsp cracked white pepper

3 dashes of stevia powder

Directions

Heat toasted sesame oil over med-high heat. Place tofu cubes in 2 TBS Sesame Oil and let brown on one side. Before flipping, sprinkle the curry over all cubes and add crushed garlic. Flip and let cool for 1 minute. Add the cauliflower and onions, cook for 5 min, stirring occasionally. Add the garbanzo beans, cumin, sea salt, stevia, and white pepper stirring well. Cover and simmer for about 10 minutes. Add the tomatoes and simmer for another 5 minutes, covered.

Broccoli and Tofu in Garlic Sauce

Ingredients

2 lbs. Broccoli, florets

1 lb. Tofu, firm, cubed

1 Onion, medium, diced

3 TBS Garlic, crushed or minced

1 ½ tsp. Ginger, powder

1/4 tsp. Cayenne Pepper

2 cups brown rice

1/3 cup Soy Sauce or Liquid Aminos

3 TBS Corn Starch or 1/4 tsp Xanthan Gum

3 dashes Stevia powder

1 cup Water

Directions

1) Take two cups of brown rice cook in 4 cups of boiling water reduce to simmer and cook for 50 minutes. Begin cooking the rice at the same time you begin preparing this recipe.

2) Peel and dice onion, peel and crush the garlic, place in a wok or frying pan with 2 TBS Olive or sesame oil. Cook on medium heat until the onion just begins to become translucent. When using a wok, use a little water instead of oil to cook the food.

3) Wash and separate the broccoli florets and thinly slice the stems. Cube the tofu into 1/2" cubes. Add the broccoli, tofu, ginger, and cayenne pepper. Cook until the broccoli begins to get tender.

4) Mix the corn starch (or xanthan gum) and stevia into the soy sauce with about 1/2 cup of water and add to the cooking broccoli and tofu. Continue cooking and mixing continuously in the wok or frying pan. When the sauce thickens and thoroughly coats the other ingredients, remove from the heat. Add water as necessary to adjust the thickness of the sauce. Serve over a bed of brown rice and enjoy.

Spicy Chili

Ingredients

2 lbs. mixed dry beans
 (Black, Pinto, Kidney)

2 lbs. fresh organic tomatoes

1 large onion, diced

1 lb. extra firm Tofu, cubed (optional)

1 lb. Frozen Corn

1 Green Bell Pepper, diced

2 TBS Garlic, chopped or crushed

¼ tsp Stevia Powder or ½ cup Succanat
 (sugar replacement)

2 TBS Chili Powder

2 TBS Cumin

1 TBS Basil, dried leaf

5 TBS Olive Oil or Organic Butter

2-3 Chipotle Peppers, chopped

1/4 tsp. Cayenne Pepper (optional)

Directions

The chili can be prepared in a crock-pot or it can also be prepared on the stove top in a large covered pot. If using a crock pot, it is suggested that you begin cooking the beans the night before. If cooking the beans on the stove top, it is suggested to soak the beans the night before and then begin cooking first thing in the morning. This chili recipe can be made with one kind of bean or several varieties (black, kidney, pinto, or multi-bean blends). Wash and clean the beans and place in crock pot. Add 10 cups of boiling water. This speeds up the cooking process. Cook on "high" until you're ready for bed, and then turn down the heat to "low" for cooking overnight. First thing in the morning, turn the slow-cooker heat up to "high." Prepare all the other ingredients and add to the slow-cooker. Cook on "high" for another 4 to 6 hours. Add water as necessary. If cooking on the stove top, first thing in the morning begin cooking the beans. Wash and clean the beans and place in stove top pan with 10 cups water. When it begins to boil, turn heat to low and allow to simmer for 35 minutes. In the meantime prepare all the other ingredients and add to the pot after first 35 minutes of cooking. Raise the heat until the ingredients begin to boil and then lower the heat to simmer. Cook for another 4 to 6 hours. Stir often during the cooking process. If the chili begins to thicken before it is thoroughly cooked, add a little water. Serve the chili either as is, over brown rice or with fresh salad. Use the leftovers to make a chili salad.

Lentil Loaf with Barbecue Sauce

The Perfect meat substitute on sandwiches! Add avocado, sliced tomatoes and onions.

Ingredients

1-1/2 cups Lentils, uncooked

1 cup Brown Rice, uncooked

2 Onions, diced

6 TBS Tomato Puree

4 TBS Olive Oil

2 TBS Molasses, unsulphured

1 TBS Brown Mustard

1 TBS Soy Sauce or Liquid Aminos

2 cloves Garlic, pressed

2 tsp. Sage

1 tsp. Marjoram

1 tsp. sea salt

4 dashes stevia powder

1/2 cup Hot Sauce (to taste)

Directions

1) Place 3 1/2 cups of cold water in a covered glass pot, heat up until it reaches a boil. While the water is heating, rinse the lentils in a strainer, and remove any stones or other foreign matter. Add the rinsed lentils and 1 tsp sea salt to the boiling water turn to low and allow to simmer. Cook until all the water is absorbed.

2) Place 2 cups of cold water in a second pot and heat on stove until it boils. Add the rice to the boiling water, cover, and lower the heat to a simmer. Cook until all the water is absorbed.

3) While the lentils and rice are cooking, wash, peel and finely dice the onions. Sauté both onions for 2-3 minutes and add half to the lentil pot when the water is almost completely absorbed. Cook with the lentils until the water is all absorbed.

4) Prepare barbecue sauce while the lentils and rice are cooking. In a small mixing bowl thoroughly combine the tomato puree, mustard, hot sauce, olive oil, molasses, soy sauce and one half called for amount of the garlic, sage, marjoram and stevia.

5) When the lentils are cooked, place them in a large mixing bowl and coarsely mash so that most of the lentils are broken. Add the other half of the remaining garlic, sage, marjoram, onion, stevia and one half of the barbecue sauce to the mashed lentils and mix well. Add the cooked rice and, again, mix well!!

6) Firmly press the lentil loaf mix into a lightly oiled loaf pan or ceramic baking dish. Pour on the remaining barbecue sauce and evenly spread over the surface. Bake in a preheated oven at 350F for 1 hour. Cut ½ inch slices, serve open face with toasted Ezekiel bread, fresh slices of tomato and onion. You can add some Ketchup or Vegenaise (mayo) for extra flavor.

Vegetarian Lasagna

Dairy free, meat free, wheat free, sugar free, no guilt, but all the flavor.

Ingredients

1 lb. Brown Rice Lasagna
4 zucchini, sliced thin lengthwise
3 lb. Spinach, fresh
1 qt. Organic Spaghetti Sauce
2 TBS Olive Oil
1 Onion, large, diced
2 TBS fresh Garlic, crushed
2 tsp. Oregano, dried
2 tsp. Sweet Basil, dried
1 tsp. Fennel, ground

1 tsp White Pepper, ground
1 tsp sea salt
4 dashes Stevia powder
1/4 tsp. Cayenne Pepper
1 lb. Organic Firm Tofu
1/2 cup Lemon Juice
2/3 cup Nutritional Yeast
3 TBS Corn Starch
   or 1 tsp Xanthan Gum

Directions

1) Begin by preparing the sauce; place the organic spaghetti sauce, olive oil, spices, stevia, sea salt, diced onions, in a medium size pot and bring to a simmer for 3 minutes. Take the spinach, chop into 1 inch pieces, add it to the sauce, and cook until it begins to simmer. Then remove from heat and set to the side.

2) While the spinach is cooking, cook the lasagna in a separate pot until tender. Follow directions on the box. Rinse with cold water and set aside.

3) Place the tofu, lemon juice, nutritional yeast and cornstarch into a blender or food processor and blend at high speed until creamy. Slice the zucchini lengthwise into 1/8 inch thick pieces and set aside.

4) In a large 2 QT glass baking dish, place a layer of the spinach sauce, then place a layer of lasagna, followed by a thin layer of the tofu cream, and then zucchini. Repeat making successive layers in the same order until all the ingredients are used or until the baking dish is full. Try to have at least three sets of layers.

5) Bake in the oven at 350 F for 30-35 minutes. Remove and allow to cool for about 10 minutes before serving.

Veggie Burger

Note: Chick pea flour can be purchased in a health food store. This recipe will make 12 veggie burgers. These can be frozen for later use after they have been cooked. Enjoy on spelt grain or sprouted grain buns, sliced tomatoes, romaine lettuce, mustard and fruit juice sweetened ketchup.

Ingredients

1 cup Brown Rice, dry grain

1 cup Lentils, dry beans

1 cup Chick Pea/Garbanzo Flour

1 cup Oat Flour, or Quick Oats

1 TBS Sea Salt

6-oz. can Organic Tomato Paste

3 Carrots, medium , shredded

1 Potato, medium, shredded

1 Onion, medium, finely chopped

4 Garlic cloves, minced

1 TBS Oregano

2 Chipotle Peppers, finely chopped
   or 1 tsp Smoke Flavor

Hot Pepper Sauce, to taste

Corn Meal (for dusting the baking pan)

Burger Directions

1) Begin by placing 4 1/2 cups of water in a medium sized covered pot on the stovetop. When the water comes to a boil, add the brown rice and lentils, and place the cover on the pot. Reduce the heat to simmer and let cook until all the water is absorbed.

2) While the rice and lentils are cooking, wash and peel the carrots, potato, onion, and garlic. Finely shred the veggies with a food processor or a hand grater. If using a food processor, the garlic and chipotle peppers can be thrown in without mincing.

3) When the brown rice and lentils have absorbed all the water, remove from the stovetop and empty the pot contents into a large mixing bowl, add the tomato paste and thoroughly mash ingredients together. Then add all the shredded/chopped veggies into mix and continue mashing together.

4) Add a little of the chick pea flour and oat flour or quick oats and continue mashing. (Do not use cooked chick peas or the burgers will be too soft.) Continue to add more of the flour in 1/4 cup increments until all of the ingredients are thoroughly mashed and blended together.

5) Preheat your oven to 350F. Thoroughly dust the surface of a large baking sheet with corn meal. Form the veggie burger mix into the desired size using a mixing spoon and a smaller spoon, or by forming them in your hands. Place the veggie burgers on the baking sheet and flatten to the desired thickness, making sure that the burgers stay circular.

6) Bake for 1 hour and 15 minutes, if you like the outsides of the burgers slightly crispy. If you like the burgers softer on the outside you can cook them for 55 min-1 hour.

7) When the burgers are baked to the desired consistency, remove from the oven and enjoy with Ezekiel Sprouted Grain buns, sliced tomatoes, romaine lettuce and fruit juice sweetened ketchup.

Carrot & Orange Stir-Fry

Ingredients

2 TBS Sunflower or Olive Oil
1 lb. Carrots, shredded in long strips
8 oz. Leeks, shredded in long strips
2 oranges, peeled and segmented
2 TBS Fruit Sweetened Ketchup
1-2 TBS Xylitol or Succanat
2 TBS Soy Sauce or Bragg's Liquid Aminos
1 cup chopped cashews or almonds

Directions

Mix the fruit sweetened ketchup, Xylitol and soy sauce together in a small bowl. Then Heat the oil in a large wok or frying pan, until it begins to sizzle. Add the grated carrots and leeks to the wok and stir-fry for 2-3 minutes, until vegetables are softened. Add the orange segments to the wok and heat through gently for 2 min. ensuring that you do not break up the orange segments as you stir the mixture. Add this mixture to the wok and stir fry for 2 more minutes. Transfer the stir-fry to warm serving bowls and scatter with nuts. Serve immediately. Goes well with cooked halibut overtop.

Zucchini Curry Pasta

Ingredients

1 large Onion, coarsely diced

1-1/2 TBS Garlic, crushed

3-4 Carrots, medium, sliced

2 Zucchini Squash, medium

1 Yellow Squash, medium to large

1 28-oz. can Crushed Tomatoes

1 cup Raisins

1 cup Walnuts, large pieces

3 Fuji Apples, ¼ inch chunks

1 TBS Turmeric, powder

1 TBS Paprika

2 tsp sea salt

4 TBS Honey

1-1/2 tsp Cinnamon, ground

1/4 tsp. Cayenne Pepper

1 lb. Brown Rice or Kamut Penne Pasta

2 TBS Olive Oil

1 TBS Cumin, ground

Directions

1) Wash and peel the onion, carrots and garlic. Cut the onion in half from top to bottom, and coarsely dice. Stir-fry these veggies in a ¼ cup water or olive oil on medium high. Place the onions, garlic, carrots and raisin in the pan or wok. Cook until the onions begin to become translucent.

2) Wash and clean the zucchini and yellow squash, slice and cut into bite size pieces. Add all other ingredients, except the pasta and apples, and continue cooking until the veggies are tender (about 10 minutes). Mix as necessary to ensure uniform cooking.

3) While the veggies and sauce are cooking, cook the brown rice or kamut penne pasta. Follow directions on the package. After cooking, strain into a colander and add 2 TBS Olive Oil, so the noodles won't stick together.

4) Wash and cut the apples in quarters. Remove the core, and cut the large slices across into 1/4 inch thick bite size pieces.

5) When the veggies and sauce have cooked about 10 minutes, add the apples and mix well. Continue cooking until the apple is tender, but not overcooked. In a large bowl mix together the pasta and stir fried mix. Serve warm or place in refrigerator for a cold salad.

California Pizza

You can buy pre-made spelt crusts at the health food store.

Pizza Crust Ingredients

Makes two 9 " crusts, or one 18 " crust

1 TBS active dry yeast
1 ¼ cups warm water
2 TBS soy flour or
   soy milk powder (replaces corn meal)
2 TBS sunflower/ olive oil
2 TBS honey or ½ dropper of stevia
1 tsp sea salt
3 ½ cups spelt flour

Pizza Crust Directions

1) Mix ¼ cup warm water and yeast in a 1 cup measuring cup. Stir briefly and allow time to soak while you measure other ingredients.
2) Mix 1 cup warm water, soy flour, oil, honey/stevia, and sea salt in a large mixing bowl. When yeast is soft and bubbly add it to the mixing bowl.
3) Add 1 ½ cups of flour to the mixture and beat together well. Add the other cup of flour gradually and mix until there are no clumps.
4) Take out dough onto a floured board and kneed 10 min. adding flour as needed to keep the dough from sticking to board.
5) Cover in a bowl and Let dough rise in a warm place for 1 hour. While dough is rising, prepare the other ingredients.

Note on Variations: If you can't use tomato sauce, spread crust with ¼ cup Red Chile sauce by 505 Organics or use sauce of choice. If you tolerate cheese you can use raw cheeses instead of the other cheese substitutes.

Pizza Toppings Ingredients

¾ lb. Turkey Kielbasa
   (Welshire Farm™), thinly sliced
1-2 TBS olive oil
1 medium onion, chopped
8 oz sliced olives
1 ½ cup grated zucchini
½ cup pine nuts (optional)
3 cloves garlic, minced

1 cup organic tomato sauce
6 slices of tomato (optional)
1 tsp oregano & basil
½ tsp thyme
¼ tsp white pepper
2 cups grated jalapeno almond,
   rice cheese or raw cheese

Directions

1) When dough has risen, preheat oven to 400 degrees. Oil one large cookie sheet or pizza pans generously with olive oil. Heat pans in oven for a minute while you roll out the dough.

2) Divide dough in half if making two pizza's. Need out the dough into the pans arranging with fingers.

3) Cover with tomato sauce, sprinkle sea salt and other spices over sauce. First spread around vegetables, then add grated cheese, then kielbasa slices. Garnish with tomatoes and pour over 1 TBS olive oil over each pizza. Bake for 15 minutes or until crust is brown.

Mediterranean Eggplant Pasta

Ingredients

2 large eggplants
1 tsp. Sea salt
¼ cup Olive Oil
Juice of 2 lemons
½ lemon rind
4 TBS Maple Syrup
2 TBS Capers, rinsed (optional)

1 can pitted black olives
2 cloves garlic, chopped
4 TBS Fresh parsley, finely chopped
2 tsp Sea salt
1 tsp ground white pepper
1 lb of Spiral Brown Rice Noodles

Directions:

Cut eggplant into 1 inch cubes. Optional, but pulls out the bitter flavor; Place the cubes in a colander and sprinkle with sea salt. Set aside for 30 minutes, then rinse the eggplant and pat dry. Heat up the olive oil, 2 tsp sea salt, garlic, pepper in large frying pan, then place the eggplant cubes in pan over medium heat for 8-10 minutes, toss regularly, until golden brown and softened. You may need to do this in two batches to ensure all gets cooked. Place eggplant cubes in a large serving bowl and toss with the lemon juice, capers, olives, maple syrup, ½ tsp sea salt, parsley and grated lemon rind. Cook 1 bag of Spelt or Brown Rice spiral Noodles, follow directions on box, strain, then mix together with all other ingredients. Serve warm or cold.

Roasted Baby Vegetables

Ingredients
1 eggplant
1 red onion
2 zucchinis
2 cups mushrooms
1 cup grape tomatoes
2 red bell peppers

Mix Herbs in ½ cup Olive Oil:
1 tsp parsley
1 tsp rosemary
1 tsp thyme
½ tsp white pepper
4 dashes stevia (optional)
3 cloves garlic, pressed
1 ½ tsp sea salt
4 TBS BBQ Sauce

Directions
Preheat oven to 400F. Cut the eggplant, onion and zucchini into ½ inch full moon slices. Cube the bell pepper into bite-size pieces. In a medium size bowl, mix together the herbs, olive oil, and BBQ sauce. Brush olive oil onto 2 flat baking dishes. Place vegetables on a flat baking dish, and brush on Oil Herb Mixture over the vegetables. Pour any remaining Oil Herb mixture over the vegetables. Bake side by side in the oven, or one at a time, for 10 minutes or until tender.

Asparagus Egg Tart

Ingredients for Piecrust
6 TBS Organic butter/Coconut oil
1 ½ c. spelt flour
pinch of sea salt
¼ cup water

Ingredients for filling
8 oz. Asparagus
3-4 eggs, beaten
1 cup Pepper Jack Soy Cheese
3 TBS Keifer or plain yogurt
Sea Salt and white pepper

Directions
Preheat oven to 400 F. For the crust, rub the butter into flour and salt. Stir in ¼ cup or more of cold water to form smooth dough, knead lightly on a floured surface for a few minutes. Roll out piecrust pastry into a 9-inch pie pan. Press into pan and pinch the edges. Bake for 10 minutes, until it is firm but still pale. Remove from oven turn down to 350 F. Cut the asparagus 2 inches from the top then cut the remaining into 1-inch strips to mix into the filling, tops of asparagus on top of the tart. Beat together the eggs, yogurt and grated soy cheese. Season stir in the asparagus stalks and pour into the pastry shell. Place tips on top. Bake for 35-40 min. until golden. Serve hot or cold. Serves 4.

Raisin Nut Acorn Squash

Ingredients

1 Acorn Squash
   (2 servings per Squash)
1 cup Onions (diced)
1/2 cup Walnuts (pieces)
1/2 cup Raisins
1 tsp. Cinnamon (ground)

1/2 tsp. Ginger (ground)
1/4 tsp. Cloves (ground)
½ tsp sea salt
4 TBS maple syrup
1 cup Brown or Basmati Rice
2 cups of water

Directions

1) Begin by boiling 2 cups water in a covered pot. Add the spices and sea salt and rice and lower the temperature to simmer for 50 minutes. After 40 minutes of cooking add the remaining ingredients to the rice.

2) In the mean time wash the acorn squash. Lay the squash on its side and cut in half along its length (top to bottom). Scoop out the seeds (save them for roasting, if you desire) and bake in a covered roasting pan at 375 F for 1 hour 10 min or until the squash is tender.

3) Add the rice mixture to the acorn squash at 55 minutes. Continue to cook until you reach 1 hour 10 min.

4) Remove from oven allow to cool for 10 minutes. Accompany it with Butternut soup made by Pacific™.

Stuffed Butternut & Walnut Squash

Ingredients

1 Butternut Squash
1 Apple
1/2 cup papaya chunks or apricots (in quarts)
1/2 cup pecans, pieces
4 TBS Maple Syrup
2 tsp. Cinnamon, ground
1 tsp sea salt

Directions

1) Wash the butternut squash and cut in half lengthwise. Scoop out the seed, pierce each side of squash with a fork 4-6 times, and set the squash inside glass baking dish and fill up with 1 inch level of water. Place in oven at 400 F for 1 ½ hours or until the center is tender.

2) Wash the apple and cut lengthwise into eight wedges. Cut wedges across into small pieces and place in mixing bowl. Add the papaya, pecans, maple syrup, and cinnamon, and mix well.

3) Pull the Squash out of oven after 1 hour of cooking and stuff each cavity with apple mixture. Cover the baking dish for another 30 minutes, until you reach 1 ½ hours cooking time. Allow to cool for 15 minutes and serve with Roasted Lamb or oven roasted turkey.

Desserts

Other Recipes

Chocolate Crêpe & Strawberry Walnut Filling

Note: This recipe can be substituted with other fillings.

Dry Ingredients
3 TBS cocoa powder
  or carob powder or
  2 oz baker's chocolate
½ TBS cardamom
½ TBS baking soda
1 cup brown rice flour
3 TBS succanat or xylitol

Wet Ingredients
3 TBS organic butter
  or oil
1 ½ cups almond milk
3 eggs, beaten
2 TBS maple syrup

Strawberry Maple Filling Ingredients
4 cups strawberries, sliced,
  fresh or frozen
5 TBS maple syrup
1 TBS butter or oil
½ cup walnut
3 TBS Silk® creamer or
  soy milk
½ tsp xanthan gum

Crêpe Directions

Melt butter, 2 TBS cocoa powder, cardamom and maple syrup in sauce pan, stir together. Combine the almond milk and eggs in a separate bowl. Combine dry ingredients. Then alternate pouring and mixing with the cocoa mix, and the almond milk mixture into the dry ingredients. Allow the batter to sit for ½ hour before cooking. Then using a greased griddle or large frying pan on medium high, pour over 3-4 TBS of mixture at a time and spread evenly making a round shape. Flip the crêpe after 1 minute or when opposite side is slightly browned, then only heat side for a 10 seconds. Remove From heat, place on dish with wax paper in between each crêpe so they do not stick. Our in filling and wrap like a tortilla.

Filling Directions

Place all ingredients (except the xanthan gum) in a pan on medium heat, bring to a simmer, then slowly stir in the xanthan gum until thickened. Keep warm until served.

Raw Berry Pie with Almond Crust

Note: Agar- Agar is a clear tasteless seaweed- a healthy replacement for gelatin.

Ingredients

1 basket of Strawberries
   stems trimmed
1 basket of Raspberries
1 cup fruit juice (Mango, Orange
   or Raspberry)

1 TBS Agar-Agar flakes
3 TBS Agave Nectar (honey substitute)
One recipe Almond Pie Crust (see below)

Directions

Trim and wash the berries, put them on paper towels to drain. Arrange on the Almond Pie Crust. Mix the fruit juice with agar-agar flakes in a small pot, bring to a boil for 1 minute, then simmer for another minute. Let stand a couple of minutes before poring over the fruit. After poring over the fruit, place in refrigerator and allow to set for another 30 minutes. Serves about 6, this can be served with frozen mango cream or eaten alone.

Almond Pie Crust

Ingredients

1 cup soaked almonds
1/3 cup raisins

2 TBS Tahini
1 tsp vanilla extract

Directions

1) Soak 1 cup of almonds in 2 cups of purified water overnight.
2) Pulse chop ingredients together in a food processor You may need to stop and scrape down the sides of the food processor and add 1-2 TBS of water a couple times while processing. This will be a very thick consistency, and may ball up in the processor, just work it down so the ingredients are thoroughly mixed together.
3) Spread into a 9 inch pie dish, using wet fingers. Freeze the pie crust for one hour to set, or you can bake at 250 F for 30 minutes, then, fill the crust with desired ingredients. Yields one 9 inch pie crust.

Mango Cream

Ingredients

8 oz. frozen mango chunks
5 TBS vanilla soy milk/rice milk
Sweetener to taste

Directions

Pulse chop mangos in your food processor with 2 TBS of soy milk and sweetener (if desired). When softened, add rest of milk and purée until creamy. Store in freezer or serve immediately. Serves 2

Chocolate Chip Cookies

Note: Tahini is hulled sesame butter available at health food stores and local Grocery stores.

Ingredients

¼ cup Tahini
¼ cup Water
1/3 cup Whole spelt flour
1/3 cup Applesauce
1/2 cup Granola of choice

1 tsp Vanilla extract
1/2 cup Granola (yes another cup)
1/2 cup Walnuts, finely chopped
1/2 cup Chocolate or Carob chips

Directions

1) Put the first six items in the food processor and blend for a few seconds until creamy. Scrap mixture into a medium bowl.
2) Stir in the granola, walnuts and chocolate chips. Drop cookie dough in tablespoonfuls onto a baking sheet and press down. Bake at 350F for 18 minutes. Yields 10 cookies

Oatmeal Cookies

Ingredients

½ cup butter or sunflower oil
1 cup Succanat or Xylitol
1 egg
1/3 c rice or soy milk
1 ½ c spelt flour
1 tsp cinnamon
½ tsp Vanilla extract

½ tsp baking soda
½ tsp sea salt
2 ½ cups rolled oats
¾ cup raisins, chocolate chips,
   or carob chips
½ cup chopped walnuts (optional)

Directions

Preheat oven to 350 F. Mix sugar, vanilla, oil or butter together. If using butter make sure it is soft before mixing with sugar. Cream together in a medium-mixing bowl. Add egg and rice milk, beat until well mixed. Mix dry ingredients together in another bowl. Sift together flour, soda, salt and cinnamon. Then gradually add this to the oil and sugar mixture, mixing well. Then stir in the rolled oats, raisins or chocolate chips. Grease cookie sheet, place dough on sheet and cook for 10-12 min until done.

Cashew Whipped Cream

Ingredients

1 cup almonds or cashews
¾ cup water

1 TBS. maple syrup (optional)
½ tsp. vanilla (optional)

Directions

Soak 1 cup of almonds or cashews in 2 cups of water overnight. If you're in a very warm climate, soak them in your refrigerator. After 8-12 hours, discard the soaking water and rinse the nuts. In a blender, place the nuts and enough fresh water to allow the blender to operate. Blend gradually, adding enough water to achieve a smooth consistency. Yields 1 ½ cups.

Pineapple Tofu Crème

Note: A creamy whipped topping, delicious over any cake or on top of chilled fruit, or chilled fruit soup.

Ingredients

10 oz Soft Silken Tofu
2 TBS Tofu Mayonnaise
4 TBS Pineapple Juice Concentrate, frozen
2 TBS Lime Juice
2 TBS Maple Syrup or stevia to taste

Directions

Place all ingredients into blender or a food processor, mix together until creamy smooth, then refrigerate to chill.

Fudge Drops

Ingredients

1/4 cup honey
3 TBS sunflower oil
3 TBS apple juice
1 tsp pure vanilla extract
1 cup spelt flour

1/3 cup raw or toasted carob powder
1 tsp cream of tartar or lemon juice
½ TBS baking soda
1/3 chopped cashews

Directions

Combine the honey, oil, apple juice, in a medium saucepan, heat briefly to melt honey, remove from heat and stir in vanilla. In a separate bowl sift together the flour, carob powder, cream of tartar or lemon juice and baking soda. Then stir in the nuts and wet ingredients slowly into the flour mixture. Drop rounded teaspoonfuls onto cookie sheets. Bake at 325 F for 15-18 minutes. Cool and eat. Store in refrigerator or use within a couple of days.

Creamy Carrot Cake

Ingredients

1 ¾ cup spelt flour
    or brown rice flour
2 tsp baking soda
2 tsp cinnamon
½ tsp nutmeg
¼ tsp cloves
2 dashes stevia powder
2 ½ cups carrots, grated
8 oz. pineapple, crushed

1 cup raisins
½ cup shredded coconut
3 eggs
¾ cup honey
½ cup sunflower oil
½ cup walnuts, chopped
1 Creamy Maple Frosting Recipe
   (next page)

Directions

Sift the flour, baking soda, cinnamon, nutmeg, cloves, stevia into a bowl. Resift and set aside. In a large bowl, combine the carrots, un-drained pineapple, raisins, and coconut. Set aside. In a medium mixing bowl, beat the eggs with an electric mixer until very light. Add the honey in a thin stream while beating. Beat until the mixture is very light and frothy. Add the oil in a thin stream while beating. Pour the egg mixture into the carrot bowl. Stir gently to combine. Sift half of the flour mixture over the bowl and gently fold in. repeat with the remaining flour. Fold in the walnuts. Pour into a butter greased 7 ½ ' x 11 ¾ ' baking pan or in two 8' – 9' round cake pans (for a double layered carrot cake). Bake at 325F for 50 minutes (for the large pan) or 35-40 minutes (for the layered round cake pans.) Allow to cool in pans for 10 minutes, then turn out onto wire racks and allow to completely cool. Spread Creamy Maple Frosting between the layers and on top of the cake.

Creamy Maple Frosting

Ingredients

2 (10.5oz) silken tofu packages
1/3 cup raw cashews (or other nuts)
6 TBS Maple Syrup
2 dashes stevia
1 tsp Vanilla
½ tsp cinnamon

Directions

Remove the tofu from packages and cut into slices. Place then in a steamer basket in medium size saucepan and steam for 5 minutes. Drain all excess water in tofu, between several layers of paper towels for at least 10 minutes. Put cashews, maple syrup, stevia, vanilla, and cinnamon in blender, and mix until very smooth. Add the tofu a little bit at a time, blending until the mixture is very smooth and creamy. Scrape the sides of the container so mixture doesn't stick. Chill before spreading on cake. Makes enough frosting for a 2 layer cake. Refrigerate any leftover.

Toasted Coconut Ice Cream

Ingredients

1 cup sweetened shredded or flaked coconut

1 cup rice milk or almond milk

4 cups canned unsweetened coconut milk

1 can organic chocolate syrup

2 tsp cornstarch

1 cup xylitol or succanat

1 large egg

1 large egg white

Directions

1) Preheat the oven to 325 F. Spread the coconut in a thin layer on a rimmed baking sheet and toast in the middle of the oven, stirring
frequently, until lightly golden, about 5 minutes. Set aside to cool.

2) Whisk the rice milk and cornstarch in a large saucepan until blended.

3) Add the Xylitol or Succanat and eggs, and cook over medium-low heat, whisking constantly, until the sugar is dissolved and the mixture is slightly thickened, about 8 minutes, taking special care not to boil the custard.

4) Remove from heat and allow the custard to cool slightly.

5) Whisk the coconut milk and toasted coconut into the custard until well blended.

6) Transfer the mixture to a large metal bowl. Set the bowl in a basin of cold ice water and let stand until cooled to room temperature, stir mixture occasionally.

7) Cover and place in freezer for at least 6 hours or overnight, to allow the flavors to fully develop. Then stir the mixture and process the custard in an ice cream maker according to the manufacturer's directions.

8) Store in a plastic container with a tight fitting lid. Place a piece of plastic wrap on top of the ice cream, cover, and freeze. Drizzle on Organic Chocolate Syrup to taste.

Healthy Infant Formula Recipe

Base formula Includes

For 1 Quart of goat's milk you add the rest of the following ingredients:

- ✓ 1 Quart (4 cups) Fresh or Powdered Goat Milk (Full-Fat)
- ✓ 1 cup purified water
- ✓ 1-2 tsp. Nutritional Yeast
- ✓ 1-2 tsp. Black Strap Molasses
- ✓ ¼ tsp. of kelp
- ✓ ½ to ¾ capsule of Probiotic (AIM company)
- ✓ 1-2 TBS. Pure maple syrup

Directions

Mix all the ingredients in a blender for 1 minute.

Additional Nutrients to add

- ✓ 1 TBS. Total of any of the following Oil (Only: Extra Virgin Olive Oil, Cod Liver Oil, Flax seed Oil) to above recipe
- ✓ 1/8- 1/4 cup whey protein: This can be taken every day for protein source. Best brands to buy- Goatein by Garden of Life™ or Designer Whey Protein™ (vanilla).

Baby Food Recipe's

Note: these recipes can be kept for 3 days in the fridge.

Solomon's Meal
Note: Blend all these ingredients together

¼ Mashed Avocado
½ cup Goat Yogurt (plain or vanilla) or Kefir (by Lifeway™)
1 tsp. Black Strap molasses
¼ cup Brown rice or oatmeal

Blended Fruit Medley
Note: Blend all these ingredients together

1 Pear or ½ cup strawberries/ blueberries.
3 black mission figs, re-hydrated in water overnight.
½-Banana

Sauces, Dips, Spreads & Salad Dressings

SAUCES, DIPS, SPREADS & SALAD DRESSINGS

The recipes for some of the dressings are left with an open amount for the spices so you can add more or less according to your taste. Feel free to add as many spices as you want, the more the better, except for hot spices like cayenne, red pepper, and white pepper. If you want to reduce the overall calorie and sugar amount substitute Honey/Succanat/Agave Nectar with Stevia. Olive Oil/Sunflower Oil/Sesame Oil can be substituted with ½ cup applesauce per ¼ cup oil used. If you are unsure what some of the ingredients are refer to the Food Beautiful Shopping List or the Fabulous Food Replacement Section.

LAVENDER-LEMON CREAM

Ingredients
½ cup silken tofu or cream
½ cup rice/tofu cream cheese
2 TBS Succanat/Xylitol
     or other sweetener

2 tsp organic lavender buds
¼ tsp sea salt
Zest of 1 lemon

Directions
Beat silken tofu and rice cream cheese together. Take 2 TBS succanat and place in small pan on low, allow to melt, then add the lavender buds and stir until coated. Remove from the heat and press the buds with a spoon until finely ground. Take this mixture and fold it into the cream mixture with the grated zest of one lemon. Allow to sit for a couple hours to pull out the oils. Spread over bagels or sugar cookies! To use as a sauce dilute with ¼ cup water and mix together on medium low heat, pour over lamb or chicken.

ROYAL FLAVOR

½ cup tahini (sesame butter)
¼ cup lemon juice
¼ cup rice milk or water
1 TBS poppy seed
½ tsp red pepper flakes
½ tsp ground white pepper
¼ cup parsley or cilantro (finely chopped)
1 tsp sea salt
2 dashes powdered stevia

-----DIRECTIONS------

Mix all ingredients in a pan. Heat on medium until creamy. Serve with Roasted Vegetables.

STRAWBERRY SWEET

1 cup strawberries (fresh or frozen)
¼ cup sunflower oil
1/2 tsp. sea salt
2TBS maple syrup

-----DIRECTIONS------

Blend together until smooth. Mix over a bed of greens add fresh strawberries, walnuts, and raw sharp cheddar cheese.

SWEET SOUR PINEAPPLE SAUCE

¼ cup pineapple chunks
  with half the juice
2 TBS fruit sweetened ketchup
2 TBS red wine/ sherry
1 tsp cornstarch or thickeners of choice
2 TBS paprika
2 TBS Bragg's Liquid Aminos™
  (soy sauce replacement)
4 TBS Sunflower Oil

-----DIRECTIONS------

Mix together. Heat up until slightly thick. Serve over meat and vegetables.

TAHINI MINT

Note: Miso is a fermented brown rice spread, found in refrigerator section.

2 TBS tahini
2 Garlic cloves, pressed
1 TBS dried mint
½ c pure water
1 TBS lemon/lime juice
1 tsp. white miso
1 TBS apple cider vinegar
¼ cup sesame oil

-----DIRECTIONS------

Blend until smooth and chill

CURRIED DRESSING

½ cup Sunflower seeds
1 cup water
1 Lemon, peel, shop flesh
1 tsp sea salt
1 tsp Curry paste
½ TBS Bouillon
3 dashes Cayenne
½ tsp Cumin powder
1 cup Tomato juice blend
½ Green onion, chopped

-----DIRECTIONS ------

Soak seeds in water overnight. Strain.
Put into blender with water until smooth.
Peel lemon. Add to blender, along with rest
of ingredients. Blend Well. Serve hot or cold
over roasted or steamed veggies.

CHILE GINGER SAUCE

4 Red Chiles (pulp no skin)
½ tsp Cumin powder
1 TBS Garlic, chopped
¾ c Pure water
½ TBS Liquid Aminos/ Soy Sauce
1 TBS Ginger, juiced or grated
10.5 oz Silken soft tofu
½ tsp Honey or Stevia to taste
1 TBS Orange Juice

-----DIRECTIONS ------

Blend until creamy in blender.
Heat on low in saucepan, serve warm.

CREAMY RANCHERO

Note: Purchase Healthy Mayo (Vegenaise
by Follow Your Heart)

10 oz. silken tofu
¼ cup Onion, chopped
1 Garlic clove, pressed
1 tsp Soy Sauce
1 tsp Cumin
½ tsp Dill weed
2 TBS Lemon juice
2 TBS Vegenaise® (Mayo)

-----DIRECTIONS ------

Blend until creamy. Chill

GINGER CASHEW SAUCE

2 TBS Cashew Butter
3 TBS Fresh Lemon Juice
1 TBS Soy Sauce (or Tamari)
1 ½ TBS Fresh ginger, skinned and chopped
¼ tsp Hot Pepper sauce or cayenne to taste
1 TBS Toasted sesame oil
3 tsp honey or add stevia to taste

-----DIRECTIONS ------

Blend until smooth and creamy. Serve this
over Asian Salads or Asian Noodles.
Makes 1 cup.

RED ROGUE VINIGARETTE

1 cup fresh tomatoes, chopped
2 TBS nutritional yeast flakes
¾ c water
3 TBS olive oil
½ tsp sea salt
½ tsp thyme
½ tsp dill weed
2 garlic cloves, chopped
½ tsp freshly cracked white pepper
3 dashes powdered stevia

-----DIRECTIONS------

Blend all ingredients in a blender until smooth and creamy. Keep leftovers bottled in fridge. Great with leafy greens and pasta salads Makes 2 cups.

TOMATOE VINAIGRETTE

1 tsp Fruit Sweetened Ketchup
1 tsp Soy sauce
2 tsp Olive Oil
¼ c Brown Rice Vinegar
½ TBS Roasted Red Pepper sauce
2 tsp honey or use stevia to taste
1 c Tomato, seeded and finely chopped
1 TBS Parsley, minced

-----DIRECTIONS------

Whisk together the first six ingredients, Then mix in tomato and parsley.
Chill and Serve. Makes 1 ½ cups

AVOCADO LIME SAUCE

Note: Purchase Healthy Mayo
(Vegenaise by Follow Your Heart®)

1/3 cup Avocado, mashed
2 TBS Apple Cider Vinegar
½ cup Limejuice
2 Garlic cloves, minced
1 Serrano Chile, chopped and seeded
3 TBS Healthy Mayo
½ cup pure water
Sea Salt and White Pepper to taste
2 dashes of Stevia

-----DIRECTIONS------

Blend until smooth. Makes 1 ½ cups

CUCUMBER DRESSING

½ cup Cucumber, skinned, chopped
   and seeded
2 TBS Sunflower Oil
½ TBS Bragg's Liquid Aminos
   or Soy Sauce
½ cup Healthy Mayo
4 Dill Pickles with
2 TBS Pickle Juice
2 TBS Lemon Juice

-----DIRECTIONS------

Put in blender puree until creamy
Makes 1 ¼ cups.

PAPAYA LIME DRESSING

1 cup ripe papaya (½ papaya)

2 ½ TBS lime juice

1 tsp Dijon mustard

½ tsp cracked white pepper

1/8 tsp. sea salt

2 TBS water

2 TBS Agave nectar or stevia to taste

----DIRECTIONS----

Cut Papaya, scoop out seeds, peel away skin, and shop flesh. Place all ingredients into blender, mix until creamy.

Makes 1 1/3 cups

COLE SLAW DRESSING

½ cup healthy mayonnaise

3 TBS orange juice

¼ cup olive oil/sesame oil

2 dashes cayenne pepper

2 TBS orange oil

2 TBS poppy seeds

1 dash cinnamon

1 tsp sea salt

½ c honey or stevia powder (to taste)

-------DIRECTIONS -------

Blend until smooth and chill

FRESH FROM GARDEN

1 cup plain yogurt/kefir

¼ cup lemon juice

¼ cup olive oil/sesame oil

1 tsp basil

1 tsp thyme

1 tsp oregano

4 TBS Agave Nectar (to taste)

1 tsp Sea salt

------DIRECTIONS ------

Blend until smooth and chill

NO CHEESE-CHEESE SAUCE & DIP

INGREDEINTS

3 cup Water
½ cup Rolled Oats
½ cup Nutritional Yeast Flakes
¼ cup Tahini
¼ cup Arrowroot Powder (thickener)
2 TBS Lemon Juice
1/8 tsp Turmeric Powder

2 TBS Onion, minced
½ TBS Tamari or Soy Sauce
1 tsp Basil
½ tsp thyme
3 dashes Cayenne
1 Garlic Clove, minced

DIRECTIONS

Blend all ingredients until smooth. Pour into small saucepan and heat until it reaches a boil, stirring with a whisk, keep stirring on low until thick. Yields 4 cups.

LEMON BALM & HYSSOP FUSION

Ingredients

3 TBS Cilantro, fresh
1 tsp Lemon Grass
1 tsp Hyssop or fresh Thyme
1 tsp Basil
1/8 tsp Paprika

1/8 tsp Cinnamon
¼ tsp Xanthan Gum
2 tsp Bragg's Liquid Aminos®
1 TBS dried Red Bell Peppers
3 TBS Mango Juice
¼ cup Kefir or plain yogurt

Directions:

Mix all ingredients, except the xanthan gum in a food processor for 3 minutes, while mixing pour in the xanthan Gum. Chill and serve. Goes great on salads or steamed veggies containing zucchini, sautéed onion and broccoli!!

GINGER CASHEW PESTO

Note: Can be spread over spelt crust pizza with 2 cups grated zucchini and 1 ½ cups grated goat cheese or mozzarella rice cheese. Place in oven for 10-12 minutes at 425F.

Ingredients

½ cup raw cashews
1 cup cilantro leaves
3 TBS lime juice
3 TBS honey
¼ cup toasted sesame oil

2 garlic cloves, minced
2 tsp ginger root peeled and
1-2 dashes cayenne
1 tsp sea salt & paprika

Directions

Place everything in a blender or food processor (using the "S" blade) pulse chop to slightly chunky. Place in refrigerator and chill until served.

FIRE ROASTED HUMMUS

Note: You can make this raw hummus by soaking 2 cups of dry garbanzo beans for 24 hours, then process just like recipe below.

Ingredients

14 oz can garbanzo beans
5 TBS Tahini
3 cloves garlic, minced
Juice of 1 lemon, ½ the peel
2 pinches cayenne pepper
½ cup Olive Oil

1 ½ tsp sea salt
2 fire roasted red peppers
¼ tsp ground white/black pepper
2 TBS paprika
3 dashed stevia powder
¼ tsp ground cumin

Directions

Using a food processor or blender, puree the garbanzo beans, roasted red pepper, lemon peel, and olive oil until smooth. Then add to mixture; Tahini, garlic, lemon juice, paprika, cayenne, cumin, sea salt, pepper and stevia (to taste). If to thick you can add 2 –3 TBS water. Serve with warmed sprouted grain Pita Bread, baby carrots or chips.

THAI RED CURRY SAUCE

Ingredients

2 garlic cloves, minced

2 roasted red bell peppers chopped

1 TBS ginger root, chopped or pressed

2 TBS fresh mint, roughly chopped

¼ onion, chopped

¾ cup lime juice

1 tsp ground cumin

2-3 pinches ground cloves

cayenne pepper, to taste

¾ tsp. paprika

14 oz. coconut milk

2 TBS red curry from
   Thai Kitchen®

½ cup xylitol or succanat

Directions

In a food processor or blender mix together garlic, roasted bell peppers, ginger, mint, onion, lime juice, cayenne, cumin, cloves and paprika. Set aside. In a large saucepan simmer coconut milk then add the red curry sauce with blended herbs, and honey for 5 min. Pour over a bed of brown rice topped with steamed broccoli, cabbage, carrots and baby corn veggies. You can also serve with white fish or other organic white meat!

GREEN CURRY SAUCE

Ingredients

4 garlic cloves, minced

2-3 mild chilies, chopped

1 TBS ginger root, chopped or pressed

2 dashes cayenne pepper

1 tsp ground cumin

2-3 pinches ground cloves

1 pinch cinnamon

¼ onion, chopped

½ cup lemon juice

14 oz. coconut milk

2 TBS green curry from
   Thai Kitchen®

½ cup honey

1 TBS fish sauce (optional)

Directions

In a food processor or blender mix well the garlic, ginger, chilies, onion, lemon juice, cayenne, cumin, cloves, and cinnamon. Set aside. In a large saucepan simmer coconut milk then add the green curry sauce with blended herbs and honey, stir occasionally for 5 min. Best served hot over veggies or use for dipping!

Recipes for Juicing

OPTIMAL JUICING

Clean the vegetables thoroughly and cut them into small enough pieces to fit through the mouth of the juicer. Drinking the virgin juice can be hard on the stomach and may cause gas so it is recommended to dilute the juice with 1/3 the amount with water. For example if you have 12 oz. of fresh juice add 4 oz. of water. It is suggested on the first two sips to swish it around in the mouth for 15 seconds to activate your digestive enzymes. This can prevent the stomach from experiencing any access stress. For those who take calcium supplements, they can be taken with the juice as the juice helps in the absorption and utilization of the calcium supplement. Each recipe will yield about 12-16 oz. of juice. You can save time juicing everyday by making 1 large batch and freezing the juice in glass jars. Make sure to dilute the juice and leave about 1 inch space between the juice and the lid, so the glass doesn't break. Enjoy the recipes and feel free to get creative with it.

GREEN MACHINE	COLOR ME A RAINBOW
2 large handfuls spinach	½ beet
1 large handful parsley	1 apple
½ cucumber	2 celery ribs
2 celery ribs	2 carrots
1 apple	1 handful parsley
	2 cups red cabbage
THE REAL V-8 JUICE	**CARROT LEMON JUICE**
2 tomatoes	4 carrots
2 celery stocks	3 celery ribs
1 clove garlic	½ lemon
¼ yellow onion	1 apple
2 handfuls parsley or cilantro	1 handful spinach

GINGER WITH GREENS

½ cucumber
¼ beet 2 handfuls spinach
1" slice of fresh ginger
1 apple

A FULL SALAD JUICE

1 tomato
6 leaves of romaine lettuce
2 celery stocks
2 carrots
2 handfuls spinach
¼ onion
1 clove garlic

BEET SWEET

½ beet, with top
1 sweet potato
1 apple
2 celery stocks

TUMMY TONIC

¼ inch slice of ginger
½ cup peppermint or spearmint
½ pineapple with skin

OH SO GREEN

4 celery ribs
½ cucumber
Handful of spinach
Handful of parsley
1 apple

SWEET AS EVER

1 apple
5 carrots
3 celery ribs

BROCCOLI & CARROT

1 broccoli spear
3 carrots
1 apple
1 handful parsley
3 celery ribs

CLEAN AS A WHISTLE

4 carrots
1 handful parsley
½ onion
2 clove garlic
1 apple

CABBAGE DELIGHT

½ head red cabbage
3 carrots
2 celery ribs

BODY COOLER

1 tomato or apple
1 cucumber
3 celery ribs
½ cup peppermint (optional)

FRUITS FOR IMMUNE POWER

1 orange, peeled
1/8 of the orange zest
½ pineapple with skin
½ cup strawberries
1 banana, peeled
Juice the first 4 ingredients
Then place banana and
juice in a blender until liquefied.

MEXICALI JUICE

1 jicama
4 carrots
1 apple
2 celery ribs

FRUIT POTASSIUM PUNCH

1 peach, pitted
½ papaya
2 oranges, peeled
1 banana

Juice first 3 ingredients,
then add banana and juice
 into blender. Mix until liquefied.

KIDNEY TONIC

½ lemon
¼ lemon zest
20 grapes
1 cup cranberries
2 apples

VEGGIES IMMUNOPOWER

1 cup Jerusalem artichoke
2 carrots
Handful of parsley
2 cloves garlic
¼ inch slice ginger
1 apple

FENNEL TUMMY TONIC

1 handful of peppermint
   or spearmint
1 rib of fennel
2 apples

MELON-AID

½ of a cantaloupe
½ of lemon
¼ lemon zest
1 apple
1 kiwi

You can replace with
any melon of choice.

LIVER TONIC

6 dandelion leaves
½ beet with top
1 apple
3 carrots

VEGGIE POTASSIUM

Handful of parsley
3 carrots
3 celery ribs
Handful of spinach
1 tomato

GINGER ALE

5 oz. ginger ale
1 lemon wedge with peel
¼ inch of ginger
1 green apple

GINGER-PINEAPPLE

½ pineapple
¼ inch of ginger
½ cup wheatgrass/parsley

SKIN TONIC

1 apple
¼ head of cabbage
2 celery ribs
1 handful of parsley

CLEANSING COCKTAIL

1 apple
4 carrots
½ beet
2 celery ribs

NOTES

1. Graimes, Nicola. *The Best-Ever Vegetarian Cookbook.* New York, NY :Hermes House, 2002.

2. Baird, Lori. and Rodwell, Julie. *The Complete Book of Raw Food.* New York, NY: Healthy Living Books, 2004.

3. Levin, James, MD., and Cederquist, Natalie. *A Celebration of Wellness.* San Diego, CA: GLO Inc.,1992.

4. Haas, Elson M., M.D., *The Detox Diet.* Berkely, CA: Celestial Arts Publishing, 1996.

5. Dufty, William. *Sugar Blues.* New York: Warners, 1996.

6. Murray, Michael T., N.D. *The Complete Book of Juicing.* United States: Murray, Michael T. 1998.

7. Murray, Michael T., N.D *The Encyclopedia of Healing Foods.* New York: Atria Books, 2005.

8. Pitchford, Paul. *Healing with Whole Foods-3rd Edition.* Berkeley, California: North Atlantic Books, 2002. 456-553

9. Balch, Phyllis A., CNC, and Balch, James F., M.D. *Prescription for Nutritional Healing 3rd Edition.* New York: Penguin Putnam Inc., 2000.

10. Lerner, Ben, D.C., *Body By God.* Tennessee: Thomas Nelson Publishers, 2003

11. Furman, Joel, M.D., *Eat To Live.* Boston: Little, Brown and Company, 2003.

12. Rubin, Jordan S., N.M.D., Ph.D. *The Maker's Diet.* Florida: Siloam, 2004.

13. Young, Shelly L.M.T., Young, Robert O., Ph.D., D.Sc., *Back To The House of Health.* Utah: Woodland Publishing, 1999.

14. Mark and Patti Virkler, *Eden's Health Plan-Go Natural!* Pennsylvania: Destiny Image Publishers, 1994.

FOREWORD

As an education and training organization within the IT Service Management (ITSM) industry, we have been impressed by the positive changes introduced by the ITIL® 2011 edition of the ITIL® framework. The evolution of the core processes and concepts provided by the framework provides the more holistic guidance needed for an industry that continues to mature and develop at a rapid pace. We recognize, however, that many organizations and individuals who have previously struggled with their adoption of the framework will continue to find challenges in implementing ITIL® as part of their approach for governance of IT Service Management practices. In light of this, one of our primary goals is to provide the quality education and support materials needed to enable the understanding and application of the ITIL® framework in a wide-range of contexts.

This comprehensive book is designed to complement the in-depth accredited eLearning ITIL® Foundation Certificate in IT Service Management program provided by The Art of Service. The interactive eLearning program uses a combination of narrated presentations with flat text supplements and multiple choice assessments. This book provides added value to the eLearning program by providing additional text and real life examples to further cement your knowledge. Your learning and understanding will be maximized by combining these two study resources, which will ultimately prepare you for the APMG ITIL® Foundation Certificate in IT Service Management exam. This fourth edition also includes appropriate alterations based on the recent review of the framework and the ITIL® 2011 edition Foundation syllabus and associated exams. We have also used student feedback to include improvements to the format and material, including additional content and sample exam questions.

We hope you find this book to be a useful tool in your educational library and wish you every success in your IT Service Management career!

The Art of Service

This publication is to be used only in conjunction with the online eLearning program relevant.

HOW TO ACCESS
THE eLEARNING PROGRAM

- Direct your browser to: www.theartofservice.org
- Click 'login' (found at the top right of the page)
- Click 'Create New Account'
- Follow the instructions to create a new account. You will need a valid email address to confirm your account creation. If you do not receive the confirmation email, check that it has not been automatically moved to a Junk Mail or Spam folder.
- Once your account has been confirmed, email your User-ID for your new account to key11@theartofservice.com
- You will receive a return email with an enrolment key that you will need to use in order to access the eLearning program. Next time you log in to the site, access the program titled: *ITIL® 2011 Foundation eLearning Program*

Minimum system requirements for accessing the eLearning Program:

Processor	Pentium 4 (1 GHz) or higher
RAM	256MB (512 MB recommended)
OS	Windows XP, Vista, 7, MCE, Mac OSX
Browser	Mozilla Firefox 3+ (recommended), Internet Explorer 6.x or higher, Safari, Opera, Chrome, all with cookies and JavaScript enabled
Plug-Ins	Adobe Flash Player 8 or higher
Internet Connection	Due to multimedia content of the site, a minimum connection speed of 512kbs is recommended. If you are behind a firewall and are facing problems in accessing the course or the learning portal, please contact your network administrator for help.

Kuotai Wu

Over1234

If you are experiencing difficulties with the Flash Presentations within the eLearning Programs, please make sure that:

1. You have the latest version of Flash Player installed, by visiting http://get.adobe.com/flashplayer/

2. You check that your security settings in your web browser do not prevent these flash modules from playing

3. For users of Internet Explorer 7, a solution involves DESELECTING "Allow active content to run files on my computer" in Internet Explorer -->Tools, Options, Advanced, Security settings.

CONTENTS

INTRODUCTION

Looking back on a period where corporate giants fell and government bailouts were measured in the billions, not to mention the overwhelming natural disasters that have occurred all over the world, the challenges faced by a typical IT Service Provider may seem of low priority. But now that IT budgets have come under more financial scrutiny than ever before, the value provided by managing IT with controlled, repeatable, and measurable processes has become all the more obvious. So, for the modern Chief Information Officer (CIO), employing quality IT Service Management (ITSM) practices can often help in achieving a quality sleep each night.

The term IT Service Management is used in many ways by different management frameworks and the organizations that seek to use them. While there are variations across these different sources of guidance, common elements for defining ITSM include:

- Description of the **processes** required to deliver and support IT Services for customers
- A focus on delivering and supporting the **technology or products** needed by the business to meet key organizational objectives or goals
- Definition of roles and responsibilities for the **people** involved, including IT staff, customers, and other stakeholders
- The management of **external suppliers (partners)** involved in the delivery and support of the technology and products being delivered and supported by IT

The combination of these elements provide the capabilities required for an IT organization to deliver and support quality IT Services that meet specific business needs and requirements.

The official ITIL® definition of IT Service Management is found within the Service Design volume (Service Design, page 16), and defines ITSM as *The implementation and management of quality IT services that meet the needs of the business. IT service management is performed by IT service providers through an appropriate mix of people, process and information technology.* Organizational capabilities are influenced by the needs and requirements of customers, the culture that exists within the service organization, and the intangible nature of the output and intermediate products of IT services.

However, IT Service Management comprises more than just these capabilities alone, being complemented by an industry of professional practice and wealth of knowledge, experience, and skills. The ITIL® framework has developed as a major source of good practice in Service Management and is used by organizations worldwide to establish and improve their ITSM practices.

Benefits of ITSM

WHILE THE BENEFITS OF APPLYING IT Service Management practices vary depending on the organization's needs, some typical benefits include:

- Improved quality service provision
- Cost-justifiable service quality
- Design of services that meet business, customer, and user demands
- Integrated and centralized processes
- Transparency of the roles and responsibilities for service provision
- Continual improvement, incorporating lessons learnt into future endeavors
- Measurable quality, performance, and efficiency attributes

It is also important to consider the range of stakeholders who can benefit from improved ITSM practices. As perspectives will differ for each stakeholder, the benefits provided by enhanced ITSM practices may apply to one or more of the following parties:

- Senior management
- Business unit managers
- Customers
- End users
- IT staff
- Suppliers
- Shareholders

Business and IT Alignment

A COMMON THEME IN ANY IT Service Management framework is to enable and demonstrate business and IT alignment. When staff members of an IT organization have only an internal focus on the technology being delivered and supported, they lose sight of the actual purpose and benefit that their efforts deliver to the business and customers. A way in which to communicate how IT supports the business is using Figure 1.A (on page 14), which demonstrates business and IT alignment.

Figure 1.A divides an organization into a number of supporting layers that work towards meeting a number of organizational goals. These layers are communicated by the following:

Organization	What are the key strategic goals and objectives for the organization? These objectives define who we are as an organization and where we want to be in the future.
CORE Business Processes	These are represented by the repeatable business activities that produce desirable results for the business. Without these results, the organizational objectives defined above would not be supported or achieved.
IT Service Organization	Defines the IT Services and supporting infrastructure that is required to enable the effective and efficient execution of the business processes above. IT Services are used by the business to facilitate and enhance outcomes, including improved efficiency of operations or ensuring accuracy in the records and information being managed.
IT Service Management	Made up by the repeatable, managed, and controlled processes used by the IT department that enable quality and efficiency in the delivery and support of the IT Services above.
IT Technical Activities	The actual technical activities required as part of the execution of the ITSM processes above. ITSM is utilized to ensure that any resources and effort spent performing the technical activities are optimized according to the greatest business need or reward. As these activities are technology specific (e.g., configuring application server), they will not be a focus of this book's content.

© **Crown** Copyright 2011 Reproduced under license from the Cabinet Office

Each layer within this structure is utilized to support the layer(s) above. At the same time, each layer will in some way influence the layer below it. For example, a business process that is required to be executed at all times without disruptions (e.g., emergency health services) would result in highly resilient IT services being implemented, supported by ITSM processes that reduce the risk and impact of disruptions occurring.

OUR BUSINESS: A FASHION STORE

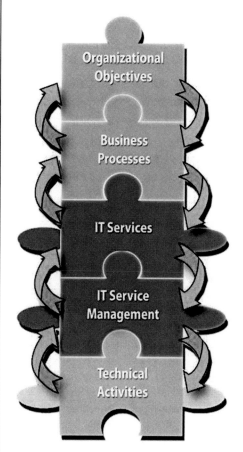

What are some of our organization's objectives or strategic goals?
- We want to increase profits by 15 percent each year
- We want to have a good image and reputation with a loyal customer base

What Business Processes aid in achieving those objectives?
- Retail/sales
- Marketing
- Manufacturing
- Procurement, HR, finance etc.

What IT Services are these business processes dependent on?
- Websites (internal and external)
- Communication services (email, video conferencing)
- Automatic procurement system for buying products
- Point of Sale Services

Figure 1.A—Business and IT Alignment

We have ITSM in order to make sure that IT Services are:
- What we need (Service Level Management, Capacity Management etc.)
- Available when we need it (Availability Management, Incident Management etc.)
- Provisioned cost-effectively (Financial Management, Service Level Management)

If we don't manage the IT Services appropriately, we cannot rely on these services to be available when we need them. If too many disruptions occur, we cannot adequately support our business processes effectively and efficiently. If the business processes are not operating as they should, we will ultimately fail to support and achieve our overall organization's objectives!

Also note the relationship between IT Service Management processes and the technical activities below. Used properly, ITSM processes can optimize the time, effort, and other resources spent performing technical activities, ensuring that all staff actions are working in accordance to agreed business priorities and objectives.

This is just a simple example used to illustrate the relationship between ITSM and the organization. Any approach used to improve ITSM practices should always be carefully considered to ensure that the plans suit the organization in terms of:

- Size (number of staff, customers, IT devices etc.)
- Geographical dispersion
- Culture and ethos
- Current maturity and capability levels

What is ITIL®?

ITIL® STANDS FOR THE INFORMATION Technology Infrastructure Library. ITIL® is the international de facto management framework describing best practices for IT Service Management. The ITIL® framework evolved from the UK government's efforts during the 1980s to document how successful organizations approached service management. By the early 1990s, they had produced a large collection of books documenting the best practices for IT Service Management. This library was eventually entitled the IT Infrastructure Library®. The Office of Government Commerce in the UK continues to operate as the trademark owner of ITIL®.

ITIL® has gone through several evolutions and was most recently refreshed and reviewed with the release of the 2011 edition. Through these evolutions, the scope of practices documented has increased in order to stay current with the continued maturity of the IT industry and meet the needs and requirements of the ITSM professional community.

ITIL® is only *one of many* sources for ITSM best practices and should be used to complement any other set of practices being used by an organization.

Five volumes make up the ITIL® 2011 Edition:

- Service Strategy
- Service Design
- Service Transition
- Service Operation
- Continual Service Improvement

Each volume provides the guidance necessary for an integrated approach and addresses capabilities' direct impact on a service provider's performance. The structure of the ITIL® framework is that of the service lifecycle. It ensures organizations are able to leverage capabilities in one area for learning and improvements in others. The framework is used to provide structure, stability, and strength to service management capabilities with durable principles, methods, and tools. This enables service providers to protect investments and provide the necessary basis for measurement, learning, and improvement.

In addition to the core publications, there is also *ITIL® Complementary Guidance*. This consists of a complementary set of publications with guidance specific to industry sectors, organization types, operating models, and technology architectures. At present, this complementary guidance is available by subscription from http://www.bestpracticelive.com.

Best practices

IGNORING PUBLIC FRAMEWORKS AND STANDARDS *can needlessly place an organization at a disadvantage. Organizations should seek to cultivate their own proprietary knowledge on top of a body of knowledge developed from using public frameworks and standards* (Service Strategy, Page 20).

Public frameworks (ITIL®, COBIT, CMMI etc.): Frameworks are scaled and adapted by the organization when implemented, rather than following a prescriptive set of practices (standards). Examples of public frameworks for ITSM include:

- ITIL®
- COBIT—The Control Objectives for Information and related Technology
- Capability Maturity Model Integrated (CMMI) for IT Services

Standards: Usually a formal document that establishes uniform engineering or technical criteria, methods, processes, and practices. Unlike frameworks, they are prescriptive in declaring mandatory elements that must be demonstrated. Examples of standards relating to ITSM are:

- ISO/IEC 20000—International Standard for IT Service Management
- ISO/IEC 27001—International Standard for Information Security Management Systems
- ISO/IEC 38500—Corporate governance of information technology standard

Proprietary knowledge of organizations and individuals: Specific expertise developed for internal purposes or developed in order to sell to other organizations (e.g., Gartner).

Generally, best practices are defined as those formalized as a result of being **successful in wide-industry use**.

COMMON TERMINOLOGY

C ritical to our ability to participate with and apply the concepts from the ITIL® framework is the need to be able to speak a common language with other IT staff, customers, end-users, and other involved stakeholders. This chapter documents the important common terminology that is used throughout the ITIL® framework.

Care should be taken when attempting the ITIL® Foundation exam, as there will be a number of questions that seek to ensure the candidate has an effective grasp of the terminology used throughout the framework.

A full glossary has been included at the back of this book for terminology and acronyms that are covered under the ITIL® 2011 Foundation syllabus. The following introductory glossary is provided as an introduction to the common terms found within the framework. Throughout the book, relevant terms will be discussed in more detail in the context of their corresponding process or lifecycle stages.

Terminology	Explanations
Baselines	*(ITIL® Continual Service Improvement) (ITIL® Service Transition)* A snapshot that is used as a reference point. Many snapshots may be taken and recorded over time but only some will be used as baselines. For example: • An ITSM baseline can be used as a starting point to measure the effect of a service improvement plan • A performance baseline can be used to measure changes in performance over the lifetime of an IT service • A configuration baseline can be used as part of a back-out plan to enable the IT infrastructure to be restored to a known configuration if a change or release fails
Business Case	A decision support and planning tool that projects the likely consequences of a business action. It provides justification for a significant item of expenditure. Includes information about costs, benefits, options, issues, risks, and possible problems.
Capabilities	The ability of an organization, person, process, application, CI, or IT service to carry out an activity. Capabilities can be described as the functions and processes utilized to manage services. These are intangible assets of an organization that cannot be purchased but must be developed and matured over time. The ITSM set of organizational capabilities aims to enable the effective and efficient delivery of services to customers.
External Service Providers	Service provider that provides IT services to external customers, **e.g.,** providing internet hosting solutions for multiple customers.
Functions	A team or group of *people* and the tools they use to carry out one or more processes or activities. Functions provide units of organization responsible for specific outcomes. *ITIL® Functions covered include*: • Service Desk • Technical Management • Application Management • IT Operations Management
Internal Service Providers	An internal service provider that is embedded within a business unit, e.g., one IT organization within each of the business units. The key factor is that the *IT services provide a source of competitive advantage* in the market space the business exists in.
IT Service Management	A set of specialized organizational capabilities for providing value to customers in the form of services.

Terminology	Explanations
Process	A set of *coordinated activities* combining and implementing resources and capabilities in order to produce an outcome and provide value to customers or stakeholders. Processes are *strategic assets* when they create competitive advantage and market differentiation. They *may* define roles, responsibilities, tools, management controls, policies, standards, guidelines, activities, and work instructions if they are needed.
Process Owner	The person/role responsible for ensuring that the process is fit for the desired purpose and is accountable for the outputs of that process. **Example**: The owner for the Availability Management Process
Process Manager	The person/role responsible for the operational management of a process. There may be several managers for the one process. They report to the Process Owner.
Resources	A generic term that includes IT infrastructure, people, money, or anything else that might help to deliver an IT service. Resources are also considered to be tangible assets of an organization.
Service	A means of delivering value to customers by facilitating outcomes customers want to achieve without the ownership of specific costs or risks. The role of the service provider is to manage these costs and risks appropriately, spreading them over multiple customers if possible.
Service Owner	The person/role accountable for the delivery of a specific IT Service. They are responsible for continual improvement and management of change affecting services under their care. **Example**: The owner of the Payroll Service
Shared Service Providers	An internal service provider that provides shared IT service to more than one business unit, e.g., one IT organization to service all businesses in an umbrella organization. IT Services for this provider do not normally provide a source of competitive advantage but, instead, *support effective and efficient business processes* across an organization.

© **Crown** Copyright 2011 Reproduced under license from the Cabinet Office

What are Services?

THE CONCEPT OF **IT SERVICES** as opposed to *IT components* is central to understanding the Service Lifecycle and IT Service Management principles in general. It requires not just a learned set of skills but also a way of thinking that often challenges the traditional instincts of IT workers to focus on the individual components (typically the applications or hardware under their care) that make up the IT infrastructure. The mindset requires, instead, an alternative outlook to be maintained, incorporating the end-to-end service perspective for what their organization actually provides to its customers.

The official definition of a service is *a means of delivering value to customers by facilitating outcomes customers want to achieve without the ownership of specific costs or risks* (Service Strategy, Page 13). But what does this actually mean? The following analogy explains some of the key concepts in a way that most (food lovers) will understand.

While most people do enjoy cooking, there are often times when they wish to enjoy quality food without the time and effort required to prepare a meal. If they were to cook, they would need to go to a grocery store, buy the ingredients, take these ingredients home, prepare and cook the meal, set the table, and, of course, clean up the kitchen afterwards. The alternative is that they can go to a restaurant that delivers a service that provides them with the same outcome (a nice meal) without the time, effort, and general fuss required if they were to cook it themselves.

Now consider how that person would identify the quality and value of that service being provided. It is not just the quality of the food itself that will influence their perceptions, but also:

- The cleanliness of the restaurant
- The friendliness and customer service skills of the waiters and other staff
- The ambience of the restaurant (lighting, music, decorations etc.)
- The time taken to receive the meal (and was it what they asked for?)
- Did they offer a choice of beverages?

If any one of these factors does not meet the person's expectations, then ultimately the perceived quality and value delivered to them as a customer is negatively impacted. Now, relate this to an IT staff member's role in provisioning an IT Service. If they focus only on the application or hardware elements provided and forget or ignore the importance of the surrounding elements that make up the end-to-end service, just like in the example of the restaurant, the customer experience and perceived quality and value will be negatively impacted.

But if they take a service-oriented perspective, they also ensure that:

- Communication with customers and end users is effectively maintained
- Appropriate resolution times are maintained for end user and customer enquiries
- Transparency and visibility of the IT organization and where money is being spent is maintained
- The IT organization works proactively to identify potential problems that should be rectified or improvement actions that could be made

Using these principles, every phone call to the Service Desk or email request for a password reset presents an opportunity to demonstrate service excellence and a commitment to our customers.

To ensure that a service is managed with a business focus, the definition of a single point of accountability is absolutely essential to provide the level of attention and focus required for its delivery.

The service owner is accountable for the delivery of a specific IT service. The service owner is responsible to the customer for the initiation, transition, and ongoing maintenance and support of a particular service and accountable to the IT director or service management director for the delivery of the service. The service owner's accountability for a specific service within an organization is independent of where the underpinning technology components, processes, or professional capabilities reside.

Service ownership is as critical to service management as establishing ownership for processes that cross multiple vertical silos or departments. It is possible that a single person may fulfill the service owner role for more than one service. The service owner is responsible for continual improvement and the management of change affecting the service under their care. The service owner is a primary stakeholder in all of the underlying IT processes that enable or support the service they own. (Service Strategy, Page 330)

Processes and Functions

Defining Processes

PROCESSES CAN BE DEFINED AS *a structured set of activities designed to accomplish a specific objective. A process takes one or more defined inputs and turns them into defined outputs (Service Strategy, Page 20).*

Every process has four attributes: trigger, activity, dependency, and sequence. Processes are triggered by some occurrence or event, such as a customer call to the Service Desk, an alert through IT Operations, a missed service level in a report, etc. Once a trigger is made, the process is a series of actions that will take any inputs to the process and create an output. The trigger could provide information about the event that will be used by the process, or additional information may be required. This information is the basis for determining the dependencies on the process and is the output from other processes. The actions themselves are pre-defined and ordered to obtain a specific result.

Let's return to the dining analogy previously used. Consider "providing dining experience" as the process of the waiter. The process is triggered when the customer is seated at the table. The waiter takes action to ensure the customer has great experience during dinner. Along the way, the waiter obtains information that will allow the customer's needs to be known and delivered: some information will be tangible, such as the customer's order, while other information will be perceived, such as the customer's mood or disposition. This information will change from one customer to the next, but will generally be the similar across all customers (i.e. all customers will order from the menu, but not every customer will order the same thing).

In order to deliver the desired experience, the waiter is dependent on the capabilities of several other roles and processes, such as the cook, the bartender, and the restaurant manager. The sequence of activity provided by the waiter is even under scrutiny: should drink orders be taken before ordering off the menu? Should the drinks be delivered with the appetizer? How many times should the waiter return to the table? When should dessert be served?

How the processes are defined will impact productivity within the organization and functions. Some organizations use processes as strategic assets because they set the organization apart from others in the market place. The "dining experience" process is nearly the same from restaurant to restaurant, but you, as a customer, have a favourite restaurant because of how the restaurant staff executes the process. A well-defined process will have the following characteristics:

- The process can be measured. While the most important measurement of a process is performance, other measurements may be desired. Some managers will seek measurements related to cost, quality, and other variables. People performing the process, called practitioners are focused on duration and productivity.

- The process provides a specific result. This result is usually pre-defined and each instance must be recognizable within its definition. The result must be countable. The end result of the waiter's process in a restaurant could be the customer pays for their meal. At the end, the waiter can determine the success of their process execution by adding up the number of paying customers to the number of total customers.
- The process meets the customer's expectations. If the process does not meet the needs of the customer, it does not provide value and can be considered inadequate. Customers may be internal and external to the organizations: they can be a single individual, several individuals, or even another process. Whatever the characteristics of the customer, the process must meet their expectations: so understanding the expectations in the early part of the process or before it is triggered is paramount in delivering the desired result.
- The trigger responds to the different types of triggers appropriately. A seated customer is not the only trigger for restaurants; different restaurants are designed to initiate their processes for different triggers, such as drive-thru, carry-out, delivery, or catered events. How the process is triggered will define certain adjustments to the process to ensure a great dining experience.

In the restaurant analogy, the waiter has been the primary executer of the process. From an ITSM, the waiter is considered a process practitioner. The process practitioner is responsible for carrying out one or more process activities. The process practitioner should understand their role and how it contributes to the overall delivery of the service and creating value for the customer and the business. They should work in cooperation with other stakeholders interested in the service delivery and value of the process, such as the manager, co-workers, and customers. This cooperation ensures that everyone's contribution is consistent to produce the best result from the process.

The process practitioner is also responsible for ensuring the inputs, outputs, and interfaces are appropriate and sufficient. The best waiters will confirm the customer's order, work with the cook to fulfil the order, and quality check the order before delivering to the customer. In addition, the waiter will maintain a journal of the process that will result in a final report to the customer in the form of a receipt: many restaurants have adopted POS (point of sale) systems requiring waiters to log activities and "events" to manage the dining experience for the customer.

The waiter is not the only process practitioners in the process, nor are process practitioners the only role associated to a process. The process manager role is a person accountable for the operational management of a process. In a restaurant, this person oversees all the waiters and other process practitioners and may even be a process practitioner themselves. In a restaurant chain, several process managers may exist. For smaller organizations, the process manager role may be assigned to the person who also fulfils the process owner role.

The process owner role is accountable for ensuring a process is fit for purpose (Service Strategy, Page 331). The process owner must ensure the process is performed according to the agreed and documented standard. They must ensure the process is defined, as well as the process meets its objectives.

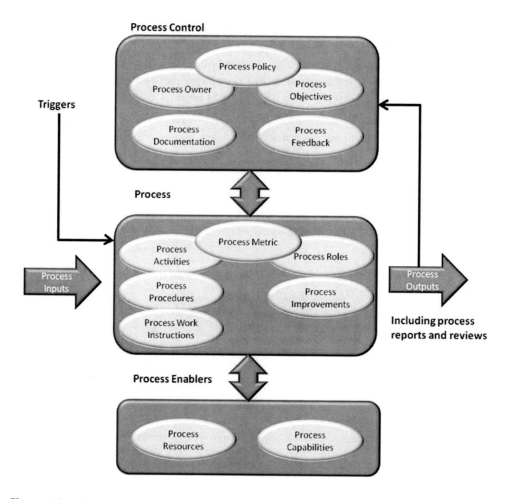

Figure 2.B—Generic Process Elements
© Crown Copyright 2011 Reproduced under license from the Cabinet Office

The previous figure defines the physical components of the process. These components are tangible and can be easily recognized and controlled. However, processes also have behavioural components, which are intangible. Behavioural components are often-times an underlying pattern within the members of the organization that impact decision-making, communication, and learning processes. Attitudes, prejudices, and work ethic are examples of behavioural components, though at an organizational level, not an individual level. At an organizational level, these components do not exist apart from the work processes, but will affect the activities of the process and its desired results.

Any well-designed process can be derailed at any point be existing negative behavioural components. Resistance to change can be considered a negative behavioural component to continuous improvement because process drives change at all times: resistance in this context is a direct adversary to improvement. Conversely, a positive behavioural component will enable a poorly-designed process to meet the desired result. A motivated workforce is considered a positive behavioural component. Ideally, an organization will want a well-designed process over a poorly-designed process: a motivated workforce will most likely ignore the poor process to ensure a better result is delivered to the customer.

When defining and designing processes, the physical and behavioural aspects of the processes should both be considered. This is done best by engaging the required stakeholders (e.g., staff members, customers, and users etc.) in the design of processes. Stakeholders will expressed, if given the opportunity, their own ideas, concerns, and opinions about how the processes are designed, implemented and improved. These communications will identify the existing behaviours related to the process, either because the stakeholders explicitly mentioned them or because of how the stakeholders expressed themselves.

Stakeholder groups are comprised of individuals performing the same tasks. Waiters are a stakeholder group. As a group, the individuals have been provided training and education relevant to their role in the process and understand the value of the process in the business. Involvement in the design of the process also empowers the stakeholder in the change, reducing the possibility of active of passive resistance when the change actually occurs within the organization

Defining Functions

FUNCTIONS ARE A LOGICAL GROUPING of roles and automation that are responsible for executing a defined process and/or a specific activity within a process. Functions are typically isolated from each other logically: it's easy to acknowledge the differences between the wait staff and the kitchen staff in a restaurant on several levels. As such, they can be considered two functions comprised of several roles within the restaurant. Although, they are isolated in their defined roles and responsibilities, functions are often dependent on the other functions to effectively perform their duties. In a restaurant, the wait staff would not be able to provide the desired dining experience without quality food: conversely, the kitchen staff would not be cooking without the wait staff interacting with the customer.

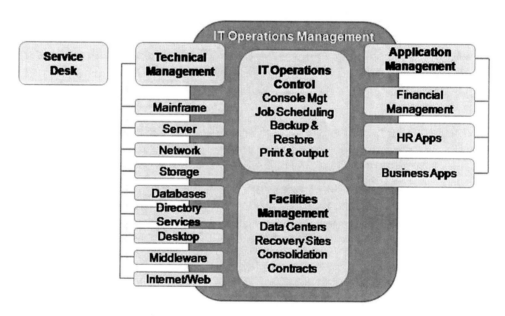

Figure 2.C—The ITIL® Functions from Service Operation

© **Crown** Copyright 2011 Reproduced under license from the Cabinet Office

RACI Model

IT IS SAID THAT PROCESSES are perfect … until people get involved. This saying comes from the perceived failure of processes in many organizations, which can frequently be attributed to misunderstandings of the people involved and a lack of clarity regarding the roles and responsibilities that exist.

A useful tool to address this issue, assisting with the definition of the roles and responsibilities when designing processes, is the RACI Model. RACI stands for:

R—Responsibility (actually does the work for that activity but reports to the function or position that has an "A" against it.)

A—Accountability (is made accountable for ensuring that the action takes place, even if they might not do it themselves. This role implies ownership.)

C—Consult (advice/guidance/information can be gained from this function or position prior to the action taking place.)

I—Inform (the function or position that is told about the event after it has happened.)

	Service Desk	Desktop	Applications	Operations Manager
Logging	RACI			CI
Classification	RACI	RCI		CI
Investigation	ACI	RCI	RCI	CI

Figure 2.D—The RACI Model

A RACI MODEL IS USED to define the roles and responsibilities of various functions in relation to the activities of Incident Management.

General rules that exist:

- Only 1 "A" per row can be defined (ensures accountability, more than one "A" would confuse this)
- At least 1 "R" per row must be defined (shows that actions are taking place) with more than one being appropriate where there is shared responsibility.

In the example RACI model given, the Service Desk is both responsible and accountable for ensuring that incidents are logged and classified, but not responsible for the subsequent investigation, which in this case will be performed by other functional teams.

THE SERVICE LIFECYCLE

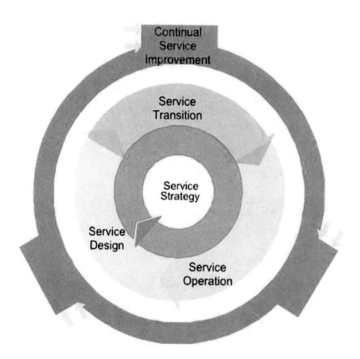

Figure 3.A—ITIL® Service Lifecycle Model
© Crown Copyright 2011 Reproduced under license from the Cabinet Office

Lifecycle: The natural process of stages that an organism or inanimate object goes through as it matures. For example, the stages that a human goes through are birth, infant, toddler, child, pre-teen, teenager, young adult, adult, elderly adult, and death.

The concept of the *Service Lifecycle* is fundamental to ITIL® 2011. Previously, much of the focus of ITIL® was on the *processes* required to design, deliver, and support services for customers. As a result of this previous focus on processes, Version 2 of the ITIL® Framework provided best practices for ITSM based around the **how** questions.

These included:
- How should we design for availability, capacity, and continuity of services?
- How can we respond to and manage incidents, problems, and known errors?

As ITIL® 2011 now maintains a holistic view covering the entire lifecycle of a service, no longer does ITIL® just answer the how questions, but also **why**?
- Why does a customer need this service?
- Why should the customer purchase services from us?
- Why should we provide (x) levels of availability, capacity, and continuity?

By first asking these questions, it enables a service provider to provide overall **strategic objectives** for the IT organization, which will then be used to direct *how* services are **designed**, **transitioned**, **supported**, and **improved** in order to deliver optimum value to customers and stakeholders.

The ultimate success of service management is indicated by the strength of the relationship between customers and service providers. The 5 stages of the Service Lifecycle provide the necessary guidance to achieve this success. Together they provide a body of knowledge and set of good practices for successful service management.

This end-to-end view of how IT should be integrated with business strategy is at the heart of ITIL's® five core volumes.

Mapping the Concepts of ITIL® to the Service Lifecycle

THERE HAS BEEN MUCH DEBATE as to exactly how many processes exist within ITIL® 2011. Questions asked include:

- What exactly constitutes a process?
- Shouldn't some processes be defined as functions?
- Why has x process been left out of this study material?

In developing this material, we have based our definitions of processes and functions, and where they fit within the lifecycle, on the guidance provided by the ITIL® 2011 Foundation syllabus produced by APMG and the Cabinet Office ITIL® 2011 Service Lifecycle suite of books. Figure 3.B demonstrates the processes and functions of ITIL®, in relation to the five Service Lifecycle stages that are covered at this foundation level.

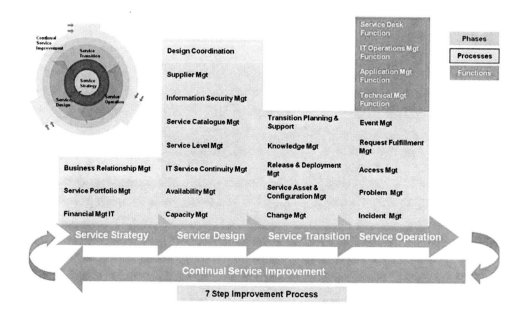

Figure 3.B—The Major Concepts of ITIL® 2011 Foundation Level
"Based on Cabinet Office ITIL® material. Reproduced under licence from the Cabinet Office"

Note:
- The Service Lifecycle stages (and ITIL® books) are shown through the arrows at the bottom
- The concepts in light shading are the ITIL® 2011 processes covered within the foundation program
- The concepts in dark shading are functions
- Processes that are not covered by the current ITIL® 2011 Foundation syllabus are not discussed fully in this book but will be referenced where necessary for understanding.

How does the Service Lifecycle work?

ALTHOUGH THERE ARE FIVE STAGES throughout the Lifecycle, they are not separate, nor are the stages necessarily carried out in a particular order. The whole ethos of the Service Lifecycle approach is that each stage will affect the other, creating a continuous cycle. For this to work successfully, the Continuous Service Improvement (CSI) stage is incorporated throughout all of the other stages. Figure 3.C demonstrates some of the key outputs from each of the Service Lifecycle stages.

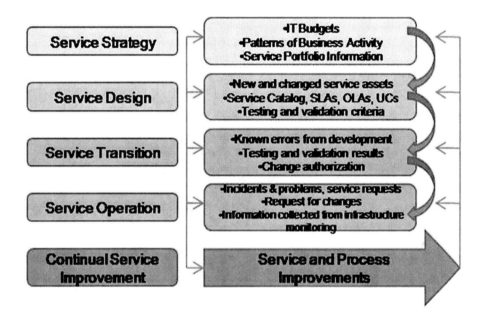

Figure 3.C—How Does the Service Lifecycle Work?

IT IS IMPORTANT TO NOTE that most of the processes defined do not get executed within only one lifecycle stage.

Service Strategy Stage: Determines the needs, priorities, demands, and relative importance for desired services and identifies the value being created through services and the predicted financial resources required to design, deliver, and support them. This stage builds the context for the service, why it exists, and what it delivers.

Service Design Stage: Designs the infrastructure, processes, and support mechanisms needed to meet the availability requirements of the customer. This stage defines how the service works within and for the context developed in the service strategy stage, specifically designing the foundation for the future state of the service.

Service Transition Stage: Validates that the service meets the functional and technical fitness criteria to justify release to the customer. The transition stage ensures that the current state of the service and its underlying IT infrastructure is moved into the future state designed in the previous stage.

Service Operation Stage: Monitors the ongoing availability being provided. During this stage, we also manage and resolve incidents that affect service availability, performance, and reliability. The primary goal of this stage is to ensure the service and its underlying infrastructure is delivering the expected results as conceived in the service strategy stage, developed in the service design stage, and verified in the service transition stage.

Continual Service Improvement Stage: Coordinates the collection of data, information, and knowledge regarding the quality and performance of services supplied and Service Management activities performed. Service Improvement Plans developed and coordinated to improve any aspect involved in the management of IT services. The purpose of the CSI stage is to continually enhance the service either to fulfil the original context of the service or exceed expectations.

SERVICE STRATEGY

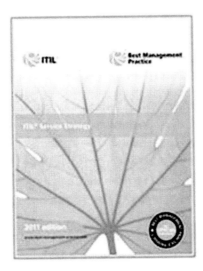

Figure 4.A—Service Strategy

"© Crown copyright 2011 Reproduced under licence from the Cabinet Office"

The Service Strategy stage is concerned predominantly with the development of capabilities for Service Management, enabling these practices (along with the IT organization in general) to become a strategic asset of the organization. The guidance provided by the volume can be summarized as:

- Understanding the principles of Service Strategy
- Developing Service Strategy within Service Management
- Developing strategies for services and services for strategies
- How strategy affects the Service Lifecycle
- Strategies for organizational and cultural change

Purpose of Service Strategy

THE PURPOSE OF THE SERVICE *strategy stage of the service lifecycle is to define the perspective, position, plans, and patterns that a service provider needs to be able to execute to meet an organization's business outcomes.* (Service Strategy, Page 331)

The objectives of service strategy include providing:

- *An understanding of what strategy is*
- *A clear identification of the definition of services and the customers who use them*
- *The ability to define how value is created and delivered*
- *A means to identify opportunities to provide services and how to exploit them*
- *A clear service provision model that articulates how services will be delivered and funded, to whom they will be delivered, and for what purpose*
- *The means to understand the organizational capability required to deliver the strategy*
- *Documentation and coordination of how service assets are used to deliver services and how to optimize their performance*
- *Processes that define the strategy of the organization, which services will achieve the strategy, what level of investment will be required, at what levels of demand, and the means to ensure a working relationship exists between the customer and service provider*

By achieving these objectives, it will ensure that the IT organization has a clear understanding of how it can better support business growth, efficiency improvements, or other strategies that need to be realized.

KEY ROLE: To stop and think about WHY something has to be done before thinking about HOW.

Benefits of Service Strategy

SERVICE STRATEGY HAS THE POTENTIAL for many significant benefits to be delivered to the IT organization and the business/customers it serves. However, in many cases, these benefits fail to be realized due to insufficient connection and interfaces with other elements of the Service Lifecycle. For example:

The IT Strategy Group from an international banking and managed investment firm has decided to address the current economic downturn by reducing investments into the IT organization and Service Portfolio. As a result, the quality of some key services fall, with the support organization struggling to respond effectively to all calls for assistance. After a few months of lowered quality of service, the organization loses a number of major customers to their primary competitors. In response to the loss of these customers, further budget reductions are planned to counter the decrease in revenue earned.

By failing to realize their customers' value perception of services through service quality, the organization became caught in a negative cycle with potentially serious long term consequences. The missing link between the decisions being made by the strategy group and the potential impact they may have on elements of service quality (in particular the support of services in this example) or service value is often a challenge when developing Service Strategy.

When developed successfully as part of a holistic IT Service Management implementation, effective Service Strategy can (Service Strategy, Page 331):

- *Support the ability to link activities performed by the service provider to outcomes that are critical to internal or external customers. As a result, the service provider will be seen to be contributing to the value (and not just the costs) of the organization.*
- *Enable the service provider to have a clear understanding of what types and levels of service will make its customers successful and then organize itself optimally to deliver and support those services. The service provider will achieve this through a process of defining strategies and services, ensuring a consistent, repeatable approach to defining how value will be built and delivered, which is accessible to all stakeholders.*
- *Enable the service provider to respond quickly and effectively to changes in the business environment, ensuring increased competitive advantage over time*

- *Support the creation and maintenance of a portfolio of quantified services that will enable the business to achieve positive return on its investment in services*
- *Facilitate functional and transparent communication between the customer and the service provider so that both have a consistent understanding of what is required and how it will be delivered*
- *Provide the means for the service provider to organize itself so that it can provide services in an efficient and effective manner*

Principles of Service Strategy

Understanding Strategy

EARLIER, WE DEFINED THE TERM "service". Now, it is appropriate to define strategy. The ITIL® Service Strategy volume defines strategy as *a complex set of planning activities in which an organization seeks to move from one situation to another in response to a number of internal and external variables.* (**Service Strategy, page 35**)

Strategy begins with the business, specifically where does the management of the business want to go and how does it know when it gets there. Within the context of Information Technology, strategy considers how the organization will use and manage technology to meet the needs of the business. Service strategy defines the role of services and service provider in achieving the business objectives of the organization through management of IT.

In 1995, Mintzberg proposed that a defined strategy will consist of four forms:

- Perspective – defines the organization's view of itself, generally communicated though the organization's vision and direction.
- Positions – defines the distinctiveness of the organization in comparison to its competitive market and identified through the minds of its customers.
- Plans – the predefined details for supporting and enhancing the organization's perspective and positions, usually identifying a potential future state for the organization and a strategic response to the state and level of investment required.

- Patterns – defines the conditions and actions that must be consistently in place and repeatable to achieve the objectives of the organization: patterns allow the organization to predict the future.

Defining a strategy using these 4 forms allows an organization to fully develop who they are, where they are going, and how they will get there. In IT Service Management, a service strategy is developed in response to the customer's business strategy. Because many companies try to have internal IT departments, it is difficult to realize that providing IT is a competitive market and other options are available. As a result, any strategic planning for an IT department should be performed such that they are competing for the customer's business.

Therefore within the context of achieving the customer's business objectives, an IT organization must define who they are (perspective), define what they can bring to the customer (position), define what the future state of the organization will be and how this future state will be achieved (plans), and what repeatable patterns need to be established or encouraged to enable successful service delivery.

Creating Service Value

PERHAPS, HISTORICALLY, BOTH PROVIDERS AND customers have used price as the focal point for communication and negotiation, but it is this path that ultimately leads to a negative experience for both parties. One of the key mantras that exist for any modern service provider (IT or otherwise) is that it is essential to clearly establish value before you can attach a price to the services offered. This ensures a few key things:

- It avoids an apples-to-oranges comparison, which usually occurs with a price focal point
- It enables the service provider to distinguish their capabilities and differentiation from their competitors
- It clearly communicates to the customer what they can expect to receive as part of the delivery service

Providers of IT services need to take special appreciation of the concept of value creation and communication due to the many misunderstandings about technology on behalf of customers (and poor communication by their IT providers). To address this issue, a central theme throughout the Service Strategy stage is value creation through services.

Value creation is a balance between the actual achievement of business outcomes, the perceptions a customer has with the service and its achievement, and the preferences of the customer. The service provider is not the determiner of value: the customer is. Because of this, the service provider has one option for creating value for the customer: identify what is valuable to the customer and do everything possible to provide it.

Let's go back to the "dining experience" and expand it to create value. The service of a "dining experience" can be provided in the home or "outsourced" to a restaurant. The business outcomes for the service delivered can vary based on need, i.e. hunger, health, socializing, etc. Cooking and eating at home can provide additional benefits, such as family time or portion control, while eating at a restaurant has other benefits.

As mentioned before, the quality of the food is not the only influence on the perceptions the customer has regarding where they eat - ambience, friendliness, and cleanliness are other factors at play. Many perceptions are achieved historically; that is, through a good experience or bad experience in the past. These perceptions can impact the preferences for the customer. A person who does not like sushi will find it difficult to find value at a sushi restaurant. Some people find more value staying home than going out to eat.

The whole of the "dining experience" is a product of getting the outcome desired, while aligning with the perceptions of the customer and catering to the customer preferences. If all customers saw value in the same way, the number and variety of restaurants would be extremely limited. As it is, not all solutions will create value for all customers. This is the same for providing IT services.

To enable a service provider to create value for a customer, a systematic approach has to be adopted. For ITIL, this approach is determining service utility and service warranty.

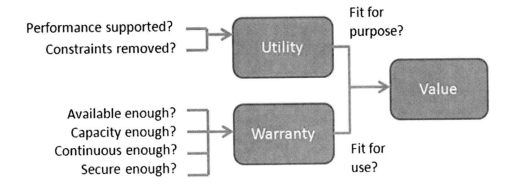

Figure 4.B—Creating Service Value
© *Crown Copyright 2011 Reproduced under license from the Cabinet Office*

Important Formula: Service Warranty + Service Utility = Service Value

Service Utility describes what a service does and its positive effect on business processes, activities, objects, and tasks. This could be the removal of constraints that improves performance or some other positive effect that improves the outcomes managed and focused on by the customer and business. Generally summarized as being fit for purpose, service utility focuses on the functional aspects of a service.

Service utility in a restaurant is the provisioning of food and drink. For IT service delivery, some examples of Service Utility are:

- Accessing networking assets and the Internet
- Enabling communication and collaboration with co-workers, colleagues, and management
- Remote access of applications and critical files

Service Warranty, on the other hand, describes how well these functions are delivered to the customer. It describes the service's attributes, such as the availability, capacity, performance, security, and continuity levels to be delivered by the provider. Importantly, the Service Utility potential is only realized when the service is available with sufficient capacity and performance.

Service Warranty in a restaurant would consist of such attributes as serving hot food hot not cold, ensuring all menu items are available when ordering, and managing the flow of the meal appropriately. For IT Service delivery, some examples of Service warranty are:

- The connection speed to the Internet
- The availability of support (e.g. 6am-10pm)
- The security controls in place for protecting confidential information

Service utility and service warranty are present for every service provided to a customer. One cannot exist without the other. By describing both Service Utility and Service Warranty, it enables the provider to clearly establish the value of the service, differentiate themselves from the competition, and, where necessary, attach a meaningful price tag that has relevance to the customer and associated market space.

Service Packages and Service Level Packages

SOME CUSTOMERS HAVE HIGH UTILITY requirements, some have high warranty requirements, and some require high levels of both. To accommodate this, service providers can seek to satisfy one or more of these types of customers by packaging different levels of Service Utility and Service Warranty and pricing these packages accordingly.

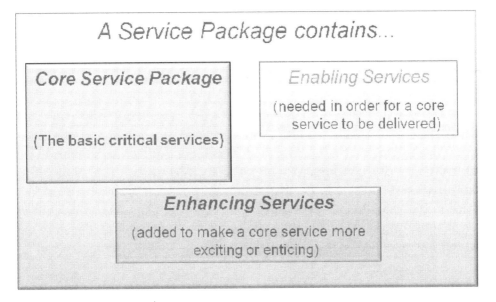

Figure 4.C—Service Package Example

"Based on Cabinet Office ITIL® material. Reproduced under licence from the Cabinet Office"

A SERVICE PACKAGE PROVIDES A detailed description of bundled services available to be delivered to customers. The package consists of one or more services used in combination to create value for the customer. The contents of a Service Package include:

- Core services – provides the basic outcomes desired by the customer, creating direct value for the business.
- Enabling services – supports the core service to ensure they provide real value to the customer. Customers may or may not see an enabling service.
- Enhancing services – does not impact the delivery of the core services, but provide an enticement to the customer to utilize the core service.

Not every restaurant is the same, but each provides a similar service package. The core services of a restaurant are cooking the food and serving the food. Without these services, a restaurant would not be operating as a restaurant. Some restaurants will adopt additional services to ensure the core services can be provided, such as equipment maintenance, dishwashing, and accounting. These additional services are enabling the core service and their sole function is to support the core services. Still more services can be added to truly distinguish the restaurant's service package from other restaurants: these services are enhancing services that add to the experience but do not directly contribute or support the core services. Enhancing services for a restaurant could consist of valet parking, reservations, entertainment, gift shop, etc.

When an IT department creates a service package, they must define the functionality required to provide the customer value for a specific business objective or process. This functionality is delivered through the provision of core services. Without these services, the customer cannot achieve their desired objectives. Assume for the moment that each of these core services require additional support to ensure availability, capacity, performance, and reliability. This support is obtained through enabling services which can be shared between the core services. To market the service and provide a unique experience, specific enticements may be included in the form of enhancing services. Together, the set of services comprise the entire service package. Some services in the set may themselves be service packages as well.

Remember, the customer determines where value exists, not the service provider. Since each customer may perceive value different, it is possible to create a different service package for each customer. However, this approach can be a highly expensive endeavour with lots of custom considerations being upheld. On the opposite spectrum, one service package can be offered to every potential customer. This approach would provide the economies of scale to allow efficiencies in delivering the service, but provides a generic package to market. A compromise of the two approaches is to predefine several levels of utility and warranty for the service package and market to different types of customers. This provides options for customer while maintaining the overall integrity of the service package.

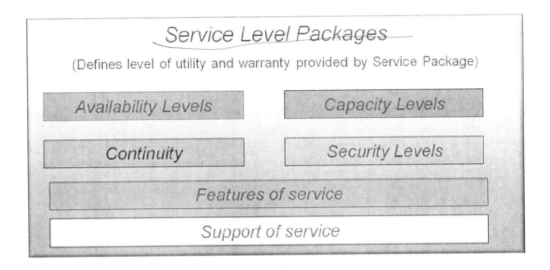

Figure 4.D—Service Level Package Example

THESE SERVICE PACKAGE OPTIONS ARE typically referred to as service level packages because they define the different service levels of the packaged set of services. Service Level Packages are effective in developing service packages with levels of utility and warranty appropriate to the customer's needs and in a cost-effective way. Usually, service level packages differ:

- Availability and Capacity Levels
- Continuity Measures
- Security Levels
- Support arrangements (e.g., hours of support)

We often see different service level packages in restaurants, such as:

- Lighter lunch fare over dinner selections
- Special considerations for large groups
- Meeting rooms
- Catered affairs, in-house and offsite

For each of these situations, the selection, price, and overall service may differ based on the customer's needs.

Most of the components of Service Packages and Service Level Packages are reusable components of the IT organization (many of which are services). Other components include software, hardware, and other infrastructure elements. By providing Service Level Packages in this way, it reduces the cost and complexity of providing services, while maintaining high levels of customer satisfaction. The use of Service Packages and Service Level Packages enables Service Providers to avoid a one-size fits all approach to IT Services, while still maintaining efficiency of operations. As a result, Service Level Packages enable service providers to offer various pricings for different levels of service and entice potential customer in procuring the available services.

Service Assets

DEFINING THE SERVICE AND ITS appropriate utility and warranty will not deliver the service to the customer. To do this, service assets are used. A Service Asset is any resource or capability used in the provision of services. They are used to create value in the form of goods and services for customers. The table below is a comparison between resources and capabilities.

Resources	Capabilities
Input to a process is consumed and manipulated to produce an output	Used to coordinate, control, and deploy resources
Easy to acquire, can typically purchase or procure	Experience-driven, information-based, needs to develop and mature over time
Tangible, often a physical product	Intangible, often made up of behaviors and experience that has developed over time
Examples: IT Infrastructure, people, or money	Examples: Teams, processes, behaviors, knowledge

© **Crown** Copyright 2011 Reproduced under license from the Cabinet Office

SO WHILE IT IS RELATIVELY easy for an organization to increase the capacity of its infrastructure, it is far more difficult and complex to improve the organization's capabilities for managing capacity and performance in a cost-effective manner. Service Strategy should seek to optimize the use and implementation of Service Assets, according to the needs and objectives of the business.

Risk

RISK IS DEFINED AS UNCERTAINTY of outcome, whether it may result in a positive opportunity or negative threat. Managing risks requires the identification and control of the exposure to risk, which, if materialized, may have an impact on the achievement of an organization's business objectives. Every organization manages its risk but not always in a way that is visible, repeatable, and consistently applied to support decision-making.

This is true for many organizations, where one of the greatest risk factors is a lack of accurate information when making decisions. The goal of risk management is to ensure that the organization makes cost-effective use of a risk framework that has a series of well-defined steps. The aim is to support better decision-making through a good understanding of risks and their likely impact.

Service Strategy should seek to maintain the appropriate balance of risk and reward in regards to investments and capabilities invested and maintained for IT.

Service Strategy Processes

THE PROCESSES INCLUDED IN THE Service Strategy lifecycle stage are:

- Financial Management
- Service Portfolio Management
- Business Relationship Management
- Demand Management
- Strategy Management for IT Services

These processes work together to enable an IT organization to maximize the value of services being provided to customers and supply quality information to other ITSM processes. Although they are primarily strategic in nature, these processes also incorporate activities that are performed through all stages of the Service Lifecycle.

The ITIL® Foundation Certificate in ITSM syllabus and the corresponding exam requirements only cover three of these Service Strategy processes, the other processes are covered in the Intermediate level of study. Therefore, this book and the corresponding eLearning program will cover the following Service Strategy processes:

- Financial Management

- Service Portfolio Management
- Business Relationship Management

Before delving into the details of each process, a very basic understanding of these processes and how they relate to each other is in order. Financial Management is an extremely important process to IT Service Management because it defines the budgeting, accounting, and charging approaches used to manage the services and deliver value to the customer. Financial management has two layers that must be performed to provide IT services: the business organization or enterprise financial management and the IT organization or financial management for IT services. For internal IT departments, financial management for IT services will often be required to adopt most aspects of enterprise financial management. For external service providers, the processes applied to each layer may differ significantly. Financial management ensures the funding is available for ongoing operations of service delivery and project-based investments.

The service portfolio is a compilation of all the provider's services, the associated business needs the service meets and a description of how the service meets those needs. The services included in the portfolio fall into three categories: future services, current services, and retired services. The service portfolio provides a representation of the investment in resources, capabilities, and funding made to provide the services. Service portfolio management is the process responsible for creating and maintaining the services and, and in this capacity, defines how services are added to the portfolio and how they are tracked throughout the service lifecycle.

To understand the requirements to the IT services provided and the value created by those services, some interaction is expected with the customer. This interaction is the responsibility of Business Relationship Management. The process has two primary roles: establish and maintain a business relationship between service provider and customer and identify the needs of the customers and the services required to meet that need over time.

Financial Management for IT

THE IT SERVICES IDENTIFIED AND delivered to the customer are in place to ensure the strategic business objectives of the organization are met. For this to happen, the IT services must be designed, developed, and transitioned into an operational environment. Additionally, optimization of the IT service to provide greater value requires improvements to be identified, designed, developed, and implemented. All these activities require one fundamental necessity: money. Usually referred to as funding, investment, or budgeting, Financial Management for IT is responsible for securing the necessary monies to provide the service to the customer.

However, Financial Management for IT provides another critical role by ensuring a balance exists between the cost of service and the quality of service. In other words, the process ensures the customer gets what they pay for. Consider all the variables in delivering the value in a service: utility, warranty, resources, capabilities, perception, and preferences. Each of these variables will impact the quality of the service. The determiner for cost is a balance between what the customer can afford and what the service provider can provide. Each of the variables to the quality of service is impacted by this balance. The goal of the customer and service provider is to obtain the highest quality at the lowest cost.

Example:

An internal service provider has been asked to provide a new service to the customer using a technology unfamiliar to the provider. As a result, the service provider is unable to quantify the costs of delivering the service. An external service provider who has some experience in this new technology has provided a plan detailing the initial investment and ongoing costs of the service, which are higher than expected. Financial management for IT has a role in the decision, because of the process' responsibility to balance cost with quality. Since the internal service provider cannot quantify the costs of service, they cannot determine if they can provide the quality required. Financial management will support the external service provider's bid in this case because the quantification is available and the quality defined.

Financial management for IT performs another critical role in maintaining the balance between supply and demand between the service provider and customer. Most services have a direct correlation between the demand on the service and the costs of providing the service. Capacity is the most prevalent of these services as an increase in demand requires more physical capacity to be procured and installed. The increased costs in response to the demand must be managed appropriately.

Ultimately, financial management provides insight into the achieved value of IT services, supporting assets, and operational processes to the business and IT. This insight, which is done in financial terms, enables clearer visibility into the services provided and positively impacts the organization's decision making capabilities. Financial management enables the organization to manage its resources and to ensure these resources are being used to achieve the organization's objectives.

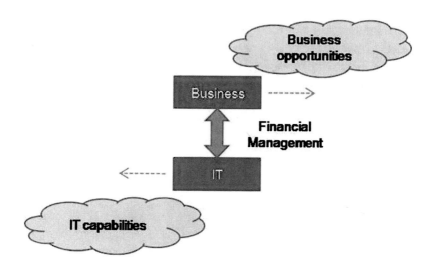

Figure 4.F—Financial Management Managing Conflicting Perspectives

WHEN IMPLEMENTED EFFECTIVELY, FINANCIAL MANAGEMENT provides the understanding and management of the distance and (sometimes) conflicting perspectives between the Business Desires/Opportunities and the Capabilities of the IT organization. It enables the business to be more IT conscious and IT to become more business - aligned.

As businesses evolve, markets change, and the IT industry matures, Financial Management is becoming increasingly adopted by IT organizations, with typical benefits including:

- Enhanced decision-making
- Increased speed of change
- Improved Service Portfolio Management
- Financial compliance and control
- Improved operational control
- Greater insight and communication of the value created by IT services

Terminology

Term	Definition
accounting	(*ITIL® Service Strategy*) The process responsible for identifying the actual costs of delivering IT services, comparing these with budgeted costs, and managing variance from the budget.
budget	A list of all the money an organization or business unit plans to receive and plans to pay out over a specified period of time. See *also* budgeting.
budgeting	The activity of predicting and controlling the spending of money. Budgeting consists of a periodic negotiation cycle to set future budgets (usually annual) and the day-to-day monitoring and adjusting of current budgets.
business case	(*ITIL® Service Strategy*) Justification for a significant item of expenditure. The business case includes information about costs, benefits, options, issues, risks, and possible problems.
charging	(*ITIL® Service Strategy*) Requiring payment for IT services. Charging for IT services is optional and many organizations choose to treat their IT service provider as a cost centre.
IT accounting	See accounting.

[handwritten note: Something that shows an action to be reasonable or necessary]

Scope

FINANCE DEPARTMENTS WILL BE FOUND in every organization. The processes used to manage finances in a business are often well-understood and established within the organization. The professional accountants in the finance department will manage these processes, set financial policies, established procedures and practices for budgeting and accounting, and define the standards used in reporting and charging.

Financial management for IT is often a separate function from the enterprise finance department. This function may report directly to either the CFO or the CIO, but have responsibilities to both. The finance department for IT is treated as a separate function because it must acquire an specialization not normally found in a typical accountant: in addition to having the understanding of business and finance, an accountant supporting IT must also have an understanding of technology. A potential hire for Financial Management for IT will benefit from more experience in cost accounting than other financial disciplines.

While Financial Management for IT is distinguished as a separate function from enterprise financial management, the policies and practices utilized by both must be consistent. The level of consistency is driven by requirements in legislation, regulations, and best practices regarding financial accountability, but also enables better communication and reporting between the business units and IT.

For internal service providers, Financial Management for IT plays the role of translator between the corporate financial systems and service management. In a typical financial relationship between business and IT, much of the operational costs for IT are recovered through the billing of business units based on demand and the pricing of service level packages. From a business manager's perspective, IT costs may be a simple line item on their yearly budget. The business may provide additional funds for investments into major improvements and new services.

The IT department receives the funding from the business and Financial Management for IT must manage the operational costs and investments separately. At times, the funding may not be enough, so Financial Management for IT must provide a justification for additional funding to the business which has the option of approving or denying. This additional funding is usually to address new services or new technologies and are introduced to the business through the use of a business case.

Financial Management is normally a well-established and well-understood part of any organization. Professional accountants manage dedicated finance departments, which set financial policies, budgeting procedures, financial reporting standards, accounting practices, and revenue generation or cost recovery rules.

Activities

THERE ARE THREE FUNDAMENTAL ACTIVITIES for Financial Management for IT Services. These are:

- Budgeting
- IT Accounting
- Chargeback

Budgeting: Predicting the expected future requirements for funds to deliver the agreed upon services and monitoring adherence to the defined budgets. This ensures that the required resources to fund IT are made available and can improve the business case for IT projects and initiatives.

IT Accounting: Enables the IT organization to account fully for the way its money is spent. The definition of Cost Models can be used to identify costs by customer, by service, by activity, or other logical groupings. IT Accounting supports more accurate budgeting and ensures that any charging method utilized is simple, fair, and realistic.

Chargeback: Charging customers for their use of IT services. Charging can be implemented in a number of ways in order to encourage more efficient use of IT resources. Notional charging is one particular option in which the costs of providing services to customers are communicated but no actual payment is required.

In a simplified form, restaurants demonstrate all three activities for each customer seated. Budgeting is usually performed before the customer enters the doors and will define the food and beverage stock available, the personnel resources required during a specific time frame, and overhead expenditures for maintenance and utilities. Each of these budgetary concerns is determined by the potential earnings for the restaurant for the given period of time.

After the customer is seated, they will order from the menu which is "accounted for" by the waiter. Each menu item has a specified cost that represents the price of the ingredients, the responsibility for the wages of the staff, the utility costs, and any waste attributed to providing the desired service. The specified cost is typically determined by the demand for the menu item and total costs are shared across customers. Each menu item has a specified price which is seen by the customer. This price must cover the actual costs associated to providing the menu item as well as increase the overall earning potential for the restaurant. The goal of the restaurant is two-fold: increase the gap between the actual costs for providing the service and the price for providing the service, as well as to have an earning potential that meets or exceeds the planned budget.

In a restaurant, charging is a simple process that is carried out by providing the customer a receipt and having them pay for the meal. In IT, charging can be more complex because the services provided are unevenly shared between business units who have different requirements for IT. The best example from the restaurant analogy is to imagine a dinner setting for ten people: does the charge for the dinner go to one person, is the bill split evenly between the 10 people, or is each person's order individually accounted for and charged independent from the other 9 people. Financial Management for IT is responsible for managing these complex situations.

Service Valuation

FINANCIAL MANAGEMENT ASSISTS IN THE role of Service Valuation, which is used to help the business and the IT service provider agree on the value of the IT service. It determines the balance demonstrating the total cost of providing an IT service against the total value offered to the business by the service. As previously described, value in services is created by the combination of Service Utility and Service Warranty.

INPUTS

THE MAJOR INPUTS TO FINANCIAL Management for IT services include (Service Strategy, Page 240):

- *Policies, standards, and practices defined by legislation, regulators, and enterprise financial managers*
- *Generally Accepted Accounting Practices (GAAP) and local variations*
- *All data sources where financial information is stored, including the supplier database, configuration management system, the service portfolio, customer agreement portfolio, application portfolio, and project portfolio, which together comprise the elements of the service knowledge management system*

- *The service portfolio provides the structure of services that will be provided, which, in turn, will be the basis for the accounting system—since all costs (and returns) will ultimately be expressed in terms of the services provided*
- *The service management processes provides information about how money is spent, what services are provided and any additional commitments made to the customer.*

Outputs

THE MAJOR OUTPUTS OF FINANCIAL Management for IT services include (ITIL® Service Strategy page 240).

- *Service valuation: This is the ability to understand the costs of a service relative to its business value.*
- *Service investment analysis: Financial management for IT services provides the information and history to enable the service provider to determine the value of the investment in a service. This information is used by the business to demonstrate the value they have realized in using the service to achieve their desired outcomes.*
- *Compliance: Regardless of the location of a service provider, or whether they are internal or external, financial data is subject to regulation and legislation. Financial management for IT services helps implement and enforce policies that ensure the organization is able to store and archive financial data, secure and control it, and make sure that it is reported to the appropriate people. IT Financial Management data specifically allows the executives of the organization to track the levels of investment in IT and ensure that the money is being used to achieve the overall organizational strategy, mitigate risks, and achieve the appropriate returns in a legal and ethical manner.*
- *Cost optimization: Cost optimization should not always be equated with cost savings. The goal of cost optimization is to make sure that investments are appropriate for the level of service that the customers demand and the level of returns that are being projected.*
- *Business impact analysis (BIA): Business impact analysis (BIA) involves understanding the effect on the business if a service were not available. This enables the business to prioritize investments in services and service continuity. Financial management for IT services contributes to BIA by providing financial data and information to quantify the potential effect on the business. It also helps to quantify and prioritize the actions that need to be taken to prevent the impact from becoming reality.*

> • *Planning confidence: Planning confidence is not a tangible output or plan— rather it refers to the level of confidence that service stakeholders have in the service provider being able to accurately forecast costs and returns. A lack of planning confidence results in a lack of confidence in the service provider, and, in many cases, an unwillingness by the business to invest in IT unless absolutely necessary.*

Business Cases

BUSINESS CASES ARE USED TO support planning and decision making activities regarding the attractiveness of a business action. Central to most business cases is a financial analysis that defines the consequences, expectations, and requirements of the business action from a financial perspective. Most business cases will start with a business objective that must be achieved and a proposed business action for achieving the objective. The business case is a detailed analysis of the benefits and impact of the business action in meeting the business objective and disrupting the delivery of other IT services.

The structure of the business case will vary from one organization to the next organization, but some common sections include:

- Introduction – provides the context for the business case, providing the business objective in question and defining clearly the business action being proposed.
- Methods and assumptions – describes the analysis being performed, often in terms of the business, finances, and technology.
  The assumptions are inputs into the analysis that will be used to determine the value of the business actions, while methods are the techniques used in the analysis. This portion of the business case establishes the scope, or boundaries, of the business case.
- Business impact – describes the results of the analysis performed in terms of financial and non-financial benefits and impact. The non-financial results of business case are just as important as the financial results since service value and service costs are not always equal.
- Risks and contingencies – every business action will have some form of risk: this section provides an opportunity to communicate those risks and provide contingencies for addressing those risks.

- Recommendations – provides the means to sanction the proposed business action and communicate any conditions or guarantees that should be placed on the proposal before acceptance.

While the business case is generally recognized as a tool to define the financial aspects of a proposed investment, they are used to communicate the business and technological benefits of a proposed solution. Because of this, the business case is also a component of service portfolio management and business relationship management.

Service Portfolio Management

THE PURPOSE OF SERVICE PORTFOLIO Management is to *ensure that the service provider has the right mix of services to balance the investment in IT with the ability to meet business outcomes. It tracks the investment in services throughout their lifecycle and works with other service management processes to ensure that the appropriate returns are being achieved. In addition, it ensures that services are clearly defined and linked to the achievement of business outcomes, thus ensuring that all design, transition, and operation activities are aligned to the value of the services* (Service Strategy, Page 170).

A medium sized company, ABC Associates, has recently started the adoption of IT Service Management to the business. They have identified the critical and non-critical objectives and outcomes of the business and approved the funding of several services. What is required is a formal approach for managing the development and operation of these services to ensure the business objectives and outcomes are achieved. This approach is provided by the service portfolio management process and provides the following benefits:

- Tracks the services through the entire service lifecycle
- Ensures each service is well defined and associated to the business outcomes they support
- Ensures all service management processes are working together to provide business value
- Tracks the investment required to ensure each service reaches a level of value desired by the customer

Service portfolio management does not manage any services, service management processes, or service assets. Rather, service portfolio management provides a structure for collecting data and making decisions related to services, service management processes, and service assets. The focus of the service portfolio is to describe IT services in terms of business value to the customer. Fulfilling this focus requires the service portfolio to articulate the business needs and describe how the services will be used to respond to those needs.

If a service provider supports multiple customer groups, they may create several service portfolios. Each service portfolio is used to contain all service considerations related to the given customer groups. This is especially important when distinguishing services between regulated industries, such as financial companies, pharmaceutical companies, and governments to name a few. In these situations, the services must support the business outcomes as well as the regulated outcomes of the industry with investments being made in both.

Terminology

Term	Definition
retire	(*ITIL® Service Transition*) Permanent removal of an IT service or other configuration item from the live environment. Being retired is a stage in the lifecycle of many configuration items.
return on investment (ROI)	(*ITIL® Continual Service Improvement*) (*ITIL® Service Strategy*) A measurement of the expected benefit of an investment. In the simplest sense, it is the net profit of an investment divided by the net worth of the assets invested.
risk	A possible event that could cause harm or loss or affect the ability to achieve objectives. A risk is measured by the probability of a threat, the vulnerability of the asset to that threat, and the impact it would have if it occurred. Risk can also be defined as uncertainty of outcome and can be used in the context of measuring the probability of positive outcomes as well as negative outcomes.
service catalog	(*ITIL® Service Design*) (*ITIL® Service Strategy*) A database or structured document with information about all live IT services, including those available for deployment. The service catalog is part of the service portfolio and contains information about two types of IT service: customer-facing services that are visible to the business and supporting services required by the service provider to deliver customer-facing services.

service pipeline	(*ITIL*® *Service Strategy*) A database or structured document listing all IT services that are under consideration or development but are not yet available to customers. The service pipeline provides a business view of possible future IT services and is part of the service portfolio that is not normally published to customers.
service portfolio	(*ITIL*® *Service Strategy*) The complete set of services that is managed by a service provider. The service portfolio is used to manage the entire lifecycle of all services and includes three categories: service pipeline (proposed or in development), service catalog (live or available for deployment), and retired services.

© **Crown** Copyright 2011 Reproduced under license from the Cabinet Office

Scope

THE SERVICE PORTFOLIO CONTAINS INFORMATION about all the services being considered for delivery by the service provider, those services already being delivered to the customer, and those services no longer available to the customer for the purpose of continually generating value from the services.

The restaurant menu is a perfect example of a service portfolio, using menu items as services. The core menu is comprised of the food and drink items currently available to the customer. These typically represent the most popular items ordered by the customer and comprise the core business for the restaurant. To continually refresh the menu, certain menu items may be considered for possible inclusion in the menu. These menu items may be introduced as daily specials or "limited time offers." These specials are made to determine the actual value for the customer and, if found popular, may find themselves included in the core menu. Seasonal menus are another form of "special" where the ingredients are restricted to a certain time of year because of growth or cost. Some menu items may lose their popularity over time or become too expensive to continue offering. They are taken off the menu, but the recipe may still exist in the kitchen. At times, these retired menu items may return as "specials" because they have some level of value.

While a service portfolio is not as flexible as a restaurant menu, the primary concepts are present. The concern of the service portfolio is to generate value for the business and this is done by considering new services, maintaining the value creation of the currently provided services, and removing the services when value is no longer perceived. The service portfolio provides information about what the customer wants, how they can get it, and what is required to ensure they receive it. External service providers will also utilize the service portfolio to identify how revenue is generated.

- Services are grouped into three distinct categories in the Service Portfolio:
- Service Pipeline (services that have been proposed or are in development)
- Service Catalog (live services or those available for deployment)
- Retired Services (decommissioned services)

The information making up the Service Portfolio(s) will come from many sources, so possible implementations may make use of existing databases and other data repositories, document management systems, financial systems, project management documentation, the Service Catalog, and other relevant input areas. Where necessary, the various sources of information may be collated and communicated by means of an internet/intranet-based interface so that duplication does not occur and that appropriate levels of detail and accessibility can be controlled.

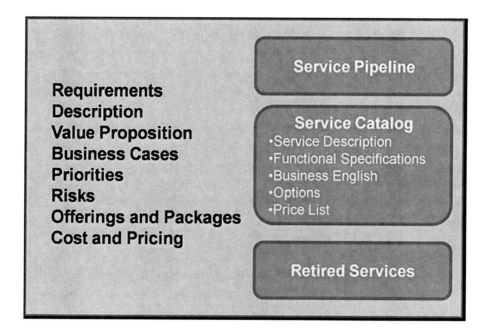

Figure 4.G—A Service Portfolio
"Based on Cabinet Office ITIL® material. Reproduced under licence from the Cabinet Office"

BY DELIVERING THE OBJECTIVES ABOVE, the Service Portfolio either answers or helps to answer the following strategic questions:

- Why should a customer buy these services?
- Why should they buy these services from us?
- What are the pricing or chargeback models?
- What are our strengths and weaknesses, priorities, and risks?
- How are resources and capabilities to be allocated?

Understanding their options helps senior executives to make informed investment decisions in service initiatives, taking into account appropriate levels of risks and rewards. These initiatives may cross business functions and may span short, medium, and longer timeframes.

Investment Categories and Budget Allocations

PERIODICALLY, THE SERVICES IN THE service portfolio will be analysed to ensure the expected value of the service is being delivered to the customer at a cost appropriate to the level of service required. This analysis could be a part of the various "checkpoints" established within the service lifecycle or as a result of a service review or some other activity designed to discern or validate service value. The results of an analysis are used by executives to determine which services will take priority when making investments.

Service Investments are split among 3 strategic categories:

Transform the Business (TTB):

TTB investments are focused on initiatives that enter new market spaces with new capabilities being developed. These investments are usually associated to services, service packages, or service package levels adopted to support a move into new market spaces. They may require different skill set in personnel, adoption of new technologies, or compliance to regulations related to the market space. The initiatives within this category will typically create new value for the business as well as additional costs.

Grow the business (GTB):

GTB investments are intended to grow the organization's scope of services or gain more customers within an existing market space. GTB investments are different from TTB investment because the concern is the existing market spaces, not new market spaces. Some of the same requirements may exist, but the focus of GTB investments is to increase the value of the services provided.

Run the business (RTB):

RTB investments are centered on maintaining service operations. This type of investment is interested in maintaining the status quo for a particular service, though some cost optimization may be performed. The importance of this level of strategic investment is to ensure the costs of the service do not increase and the value of the service does not decrease.

Each of the three strategic investment categories can be broken down into budget types available for the categories. The association between budget types and investment categories are provided in parenthesis. They are:

- Venture (TTB) – those funds in the budget set aside to create new services in new market spaces.
- Growth (GTB) – those funds in the budget set aside to create new services in the existing market space.
- Discretionary (GTB) – those funds in the budget that are available, usually to enhancing existing service, but do not need to be spent
- Non-discretionary (RTB) – those funds in the budget that must be spent to operate and maintain existing services.
- Core (RTB) – those funds in the budget set aside to operate and maintain business-critical services.

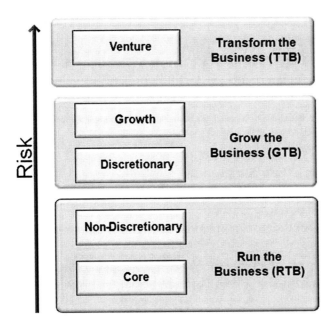

Figure 4.H—Balancing a Service Portfolio
© Crown Copyright 2011 Reproduced under license from
Cabinet Office

SERVICE RETIREMENT

AN OFTEN OVER-LOOKED INVESTMENT, this is potentially one of the largest hidden costs in a service provider's organization, particularly in a large organization with a long history. Few providers have a clear plan for retiring increasingly redundant services. This is often due to a number of reasons, including a lack of visibility of what services are actually offered and the fear that retiring a service may impact other services being offered.

Different service providers may define the "retirement" of a service in different ways. All definitions will require the service description to be removed from the service portfolio; however, some companies will maintain and manage the services delivered to existing customers while prohibiting new customers from partaking in the service. Other companies will not allow existing or new customers with the retired service. Retired services are still maintained and available should the original business requirement emerges or another business needs can be achieved by the service.

Refreshing the Portfolio

ONE THING THAT CAN BE relied on to happen is change: in the market, in business strategy, in outcomes and requirements, in technology, and in value creation. Changes occur to the conditions within every market space, invalidating previous Return on Investment (ROI) calculations. Some of these changes may be a result of:

- New competitors or alternative options entering a market
- The introduction of new compliance regulations
- Mergers and acquisitions
- New or changed public legislation
- Changes in the economic climate affecting various markets

Because of this, the attributes of a service may need to adapt in order to support the change. The methods used by the Service Portfolio Manager and other involved stakeholders seek to continually refresh the Service Portfolio, creating service investments that provide an optimum balance of risk and reward.

The role of the Chief Information Officer (or other similar roles), in this context, is to monitor, measure, reassess and, rebalance investments as the markets and associated businesses change. They will need to identify what balance is appropriate for their organization (e.g., low risk and low reward, high risk and potential high reward) and authorize service investments that match these needs.

A formal review of the service portfolio should be scheduled at least quarterly as part of continuous service improvement. This review should compare the services in the service portfolio and associated investments against the strategies for the business and IT.

Activities

EVERY SERVICE FOUND WITHIN THE service portfolio must a defined set of information used to establish the service. The information requirements should be consistent across all services. Depending on the state of the service, some information may not be available. Information commonly captured in the service portfolio for each service includes

- Requirements on the service
- Description of the service

- Description of how the service generates value
- Business case for the service, particularly the cost/benefit analysis
- Priority of the service in relation to other services in the service portfolio
- Resources and capabilities required by the service portfolio
- Risks associated with delivering the service
- Service packages and service level packages offered
- Cost and pricing of the service relative to the desired package

This information is used by Service Portfolio Management to make decisions regarding the management, development, and inclusion of the services. Service Portfolio Management consists of four main phases of activity, illustrated in Figure 4.H

Define: *This phase focuses on documenting and understanding existing services and new services. Each service must have a documented business case. Data for each service, such as which service assets are required and where investments are made, needs to be validated* (Service Strategy, Page 180). This is the activity where the service information is captured and organized within the service portfolio. The activity is initiated though efforts in strategy planning, requests from the business, opportunities in service improvement, or suggestions for services. Defining a service also includes defining the service model to demonstrate how service assets and customer assets relate to create value.

Analyze: *The analysis of services in the portfolio will indicate whether the service is able to optimize value and how supply and demand can be prioritized and balanced* (Service Strategy, page 181). An analysis of a service is an effort to connect the service to the overall strategy of the organization: for internal service providers, this connection is made to both the business strategy and IT strategy of the organization. A service analysis will clarify the investments, prioritization, and value proposition of the service.

Approve: *Every service needs to be approved and the level of investment to ensure sufficient resources to deliver the anticipated levels of service must be authorized* (Service Strategy, page 181). If the service cannot achieve the desired business outcomes for the customer, the service or changes to the service is not feasible in the existing environment. As services move through the service lifecycle, they also move through the service portfolio in one of six categories:

- Retain/build – the services are aligned with and relevant to the strategy of the organization.
- Replace – the minimum levels of technical and functional fitness required by the service are not met.
- Rationalize – the service in question is unclear in its definition, has overlapping business functionality, or supports multiple and duplicate versions of service assets providing the same functionality
- Refactor – the technical and functional fitness required for the service is present, but supports loosely defined process or system boundary
- Renew – the functional fitness of a service is achieved, but not the technical fitness, such as services reliant on new technologies that are currently being adopted but have not been adopted fully.
- Retire – services that no longer meet the objective or strategic need for the business.

Charter: *A charter is a document authorizing the project and stating its scope, terms, and references. Services are not just built on request from anyone in the organization. They have to be formally chartered and stakeholders need to be kept up-to-date with information about decisions, resource allocation, and actual investments made* (Service Strategy, page 181).

Last time we meet ABC Associates, they had come to a decision to establish the service portfolio management process to aid them in managing their IT services through the service lifecycle and ensure those services generate value for the customer. The process is in place and some work has been performed to create services within the service portfolio. Some changes have occurred in the market space, resulting in a re-evaluation of the proposed services. Before the company can move forward with designing and deploying the required services, they must define each service and their relationships between each other and the business.

As the service is defined, the service can be analysed to ensure it meets the strategic objectives of the organization. As part of this analysis, the organization can clarify the investment required to provide the service, the priority of the service with regard to meeting critical business outcomes, and the value proposition set in the business case. If feasible, a proposed change can be raised reflecting the new or changed service. The proposed change is then reviewed and approved by stakeholders, upon which a service charter is created authorizing the project to design, test, and deploy the service.

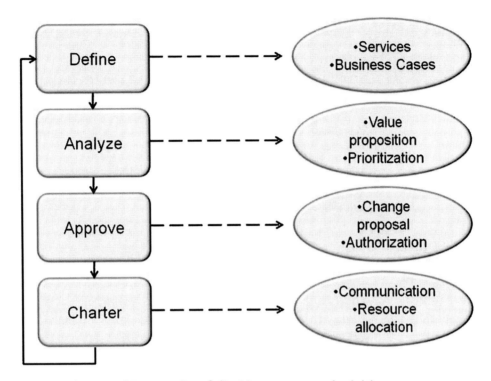

Figure 4.1—Phases of Service Portfolio Management Activities
© Crown Copyright 2011 Reproduced under license from the
Cabinet Office

Inputs

THE INPUTS TO THE SERVICE Portfolio Management will impact the individual service descriptions and provide information to make decisions in defining, analysing, and approving the services. The inputs to the process are (Service Strategy, Page 196):

- *Strategy plans*
- *Service improvement opportunities*
- *Financial reports*
- *Requests, suggestions, or complaints from the business*
- *Project updates for services in the charter stage of the process*

Outputs

OUTPUTS FROM SERVICE PORTFOLIO MANAGEMENT include (Service Strategy, Page 197):

- *An up-to-date service portfolio*
- *Service charters that authorize the work for designing and building new services or changes to existing services*
- *Reports on the status of new or changed services*
- *Reports on the investment made in services in the service portfolio and the returns on that investment*
- *Change proposals that are used to allow change management to assess and schedule the work and resources required to charter services*
- *Identified strategic risks*

Business Relationship Management

UP TO THIS POINT, WE have explored the Financial Management for IT process which ensures that the funding is in place to ensure the service can provide the desired levels of utility and warranty to the customer and the Service Portfolio Management which manages the service description and investments to the services to ensure the service has the resources and capabilities to achieve the business outcomes for the customer. The next process to explore is Business Relationship Management. It is through this process that the IT organization and the business organization with the intent to increase the service provider's understanding of the business environment and associated requirements and can validate the provided service will do so.

The defined purpose of the Business Relationship Management process from ITIL® is two-fold (Service Strategy, Page 256):

- *To establish and maintain a business relationship between the service provider and the customer based on understanding the customer and their business needs*
- *To identify customer needs and ensure that the service provider is able to meet these needs as business needs change over time and between circumstances. Business Relationship Management ensures that the service provider understands these changing needs. Business Relationship Management also assists the business in articulating the value of a service. Put another way, Business Relationship Management ensures that customer expectations do not exceed what they are willing to pay for and that the service provider is able to meet the customer's expectations before agreeing to deliver the service.*

Terminology

Term	Definition
business relationship management	(ITIL® Service Strategy) The process responsible for maintaining a positive relationship with customers. Business relationship management identifies customer needs and ensures that the service provider is able to meet these needs with an appropriate catalog of services. This process has strong links with service level management.

© **Crown** Copyright 2011 Reproduced under license from the Cabinet Office

Scope

AT THE CENTER OF THE process is the Business Relationship Manager role, which is typically filled by a senior representative from IT. Larger organizations may have several dedicated BRMs. On the business side of the relationship, senior managers are customarily serving as representatives. The relationships being built between the BRM and senior manager in the business is to ensure the activities of the service provider are aligned with the customer's business objectives.

When dealing with external service providers, the BPM role is fulfilled by dedicated account managers, with at least one assigned to each customer or group of small customers. The purpose of the relationship in this situation is to maximizing the value of contract and ensuring customer satisfaction.

Within this context, the Business Relationship Management process attempts to:

- Maintain a relationship between service provider and customer with the intent of understanding the customer and their needs.
- Understand the business outcomes desired by the customer.
- Understand the available service packages and service level packages
- Identify and appropriately respond to changes in the customer environment that may impact service delivery, levels, and demand.
- Identify technology trends that may impact service delivery, levels, and demand
- Establish and maintain a positive image of the service provider
- Ensure high levels of customer satisfaction and establish a formal process for customer complaints

The primary focus of the Business Relationship Management is to establish and maintain an interface between the IT organization and business organization. In this capacity, the process does not manage service delivery. The process is highly dependent on other service management processes and functions to fulfil their objectives. Many of the service management processes require customer input or participation, making it easy for creating independent relationships with the customer that are not controlled or managed through Business Relationship Management. This can cause confusion, especially when customer requirements are not consistently communicated or interpreted. The inherent function of the Business Relationship Management is to minimize this confusion and potential conflicts by ensuring that all communication with the customer is filtered through the Business Relationship Manager. When dealing with these service management processes requiring customer participation, clearly identified interfaces with Business Relationship Management must be in place.

Company X has never had a stable provision of IT services. All IT support is internal and must be that way because of the number of customized applications and systems that support the company. Five years ago, all IT activities were consolidated under one functional organization after years of having lines of business supporting their own IT requirements. This consolidation was a rough change for the company, but in the end, the costs for providing services dramatically decreased and several critical systems had improved performance. Despite the achievements, the services provided by IT are still relatively undefined and immature. Staff consistently communicate they are dealing with more complaints about a service than actual incidents for a service.

Several months ago, the company started implementing IT Service Management. One of the first processes formally introduced was Business Relationship Management. Since its introduction, service capabilities have increased, complaints about services have decreased, and cost of service has steadily decreased. In a recent executive meeting, the CIO recognized Business Relationship Management as the single most important achievement in improving IT services over the last year. When asked why this was the case, the response addressed these reasons:

- A dialogue between the business side of the company and the technology side of the company was created that eventually evolved into a strategic partnership with one goal in mind – increasing the productivity of each and every employee.

- The IT department was finally able to formally articulate the conflicting business requirements they were expected to fulfill, as well as the benefits and failures of the current services. This gave the business an opportunity to reevaluate and align their business requirements against the current strategy and, with the help of the IT department, approves a set of requirements that enabled consistent and reliable IT services across all lines of business.
- Old behaviours consistent with when lines of business provided their own IT support were finally broken, because a formalized point of contact outside of the service desk was established for management and business complaints against IT services. BPM enabled all such communication to be contained, analysed, and handled appropriately. The provision of a complaint and escalation process raised the business' trust and satisfaction with IT services dramatically in the first two months.

The example above shows the value of Business Relationship Management. IT services will be delivered whether or not the process is in place, but when BPM does exist, it provides the conditions for building a cooperative partnership between the business and IT, allows an opportunity to evaluate the requirements on IT against strategy, and handles conflicts arising from dissatisfaction of IT services.

Activities

THE BUSINESS RELATIONSHIP MANAGER WILL utilize two tools primarily: the customer portfolio and the customer agreement portfolio. The customer portfolio is a structured document or database used to document information about the actual and potential customers of service delivery, particularly commitments to the customer, investments relevant to the services provided to the customer, and the risks associated with the customer. The customer portfolio can be used by the service provider to determine if providing services to a particular customer is feasible, or can be used in identify new market spaces that the service provider may be successful in. Several service management processes utilize the customer portfolio which is defined and maintained by Business Relationship Management.

The customer agreement portfolio is a structured document or database capturing all the contracts or agreements between the service provider and customers. Each service will have its own contract. The customer agreement portfolio ensures

Business Relationship Management understands the services being delivered, as well as service levels and terms and conditions related to each IT service. While the tool is important to Business Relationship Management, the customer agreement portfolio is defined and maintained by the Service Level Management process.

The activities of Business Relationship Management can vary based on where a service is in its lifecycle. These activities can be consolidated into two overarching activities to describe what the BPM does. Those activities are defined by ITIIL as (Service Strategy, Page 268):

- *To represent the service provider to its customers through coordinated marketing, selling, and delivery activities*
- *To work with Service Portfolio Management and design coordination to ensure that the service provider's response to customer requirements is appropriate. Thus, the process facilitates customer advocacy throughout the Service Lifecycle.*

The first activity is simple: the BPM represents the service provider to the world of customers for the purpose of demonstrating the value of the service provider's services to the customer. The services being shown could involve new services, improved services, and adoptions of new technologies that are not currently being delivered to the customer, as well as the value of services currently being delivered.

The second activity comprises the work performed with the service provider to ensure the services designed, developed, and deployed will appropriately meet the needs of the customer. In this activity, the BPM acts on behave of the customer to communicate the requirements of the business and review the service for value.

Inputs

THE ACTIVITIES ABOVE REQUIRE THE following inputs to Business Relationship Management (Service Strategy, Page 277):

- *Customer requirements*
- *Customer requests, complaints, escalations, or compliments*
- *The service strategy*
- *Where possible, the customer's strategy*
- *The service portfolio*

- *The project portfolio to ensure that requirements are gathered in a timely fashion and that all projects include Business Relationship Management activity where appropriate*
- *Service Level Agreements*
- *Requests for change*
- *Patterns of business activity and user profiles defined by Demand Management and that need to be validated through Business Relationship Management*

Outputs

THE ACTIVITIES WILL PRODUCE THE following outputs of Business Relationship Management (Service Strategy, Page 278):

- *Stakeholder definitions*
- *Defined business outcomes*
- *Agreement to fund (internal) or pay for (external) services*
- *The customer portfolio*
- *Service requirements for strategy, design, and transition*
- *Customer satisfaction surveys and the published results of these surveys*
- *Schedules of customer activity in various service management process activities*
- *Schedule of training and awareness events*
- *Reports on the customer perception of service performance*

Service Strategy Summary

THE SERVICE STRATEGY STAGE ENABLES the organization to ensure that the organizational objectives for IT are defined and that Services and Service Portfolios are maximized for value. IT Service Strategy is used to enable excellence in service delivery through achieving balance on several levels, such as:

- Quality versus cost
- External versus internal
- Stability versus agility
- Reactive versus proactive
- Flexibility versus control
- Service provider capabilities versus customer requirements

Through the processes of the Service Strategy stage, the service provider can define and contain the desired service capabilities into an marketable package offering. Other benefits delivered through these processes include:

- Enhanced ability to predict the resources required to fund IT
- Clearer visibility of the costs for providing IT Services
- Quality information to support investment decisions in IT
- Understanding of the use and demand for IT Services with the ability to influence positive and cost-effective use of IT

As the focal point for strategy, policy, and guidelines that direct the efforts and practices of the IT organization, Service Strategy has many important interfaces with the rest of the Service Lifecycle. Some of these include:

- **Interfaces with the Service Design stage:**
  ‣ Service Archetypes and Models, which describe how service assets interact with customer assets. These are important high-level inputs that guide the design of services
  ‣ Definition of business outcomes to be supported by services
  ‣ Understanding of varying priority in required service attributes
  ‣ Relative design constraints for the service (e.g., budget, contractual terms and conditions, copyrights, utility, warranty, resources, standards, and regulations etc.)
  ‣ Definition of the cost models associated with providing services

- **Interfaces with the Service Transition stage:**
  ‣ Service Transition provides evaluations of the costs and risks involved with introducing and modifying services. It also provides assistance in determining the relative options or paths for changing strategic positions or entering market spaces.
  ‣ Request for Changes may be utilized to affect changes to strategic positions
  ‣ Planning of the required resources and evaluation of whether the change can be implemented fast enough to support the strategy
  ‣ Control and recording of service assets is maintained by Service Asset and Configuration Management

- **Interfaces with the Service Operation stage:**
  - ▷ Service Operation will deploy service assets in patterns that most effectively deliver the required utility and warranty in each segment across the Service Catalog
  - ▷ Deployment of shared assets that provide multiple levels of redundancy, support a defined level of warranty, and build economies of scale
  - ▷ Service Strategy must clearly define the warranty factors that must be supported by Service Operation with attributes of reliability, maintainability, redundancy, and overall experience of availability

- **Interfaces with the Continual Service Improvement stage:**
  - ▷ Continual Service Improvement (CSI) will provide the coordination and analysis of the quality, performance, and customer satisfaction of the IT organization, including the processes utilized and services provided
  - ▷ Integration with CSI will also provide the identification of potential improvement actions that can be made to elements of Service Strategy

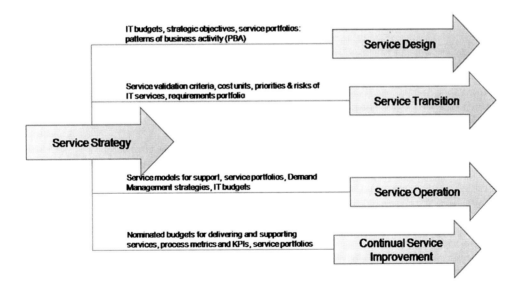

Figure 4.J—Some Service Strategy Outputs to Other Lifecycle Stages

Service Strategy Scenario

To assist with your learning and understanding of how the stages and processes work together, the following scenario will be used throughout this book.

This simplistic overview of a service gives examples of how the processes are utilized to create the service.

The business has requested that they would like to be able to use the internet for instant messaging with international offices. They are also interested in VOIP and video conferencing. We will call this new service HYPE. This scenario will continue throughout the rest of the book.

Overall Service Strategy

- It is important here to truly understand exactly what the business needs are, as well as their expectations for this service
- Value must be defined (remember that utility + warranty = value):
  - Utility considers the features of HYPE—what type of support will the business require?, what features will the business want/need?, i.e., is it fit for purpose?
  - Warranty considers the levels of service guarantee (e.g., continuity, availability, security, capacity) that the business requires to be clarified—this is set out in service level packages

- Service Level Packages:
  - Core service package—instant messaging
  - Supporting service package—added VOIP and/or video conferencing, ability to attach files
  - Service Level packages—video quality, security of transmissions, access times, service support, user access

Financial Management Considerations
- Cost to purchase/build service
- Cost of hardware (web cams, PC upgrades if necessary)
- Cost of increased internet access/bandwidth
- Charging for service?
- Budget?

Service Portfolio Management Considerations

- You have already been trialing X brand instant messenger service among the IT staff, so an entry has been added to the Service Pipeline
- Are there redundant services to retire?

Business Relationship Management Considerations
- Service portfolio and customer portfolio
- Customer satisfaction surveys and measures
- Documented business outcomes and customer requirements

By determining the above before you start to design the service, you are in a better position to ensure that HYPE will meet the customer needs (closed loop system). Remember, this is where value is agreed and Service Operation is where the value of HYPE is seen. As we all know, the level of value will more than likely be in direct correlation to the dollars the business is prepared to pay and this is why it is important to clarify this now, before we start designing.

Service Strategy Review Questions

THESE QUESTIONS ALSO COVER THE Introduction and Common Terminology Chapters.

Question 1
Which ITIL® process is responsible for developing a charging system?

a) Availability Management
b) Capacity Management
c) Financial Management for IT Services
d) Service Level Management

Question 2
What is the RACI model used for?

a) Documenting the roles and relationships of stakeholders in a process or activity
b) Defining requirements for a new service or process
c) Analyzing the business impact of an incident
d) Creating a balanced scorecard showing the overall status of Service Management

Question 3
Which of the following identifies two Service Portfolio components within the Service Lifecycle?

a) Catalog Service Knowledge Management System and Requirements Portfolio
b) Service Catalog and Service Pipeline
c) Service Knowledge Management System and Service Catalog
d) Service Pipeline and Configuration Management System

Question 4
Which of the following is NOT one of the ITIL® core publications?

a) Service Operation
b) Service Transition
c) Service Derivation
d) Service Strategy

Question 5
A Service Level Package is best described as?

a) A description of customer requirements used to negotiate a Service Level Agreement
b) A defined level of utility and warranty associated with a core service package
c) A description of the value that the customer wants and for which they are willing to pay
d) A document showing the service levels achieved during an agreed reporting period

Question 6
Setting policies and objectives is the primary concern of which of the following elements of the Service Lifecycle?

a) Service Strategy
b) Service Strategy and Continual Service Improvement
c) Service Strategy, Service Transition, and Service Operation
d) Service Strategy, Service Design, Service Transition, Service Operation, and Continual Service Improvement

Question 7
A service owner is responsible for which of the following?

a) Designing and documenting a service
b) Carrying out the service operations activities needed to support a service
c) Producing a balanced scorecard showing the overall status of all services
d) Recommending improvements

Question 8
The utility of a service is best described as:

a) Fit for design
b) Fit for purpose
c) Fit for function
d) Fit for use

Question 9
The warranty of a service is best described as:

a) Fit for design
b) Fit for use
c) Fit for purpose
d) Fit for function

Question 10
The contents of a service package includes:

a) Base Service Package, Supporting Service Package, Service Level Package
b) Core Service Package, Supporting Process Package, Service Level Package
c) Core Service Package, Base Service Package, Service Support Package
d) Core Service Package, Supporting Services Package, Service Level Package

SERVICE DESIGN

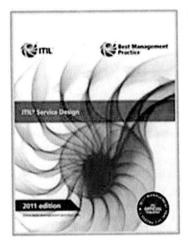

Figure 4.K—Service Design

"© Crown copyright 2011 Reproduced under licence from the Cabinet Office"

The Service Design stage is concerned predominantly with the design of IT Services, as well as the associated or required:

- Processes
- Service management information systems and tools
- Service solutions
- Technology architectures
- Measurement systems

The driving factor in the design of new or changed services is the support of changing business needs. Every time a new service solution is produced, it needs to be checked against the rest of the Service Portfolio to ensure that it will integrate and interface with all of the other services in existence.

The focus of Service Strategy seems to be on working with customers to identify their requirements on IT services and working with the service provider to identify the service packages and service levels needed to meet the customer's requirements. All of this information is documented and agreed by both parties, but it is conceptual in form because there are no services being delivered or any existing services have not been verified to meet customer requirements. Service Design takes the next step in translating the conceptual in the form of documented requirements and agreements and creating a real construct of what the services are and how they should be delivered.

Purpose and Value

ITIL® 2011 DESCRIBES THE PURPOSE of the Service Design stage as *design IT services, together with the governing IT practices, processes, and policies to realize the service provider's strategy and to facilitate the introduction of these services into supported environments, ensuring quality service delivery, customer satisfaction, and cost-effective service provision.* (Service Design, page 4).

The fundamental principle of IT Service Management is to focus on supporting business processes and providing business value. This focus requires the organization to monitor the influence between the business and technology: specifically to evaluate how changes in technology will impact the business and how changes in the business will impact technology. The foundation of this capability to monitor both business and technology is the Service Catalog – a portion of the Service Portfolio containing the active services being provided to the customer and consisting of related information such as business units, processes, and services, their relationships and dependencies on IT services, technology, and components. All aspects of Service Design are vital elements in supporting and enhancing the capability of the IT service provider, particularly the design of the service portfolio, the service catalog, and the individual IT services. All of these activities will also improve the alignment of IT service provision with the business's goals and its evolving needs.

Approaches in service design which are standardized and consistent across the IT organization will benefit both the organization and their customers. Those benefits include:

- Reduction in total cost of ownership (TCO)
- Improved quality of service
- Improved consistency of service
- Easier implementation of new or changed services
- Improved service alignment
- Improved service performance
- Improved IT governance
- Improved effectiveness of service management and IT processes
- Improved information and decision-making
- Improved alignment with customer values and strategies

The Four Perspectives (Attributes) of ITSM

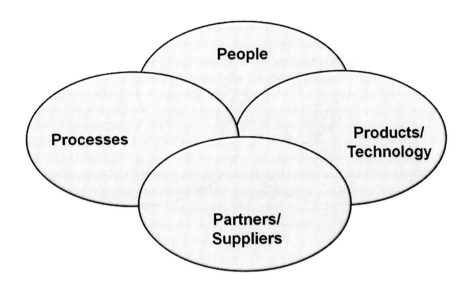

Figure 5.B—Four Perspectives (Attributes) of ITSM

"© Crown copyright 2011 Reproduced under licence from the Cabinet Office"

THERE ARE FOUR PERSPECTIVES (4P's) or attributes that are important to consider in order for IT Service Management to be successful.

Partners/Suppliers Perspective: Takes into account the importance of Partner and External Supplier relationships and how they contribute to Service Delivery. It will help to ensure that suppliers deliver value for money and provide services that are clearly aligned to business requirements.

People Perspective: Concerned with the soft side of ITSM. This requires IT staff, customers, and other stakeholders to understand the purpose of ITSM and how it should be used within the organization. Training and education should be provided to ensure staff members have the correct skills, knowledge, and motivation to perform their roles.

Products/Technology Perspective: Takes into account the quality of IT services themselves and all technology architectures (hardware and software) required to provision them. Technology should be leveraged to both support and drive strategic opportunities for the business.

Process Perspective: Relates to the end-to-end delivery of services based on process flows. By having clearly established processes (with documentation, guidelines, and other supporting tools), it will enable a more consistent, repeatable, and measurable approach to the management of services.

Again, the restaurant business is a simple example for us to illustrate the importance of the 4Ps. A restaurant is in the business of serving customers food and drink: with some exceptions, most restaurants do not grow their own food, butcher their own animals, distill their own drinks, etc. These actions are done through partners or available through suppliers. Without partners and suppliers, restaurants would have nothing to serve their customers. Additionally, restaurants utilize people to perform the activities of the restaurant required to get the food and drink to the customer. Additionally, the customer is part of the service through their compliments, complaints, and return visits.

Especially in franchised restaurants, products, technology, and processes are very important to maintain the exact image and confidence in quality from one restaurant to the next. The quality of the raw materials, ingredients, and cleaning supplies are carefully evaluated and applied appropriately according to defined process and procedures that have been designed to provide quality consistently and reliably under diverse conditions. Many restaurants adopt specifically designed equipment and timers that monitor every aspect of the preparation and cooking processes. Any slip in the quality of the products use or the breakdown of the equipment can result in an inferior product to the customer. The processes in place ensure that the food and drinks get to the customer on time and as ordered. Other processes unseen to the customer ensure that every aspect of the restaurant's operations is observed, monitored, and corrected to specific standards required by owners and health authorities.

Quality IT Service Management ensures that all of these four perspectives are taken into account as part of the continual improvement of the IT organization. It is the same when designing new or modified services in that these four perspectives need to be considered and catered for in order to enable success in its design, transition, and eventual use by customers.

Major Aspects of Service Design

SERVICE DESIGN HAS A BEGINNING and an end. The beginning of the stage is the set of new or changed business requirements. These are provided by through the Service Strategy stage and documented within the service portfolio. The end of service design is the development of a service solution that meets these business requirements. Between these points, Service Design has to "design" the service solution. Unfortunately, this is not as simple as getting what is and only what is required in IT.

Service Design must be an integrated approach that addresses the entire IT solution, not just the service solution in question; but focuses only on the service solution being designed in the present. It is an holistic approach that takes into considerations five major aspects:

- **Service solutions for new or changed services**: Starting with the requirements for new or changed services extracted from the service portfolio, each requirement is analyzed, documented, and agreed. From these activities, a solution design is produced and compared with the strategies and constraints from Service Strategy to ensure conformity to corporate and IT policies. The design of new or changed service must consistent with all other services and the design of all other services that interface with, underpin, or depend on the new or changed service are consistent with the new service. The service solution design must also be aligned with and considered in conjunction with the other four aspects.
- **The management information systems and tools, especially the service portfolio**: These are the IT Service Management components used to monitor and manage the service solutions, specifically in the areas of availability, performance, reliability, and security. The management information systems and tools must be capable of supporting the new or changed services. A review of the systems and tools is appropriate to determine their capabilities relative to this service solution and identify what actions must be taken to resolve any issues.
- **The technology architectures and management architectures**: These are frameworks to ensure that every service solution is designed and implemented consistent to a predefined set of rules and policies. Adoption of these architectures ensures compatibility between technology and management interfaces required by the service solution when connecting to the existing infrastructure. The architectures must

be reviewed to ensure they are consistent with the new or changed service and have the capability to operate and maintain the new service. If not, then either the architectures will need to be amended or the design of the new service will need to be revised.

- **The processes required**: The processes, roles, responsibilities, and skills must be reviewed to ensure they have the capability to operate, support, and maintain the new or changed service. If not, the design of the new service will need to be revised or the existing process capabilities will need to be enhanced. The scope of this review effort includes all IT and Service Management processes.
- **The measurement methods and metrics**: The existing measurement methods must be reviewed to ensure the required metrics on the new or changed service can be provided. If not, then the measurement methods will need to be enhanced or the service metrics will need to be revised.

Take a good look at the service solution and these five aspects are logically in tune to the basic expectations of a design; asking the pertinent questions:

- What is the service solution?
- How is the service solution managed?
- How does the service solution interface with other solution?
- How is the service solution used to deliver value?
- How is the value of the service solution measured?

At the end of the Service Design stage, completion of all the activities above will ensure all of these questions are answered and minimal issues arise during the subsequent Service Lifecycle stages.

Service Design Packages

THE INFORMATION CONTAINED WITHIN A Service Design Package (SDP) includes documentation of all aspects of the service and its requirements in order to provide guidance and structure through all of the subsequent stages of its lifecycle. The information contained within it should address the five major aspects of Service Design that were previously mentioned. A Service Design Package is typically produced for each new IT service, major change, or IT service retirement.

The contents of the service design package are comprised of four major sections with several smaller, but equally important, sub-sections. The four major sections are:

- Requirements
- Service Design
- Organizational readiness assessment
- Service Lifecycle Plan

The Requirements section provides the fundamental basis for the service solution, including the scope of the service and its purpose in achieving business objectives. The section is often divided into business requirements, service applicability, and service contacts. Business requirements will comprise must of the section, providing the agreed and documented business requirements captured during Service Strategy. Service Applicability will define how and where the service will be used. The service contacts identify those groups or people who are considered stakeholders in the service and located in the business, customer base, and IT.

The Service Design section provides the actual service solution design in response to the requirements provided in the previous section. Often found in this section are the requirements for service functionality, service levels, service management, and operational management, as well as the service design and topology. The service functional requirements identify the utility aspect of the service solution, including its planned outcomes and deliverables, in the form of a Statement of Requirements (SoR). Service level requirements (SLR) identify the warranty aspect of the service solution and documented within a Service Level Agreement (SLA). Both SoRs and SLAs are documented formally, reviewed, and agreed before being accepted. The management and operation requirements of the service design identifies the supporting services and agreements, and resources required to control, operate, monitor, measure and report on the service solution.

The actual design of the service solution includes:

- Service definition and Service Model
- Packaging and options
- Service components and infrastructure
- Required documentation for the service, such as user, business, service, component, transitin, support, and operational
- Processes, procedures, measurements, metrics, and reports

- Supporting products, services, agreements and supplies

The Organization readiness assessment is a report determining the organization's current ability to accept the new or changed service solution and a plan for improving the organization's ability before final implementation. The report and plan includes information relevant to the organization and service, such as:

- Benefit to the business
- Financial assessment
- Technical assessment
- Resource assessment
- Organizational assessment
- Required skills, competences, and capabilities

The final section of the service design package is the Service Lifecycle Plan. Comprised of the service program, service transition plan, service operational acceptance plan, and service acceptance criteria, the Service Lifecycle Plan provides a guideline for how the service should be transitioned into the environment and sets expectations for managing its ongoing operations. The Service program is a plan covering all the stages of the lifecycle for the service in question and includes:

- Management, coordination and integration with other projects, improvements, and services
- Risk and issues management
- Scope, objectives, and components of the service
- Required skills, competences, roles and responsibilities
- Required processes
- Interfaces and dependencies with other services
- Requirement management of teams, resources, tools, technology, budgets, and facilities
- Management of suppliers and contracts
- Report, reviews, and revision requirements for the program
- Communication plans and training plans
- Timescales, deliverables, targets and quality targets for each lifecycle stage.

The Service Transition Plan is a detailed approached documented for execution during service transition. The plan includes the transition strategy, objectives, policies, risk assessments and plans. During the transition, the service solution will be built, integrated, and tested to ensure the solution effectively meets the business objectives it was designed to meet. Once complete, the service solution will be ready for operational mode: the Service Operational Acceptance Plan is the approach to move the service from development into operation. When migrating between lifecycle stages, the Service Acceptance Criteria is used.

Service Design Processes

THE PROCESSES INCLUDED WITH THE Service Design lifecycle stage are:

- Design Coordination
- Service Level Management
- Capacity Management
- Availability Management
- IT Service Continuity Management
- Information Security Management
- Supplier Management
- Service Catalog Management

It is important to note that many of the activities from these processes will occur in other lifecycle stages, especially Service Operation. Additionally, Service Level Management also plays an important role in Continual Service Improvement.

Like all ITIL® processes, the level to which the Service Design processes are required to be implemented will depend on many factors, including:

- The complexity and culture of the organization
- The relative size, complexity, and maturity of the IT infrastructure
- The type of business and associated customers being served by IT
- The number of services, customers, and end users involved
- Regulations and compliance factors affecting the business or IT
- The use of outsourcing and external suppliers for small or large portions of the overall IT Service Delivery

Based on these influencing factors, the design team may comprise of a single person in a small IT department or a worldwide network of business and customer oriented groups in an international organization.

Design Coordination (8/8)

ONLY THROUGH WELL-COORDINATED ACTION CAN a service provider hope to create comprehensive and appropriate designs that will support the achievement of the required business outcomes. The Design Coordination process provides a single point of coordination and control for all activities and processes within the Service Design stage of the Service Lifecycle, ensuring the goals and objectives of the Service Design stage are met.

Terminology

Term	Definition
design coordination	(ITIL® Service Design) The process responsible for coordinating all service design activities, processes, and resources. Design coordination ensures the consistent and effective design of new or changed IT services, service management information systems, architectures, technology, processes, information, and metrics.

© **Crown** Copyright 2011 Reproduced under license from the Cabinet Office

Scope

EFFORTS IN DESIGN OR REDESIGN of a service can be simple or complex, small or large, quick to handle or require some time to complete; they can be conducted as a project or managed as a change through the change management process. A significant amount of design efforts will not require any attention from the design coordination process: those efforts that do require attention are typically associated with a project, a major change, or any change the organization sees design coordination as a benefit to the success of the design effort.

What does or does not utilize design coordination is determined by criteria defined by the organization. Some organizations may decide that every project and change, major and minor, must have a design stage. Other organizations create a set of criteria that is used to determine design coordination involvement. Whatever the criteria, the end result must be that changes to services are successful in delivering the requirement business outcomes with minimal disruption or negative impact on IT or business operations. If this end result is being achieved, design coordination is being performed correctly.

From ITIL® 2011, the design coordination process includes (Service Design, page 87):

- *Assisting and supporting each project or other change through all the service design activities and processes*
- *Maintaining policies, guidelines, standards, budgets, models, resources, and capabilities for Service Design activities and processes*
- *Coordinating, prioritizing, and scheduling of all Service Design resources to satisfy conflicting demands from all projects and changes*
- *Planning and forecasting the resources needed for the future demand for Service Design activities*
- *Reviewing, measuring, and improving the performance of all Service Design activities and processes*
- *Ensuring that all requirements are appropriately addressed in service designs, particularly utility and warranty requirements*
- *Ensuring the production of service designs and/or SDPs and their handover to service transition*

The design coordination process does not include:

- *Responsibility for any activities or processes outside of the design stage of the service lifecycle*
- *Responsibility for designing the detailed service solutions themselves or the production of the individual parts of the SDPs. These are the responsibility of the individual projects or service management processes*

Activities

DESIGN COORDINATION ACTIVITIES FALL INTO two categories:

- **Activities relating to the overall Service Design lifecycle stage**: Before designing any service, process, or technology used to deliver business outcomes to the customer, it is important to design how Service Design will operate. This includes developing, deploying, and improving Service Design practices, such as coordination of design activities across projects and changes. Design of Service Design practices may be performed by design coordination process manager(s)
- **Activities relating to each individual design**: These design activities focus on ensuring that each individual effort and SDP , conforms with defined practices and produce a design supporting the required business outcomes. These activities may be performed by a project manager or other individual with direct responsibility for the project or change, with the assistance and guidance of the design coordination process manager(s).

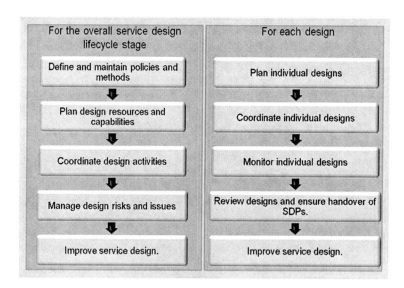

Figure 5.C—Design Coordination Activities

© **Crown** Copyright 2011 Reproduced under license from the Cabinet Office

Inputs

THE DESIGN COORDINATION PROCESS IS initiated when changes occur in business requirements and services resulting in a request for change or a new program or project. Because of the importance service design is on the viability of the service to achieve business outcomes, the more information available to support the design, the better chance the final design will require minimal improvements later on. The inputs into the process initiate, guide, and interact with the service being design

Initiating inputs are those inputs that trigger the design coordination process and provide information on the scope of the work required and set expectations for the final design. Service charters from the service strategy stage provide a framework for what the service does, why it is needed, and what requirements are to be achieved. In other parts of the service lifecycle, change requests and change records will provide detailed information about what changes are under considerations, which will serve to determine if design coordination is initiated and provide enough information to guide the design coordination activities.

Some inputs into the process are used to guide the design aspects of the solution, such as strategies, regulations, and approved approaches. In a particular design effort, requirements looking to be solved may conflict with existing requirements for other services: the design efforts must resolve this conflict and meet the new requirement. To do this, information from the business and IT strategies, plans, and policies must be considered, as well as business impact analysis results and available service packages and options. Together, the information should provide the basis for determining the proper course of action regarding the conflict, or any action during the design stage.

Governance and regulations are another form of guidance to the design, specifically establishing what must be in place and what should not be considered. The IT strategy will define the constraints and resource limitations on the service. Governance requirements may have several checkpoints in place to ensure the risky ventures are properly considered and impact to the overall service delivery is minimally impacted. Policies and requirements from corporate entities, legalities, and regulatory bodies which have been adopted provide additional opportunities and constraints on the design of the service.

Any service solution requiring integration with the existing IT environment will have to deal with the impact of the design on other services, processes, and tools used to support the service. This can range from project and change scheduled to management systems, such as the configuration management system, the architecture, and management systems, to monitoring systems for measurements and metrics. As mentioned before, not all design activities may require design coordination activities if they are simple changes with low impact and low risk; however, as risk or impact increase, the need for design coordination increases proportionally.

Outputs

THE PRIMARY OUTPUT OF THE Design Coordination process is a comprehensive and consistent set of service designs and service design packages. These are published within the service catalog and used to deliver the service in service transition and manage the service in service operations. Continual service improvement will reference the service design in order to determine the best approach for improving a service.

As mentioned before, a design effort for a particular service solution may have an impact on services, processes, and tools not within the solution. This impact is similar to the ripple effect of dropping a rock in water. In service design, the ripples should be followed to verify the impact and changes needed in other parts of service design. The result may include (Service Design, page 94):

- *A revised enterprise architecture*
- *Revised management systems*
- *Revised measurement and metrics methods*
- *Revised processes*
- *Service portfolio updates*
- *Updates to change records*

Service Level Management

Purpose

THE DESIGN COORDINATION PROCESS IS accountable for ensuring all the activities of the Service Design stage are performed appropriately and in cooperation with other design activities. A service consists of a utility aspect and a warranty aspect, so both must be incorporated into the design (it is not possible to have utility without warranty or vice versa). While utility will potentially incorporate a variety of processes in designing a solution, warranty is almost entirely designed as service levels and obtained through the Service Level Management process.

Service levels are essentially targets for the service to achieve in areas such as performance, availability, and security. Apply this to any sport, such as bicycling: the utility of the sport is the physical bicycle. Many professional bikers will work with manufacturers to design the equipment to work with the person's capabilities to achieve better performance; however, there are factors that cannot be designed in the bicycle and must be supplied by the person, such as strength, endurance, tolerance, and the like. The person can increase their individual capabilities through exercise, training, and condition. Together, they can improve their overall performance. From a coach's or sponsor's perspective, certain targets are established to demonstrate the performance is improving related to time, distance, and fatigue. Once these targets have been achieved, all future expectations are that the target will improve, not decline. If a decline is present, it indicates that a problem exists with the utility of the bicycle or the capabilities of the rider.

Service levels in IT act in the same manner. IT (coach) and business (sponsor) identify what targets should be reached by a particular service solution (bicycle) based on the current capabilities of the service provider (rider). The targets are established based on historical data from the organization and manufacturers of the service components. The expectation is that the targets will always be achieved, though improvements may be made to increase the targets. Any decline in achieving the target is an indication that the service design or service provider capabilities are lacking in some way.

The establishment, monitoring, and improvements in service levels and their achievement are the responsibility of Service Level Management. While some organizations may continue to rely on a 'best endeavors' approach to service quality, the majority have realized that there needs to be a consistent, agreed, and understandable method used for defining and reporting of IT service quality. As the modern IT organization has matured over time to be more akin to any other area of business, there has also been an increased requirement for more formal methods by which the value of funding and investments into IT are assessed and performance measured for services provided and capabilities supported. Service Level Management is the process that seeks to provide consistency in defining the requirements for services, documenting targets and responsibilities, and providing clarity as to the achievements for service quality delivered to customers.

In effect, the process seeks to manage the grey areas that are formed between customers and the IT organization, as well as ensuring that the activities performed by various IT groups are coordinated optimally to meet customer requirements. The staff involved (Service Level Management team) are fluent in both technical and business jargon, they resolve disputes between parties (but as a result are sometimes seen as a spy in both camps), and generally work to improve the relationship between the IT organization and the customers it supports.

Terminology

Term	Definition
operational level agreement (OLA)	(ITIL® Continual Service Improvement) (ITIL® Service Design) An agreement between an IT service provider and another part of the same organization. It supports the IT service provider's delivery of IT services to customers and defines the goods or services to be provided and the responsibilities of both parties. For example, there could be an operational level agreement: • Between the IT service provider and a procurement department to obtain hardware in agreed times • Between the service desk and a support group to provide incident resolution in agreed times. See *also* service level agreement.
service improvement plan (SIP)	(ITIL® Continual Service Improvement) A formal plan to implement improvements to a process or IT service.
service level	Measured and reported achievement against one or more service level targets. The term is sometimes used informally to mean service level target.
service level agreement (SLA)	(ITIL® Continual Service Improvement) (ITIL® Service Design) An agreement between an IT service provider and a customer. A service level agreement describes the IT service, documents service level targets, and specifies the responsibilities of the IT service provider and the customer. A single agreement may cover multiple IT services or multiple customers. See *also* operational level agreement.
service level requirement (SLR)	(ITIL® Continual Service Improvement) (ITIL® Service Design) A customer requirement for an aspect of an IT service. Service level requirements are based on business objectives and used to negotiate agreed service level targets.

SLAM chart	(*ITIL® Continual Service Improvement*) A service level agreement monitoring chart is used to help monitor and report achievements against service level targets. A SLAM chart is typically color-coded to show whether each agreed service level target has been met, missed, or nearly missed during each of the previous 12 months.
underpinning contract (UC)	(*ITIL® Service Design*) A contract between an IT service provider and a third party. The third party provides goods or services that support delivery of an IT service to a customer. The underpinning contract defines targets and responsibilities that are required to meet agreed service level targets in one or more service level agreements.

Scope

SERVICE LEVEL MANAGEMENT PROVIDES REGULAR communication to the customers and business managers of an organization in relation to service levels. SLM represents the IT service provider to the business and the business to the IT service provider. In this context, Service Level Management may seem to be in conflict with Business Relationship Management. This is not the case because Business Relationship Management establishes the relationship framework in which Service Level Management works within. Often times, the BRM will be involved in all customer discussions related to service levels. Service Level Management is responsible for develop the warranty aspect of the service; Business Relationship Management is responsible for both the utility and warranty aspects. Lastly, Business Relationship Management is grounded in the strategic service, while Service Level Management is grounded in the operational service: both will connect tactically.

The activities of Service Level Management are designed to manage the expectation and perception of the business, customers, and users and ensure those expectations and perceptions are matched by the quality (warranty) of service delivered by the service provider. The primary tools for doing this is the documentation and negotiation of Service Level Requirements used to develop Service Level Agreements (SLAs) for all existing services and managing those SLAs to meet agreed targets and quality measurements.

From ITIL® 2011, the SLM process should include (Service Design, page 107):

- *Cooperation with the Business Relationship Management process; this includes development of relationships with the business as needed to achieve the SLM process objectives*

- *Negotiation and agreement of future Service Level Requirements and targets and the documentation and management of SLRs for all proposed new or changed services*
- *Negotiation and agreement of current Service Level Requirements and targets and the documentation and management of SLAs for all operational services*
- *Development and management of appropriate OLAs to ensure that targets are aligned with SLA targets*
- *Review of all supplier agreements and underpinning contracts with supplier management to ensure that targets are aligned with SLA targets*
- *Proactive prevention of service failures, reduction of service risks, and improvement in the quality of service, in conjunction with all other processes*
- *Reporting and management of all service level achievements and review of all SLA breaches*
- *Periodic review, renewal, and/or revision of SLAs, service scope, and OLAs as appropriate*
- *Identifying improvement opportunities for inclusion in the CSI register*
- *Reviewing and prioritizing improvements in the CSI register*
- *Instigating and coordinating SIPs for the management, planning, and implementation of service and process improvements*

Agreements and Contracts

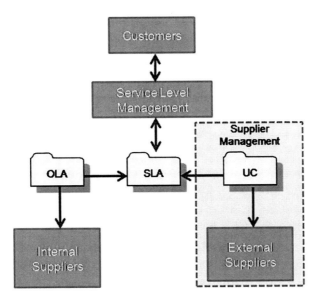

Figure 5.D—SLAs, OLAs, and UCs
"Based on Cabinet Office ITIL® material. Reproduced under licence from the Cabinet Office"

LIKE EVERY ASPECT OF THE design, service levels begin with requirements on the quality, or warranty, of the service. These requirements are derived from the Service Catalog. We will be discussing the Service Catalog in detail later, but for this discussion, the Service Catalog serves as a structured database or document for all services currently being provided to the customer and documents the utility and warranty details of the service. These warranty requirements are commonly referred to as Service Level Requirements and are entirely customer-derived, that is, these will be the minimum service levels the customer perceives they must have to fulfil their business objectives. These requirements are agreed upon by the business and IT at a strategic level.

As the design of the services utility proceeds, it may establish constraints in cost, capability, and performance that will impact the service level. The SLR should be reviewed all impacted areas of IT to validate they are reasonable and achievable. Service Level Management may have to return to the customer to communicate that the SLR cannot be met or will be met at an higher cost or more resources. This is the point where negotiation of service levels starts with the ending resulting in a Service Level Agreement.

The efforts of Service Level Management do not end with the Service Level Agreement. Additional agreements may be established to support the services in achieving the SLAs for the customer. Take the analogy of the professional bicyclists: in modern races, you find entire teams behind the rider both on and off the field. On the field, the primary rider is considered the lead and several more riders may exist to provide support, lighten the number of competitors on the field, or push the lead forward in the pack. In other words, these riders are used to enable the lead rider to perform without distraction or disruption from competing riders. Off the field, the team may be comprised of a trainer, a nutritionist, a medic, or any number of people in place to ensure the lead rider achieves and maintained their greatest potential when performing. While the lead rider and coach may have made an agreement with sponsors for a defined level of performance, each member has an agreement in place with the coach to support the lead rider.

A similar structure can also be seen in IT: a service (lead rider) is supported by other internal departments, services, and processes (riders) and external service providers (consultants). The goal of the set is to ensure that lead service is performing as it should while keeping any potential distraction or disruption to the service at bay. How these entities work together is one of the objectives of Service Design and requires some additional agreements to be in place to ensure everyone is working together. The agreements with internal service providers are called Operational Level Agreements and are the responsibility of Service Level Management to bring to fruition. Agreements with external service providers are called Underpinning Contracts and are the responsibility of Supplier Management with input from Service Level Management.

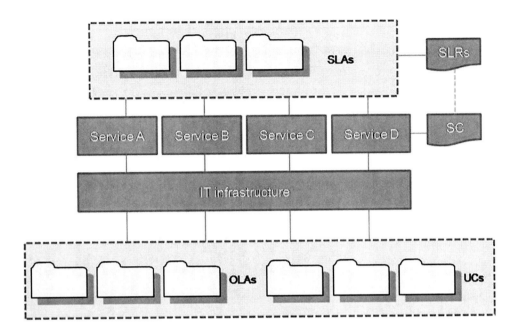

Figure 5.E—How SLAs, OLAs, and UCs Fit Together
"Based on Cabinet Office ITIL® material. Reproduced under licence from the Cabinet Office"

Question:

An organization is planning to formalize its IT Service Management practices and wants to implement Service Level Management. At present, there is very little documentation of the services currently being provided to customers.

According to the ITIL® framework, which of these documents should be developed first?

Answer: Normally the Service Catalog should be produced first because we need to define and agree what we are providing and then we can map the customer requirements to the Service Catalog to see what gaps or redundant services exist. By rushing into the creation of SLAs, it is likely they will develop into complex or inaccurate representations of service levels and not help to manage the relationship between the service provider and customers.

Although Service Level Agreements are implemented in a wide variety of fashions, the guiding principle is that they are a written agreement between an IT service provider and the IT customer(s), defining the key service targets and responsibilities of both parties.

The key word here is agreement; SLAs should not be used as a way of holding one side or the other to ransom. When SLAs are viewed in a positive way—a way of continually improving the relationship between provider and customers—mutually beneficial agreements will be developed. Viewing SLAs as just contracts can contribute to development of a blame culture by both parties.

The level of technical detail included within the SLA will also vary, depending on the type and nature of the customer. Some customers may be an IT service provider themselves; others will be purely business-focused. To be successful in all of these scenarios, SLAs must be written in such a way that they are clear and unambiguous for both parties, leaving no room for confusion or misinterpretation. They certainly won't be perfect from the moment they are developed, so a continual cycle of review and revision should seek to improve the quality and effectiveness of SLAs over time.

Service Level Agreement Structures

THERE ARE A NUMBER OF ways in which SLAs can be structured. The important factors to consider when choosing the SLA structure are:

- Will the SLA structure allow flexibility in the levels of service to be delivered for various customers?
- Will the SLA structure require much duplication of effort?
- Who will sign the SLAs?

Three types of SLA structures that are discussed within ITIL® are service-based, customer-based, and multi-level or hierarchical SLAs.

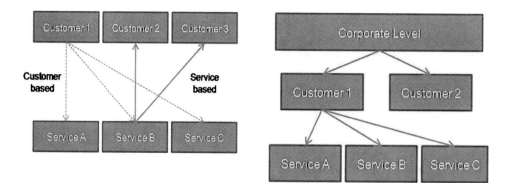

Figure 5.F—SLA Structures

"Based on Cabinet Office ITIL® material. Reproduced under licence from the Cabinet Office"

A service-based SLA structures are used when the service levels for a single service will be the same for all customers. The one-size-fits-all approach may not be as easy to implement as it may imply. Varied requirements between customers may cause or problem, as well as the constraints and capabilities of the IT infrastructure. For instance, a service requiring a network connection may implement faster LAN connections in the main office and slower WAN connections in the branch offices. As a result, a SLA based on the faster LAN may be inappropriate.

A customer-based SLA structure will apply service levels for every service being delivered to a single customer. As a result, only one service level agreement is in effect. Customers prefer this option because only one signed agreement is required.

Mutli-level SLAs can be a combination of service-based or customer-based SLAs, but are used to provide greater detail in the service level agreement the deeper into the organization the support goes. Generically, the multi-level SLA structure may have a corporate, customer, and service level. The corporate level focuses on SLAs that are relevant for every customer throughout the organization. The customer level focuses on a particular customer groups and service levels deal with a specific service relevant to the customer group. Some examples where multi-level structures can be advantageous are global/continental/country, corporate/home office/branch offices, or corporate/lines of business/functions.

Using a multi-level structure for a large organization reduces the duplication of effort, while still providing customization for customers and services (by inheritance).

The Typical Contents of SLAs

- An introduction to the SLA
- Service description
- Mutual responsibilities
- Scope of SLA
- Applicable service hours
- Service availability
- Reliability

- Customer support arrangements
- Contact points and escalation
- Service performance
- Batch turnaround times
- Security
- Costs and charging method used

The key criteria for any information to be contained within an SLA is that it must be measureable with all language used being clear and concise in order to aid understanding. As already discussed, SLAs should not only be used as legal documents for imposing penalties, otherwise it is in conflict with the goal of improving relationships between customers and the IT service provider. Another mistake made by organizations in implementing SLAs is that they become too long and technically-focused. When this occurs, there is potential for misunderstandings or for the SLA to go unread.

Service Level Management Activities

As an overview of Service Level Management, the process will generally consist of the following interrelated activities (*not necessarily in chronological order*):

1. Develop contacts and relationships
2. Design an SLA framework
3. Determine, document, and agree requirements for new services
4. Negotiate and develop SLAs
5. Review and revise SLAs, Underpinning Contracts, Operational Level Agreements, and service scope
6. Monitor service performance against SLAs
7. Produce service reports
8. Conduct service reviews and instigate improvements within an overall Service Improvement Plan (SIP)
9. Collate, measure, and improve customer satisfaction
10. Managing complaints and compliments

Service Improvement Plans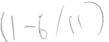

Service Improvement Plans are formal plans to implement improvements to a process or service. They are used to ensure that improvement actions are identified and carried out on a regular basis.

The identified improvements may come from:

- Breaches of Service Level Agreements
- Identification of user training and documentation issues
- Weak system testing
- Identified weak areas within internal and external support groups

Roles and Responsibilities
Service Level Manager:

- Must be senior enough to represent the organization with authority to do what is necessary
- Manages Service Catalog, SLAs, and OLAs and ensures alignment of Underpinning Contracts
- Identifies and manages improvements to services and processes
- Analyzes and reports on service level achievements

Skills: Relationship Management, patience, tolerance, resilience, and an understanding of the customer's business and how IT contributes to the delivery of that product or service.

Inputs
A NUMBER OF SOURCES OF information are relevant to the SLM process. These include (Service Design, page 120):

- *Business information*: *from the organization's business strategy, plans and financial plans, and information on its current and future requirements*
- *BIA*: *providing information on the impact, priority, risk, and number of users associated with each service*
- *Business requirements*: *details of any agreed, new, or changed business requirements*
- *The Strategies, policies, and constraints*: *from Service Strategy*
- *The Service Portfolio and Service Catalog*
- *Change information, including RFCs*: *from the Change Management process with a change schedule and a need to assess all changes for their impact on all services*
- *CMS*: *containing information on the relationships between the business services, the supporting services, and the technology*
- *Customer and user feedback*: *including complaints and compliments*
- *Improvement opportunities*: *from the CSI register*
- *Other inputs:* *including advice, information, and input from any of the other processes (e.g., Incident Management, Capacity Management and Availability Management), together with the existing SLAs, SLRs, and OLAs and past service reports on the quality of service delivered*

Outputs

THE OUTPUTS OF SLM SHOULD include (Service Design, page 121):

- **Service reports**: *providing details of the service levels achieved in relation to the targets contained within SLAs. These reports should contain details of all aspects of the service and its delivery, including current and historical performance, breaches and weaknesses, major events, changes planned, current and predicted workloads, customer feedback, and improvement plans and activities*
- **Service improvement opportunities**: *for inclusion in the CSI register and for later review and prioritization in conjunction with the CSI manager*
- **SIP**: *an overall program or plan of prioritized improvement actions, encompassing appropriate services and processes, together with associated impacts and risks*
- **The service quality plan**: *documenting and planning the overall improvement of service quality*
- **Document templates**: *standard document templates, format, and content for SLAs, SLRs, and OLAs, aligned with corporate standards*
  - **SLAs**: *a set of targets and responsibilities should be documented and agreed within an SLA for each operational service*
  - **SLRs**: *a set of targets and responsibilities should be documented and agreed within an SLR for each proposed new or changed service*
  - **OLAs**: *a set of targets and responsibilities should be documented and agreed within an OLA for each internal support team*
- **Reports**: *on OLAs and underpinning contracts*
- **Service review meeting minutes and actions**: *all meetings should be scheduled on a regular basis with planned agendas and their discussions and actions recorded and progressed*
- **SLA review and service scope review meeting minutes**: *summarizing agreed actions and revisions to SLAs and service scope*
- **Updated change information**: *including updates to RFCs*
- **Revised requirements for underpinning contracts**: *changes to SLAs or new SLRs may require existing underpinning contracts to be changed or new contracts to be negotiated and agreed*

Supplier Management

"No man is an island."

THIS PHRASE COMES FROM A longer quotation by John Donne (1572-1631). The general meaning is that human beings do not thrive when isolated from others; we are all connected and, therefore, events and changes affecting one human being affect us all.

Although abstract, this concept provides an engaging way in which a service provider should approach the management of IT services. Like the original quote, *no service provider is an island*, so events and changes affecting their customers and suppliers will in turn have some consequence for them.

What does this mean for IT Service Management? Based on this principle, we need to ensure that we carefully evaluate, select, manage, and review any suppliers who will be involved in some way in the delivery and support of IT services and be sure to develop and foster the relationship in a mutually beneficial way. As many organizations have found out recently, the death of a supplier (caused by economic downturn) may mean their own future could be short lived.

Terminology

Term	Definition
supplier	(*ITIL® Service Design*) (*ITIL® Service Strategy*) A third party responsible for supplying goods or services that are required to deliver IT services. Examples of suppliers include commodity hardware and software vendors, network and telecom providers, and outsourcing organizations. See *also* underpinning contract.
supplier and contract management information system (SCMIS)	(*ITIL® Service Design*) A set of tools, data, and information that is used to support supplier management. See *also* service knowledge management system.

underpinning contract (UC)	(*ITIL® Service Design*) A contract between an IT service provider and a third party. The third party provides goods or services that support delivery of an IT service to a customer. The underpinning contract defines targets and responsibilities that are required to meet agreed service level targets in one or more service level agreements.

Purpose

THE PURPOSE OF **IT** SERVICE Management is to generate value for the business through the delivery of services which achieve business outcomes and objectives. Up to this point, we have been focused on the internal service provider in delivering these services; and for this section, we will focus on external service providers, or suppliers. Dealing with suppliers is not a new thing for businesses or individuals. There may be several reasons why a supplier is engaged, but the most basic reason for a supplier/customer relationship is that the required service cannot be performed sufficiently by an organization given the organization's priorities and therefore the service fulfilment is passed on to another service provider.

Remember, in IT, the customer is the business and they are making arrangements with the IT department to fulfil their technology needs. The IT department is, in turn, "outsourcing" the services to a third-party supplier, in many instances, without the knowledge of the business. The desired value provided by IT services must be achieved whether the service is provided internally or externally. The cost of service must be the same or less than when provided internally. The relationship with the supplier is typically focused on the underpinning contract, an agreement where the service provider generates value in the form of a service meeting defined service levels for a negotiated price.

Within this context, Supplier Management is responsible for obtaining the value for the negotiated price from suppliers and make the service acquisition seamless to the business. IT does this by managing the underpinning contract with the supplier, as well as all other underpinning contracts with other suppliers.

The main objectives of the Supplier Management process are to (Service Design, page 207):

- *Obtain value for money from suppliers and contracts*

- *Ensure that contracts with suppliers are aligned to business needs and support and align with agreed targets in SLRs and SLAs, in conjunction with SLM*
- *Manage relationships with suppliers*
- *Manage supplier performance*
- *Negotiate and agree contracts with suppliers and manage them through their lifecycle*
- *Maintain a supplier policy and a supporting Supplier and Contract Management Information System (SCMIS)*

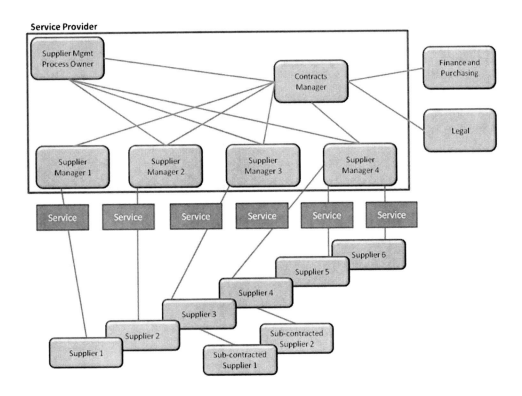

Figure 5.G—Roles and Interfaces for Supplier Management
© Crown Copyright 2011 Reproduced under license from Cabinet Office.

Scope

AT FIRST GLANCE, THE SUPPLIER Management process would seem to be simple – the whole process is about managing suppliers – but the amount of management required for each supplier may be different since not all suppliers are created equally. While Supplier Management is responsible for managing all suppliers and contracts using formal processes, those processes should be adaptable to the importance of the supplier and the underpinning contract with them. Contracts with high risk and impact, as well as high value should be given the most attention when managing the supplier. These types of suppliers are considered strategic suppliers and may have more direct involvement in the development and realization of the business strategy.

The smaller the supplier's value contribution, the more likely the supplier will be managed at an operational level with limited interaction with the business.

ITIL® 2011 states the Supplier Management process should include (Service Design, page 208):

- *Implementation and enforcement of the supplier policy*
- *Maintenance of an SCMIS*
- *Supplier and contract categorization and risk assessment*
- *Supplier and contract evaluation and selection*
- *Development, negotiation, and agreement of contracts*
- *Contract review, renewal, and termination*
- *Management of suppliers and supplier performance*
- *Identification of improvement opportunities for inclusion in the CSI register and the implementation of service and supplier improvement plans*
- *Maintenance of standard contracts, terms, and conditions*
- *Management of contractual dispute resolution*
- *Management of sub-contracted suppliers*

Activities

THE SUPPLIER MANAGEMENT PROCESS RELIES on two tools to fulfil its purpose in the organization, the underpinning contract and the Supplier and Contract Management Information System (SCMIS). The first, the underpinning contract, is the agreement between the IT organization and the external service provider (supplier) about the services provided. Each supplier should have a formal underpinning contract in place with clearly defined responsibilities and targets established. The SCMIS is a structured database or documents used to store and manage the various underpinning contracts currently in place, under consideration, or terminated.

The activities of Supplier Management revolve around these two tools and can be summarized as:

- **Definition of new supplier and contract requirements:** This activity begins with identifying the business need and preparing a business case for the service, including the reasons for obtaining a supplier. A statement of requirement (SoR) should be produced, as well as an invitation to tender (ITT). Finally, all requirements should be validated against the organization's strategy and policies.
- **Evaluation of new suppliers and contracts:** Before creating a binding contract with a potential supplier, an evaluation of the supplier should be conducted. This evaluation should consider the services rendered, the provider's capabilities, quality of service, and cost. Purchase and procurement methods may also be an important consideration. Alternative options to the solution, supplier, or even contract should be evaluated and used to compare opportunities and risks. With this information, the decision to select a supplier will be more successful. The final steps will be negotiate and award the contract. The contract should contain language relevant to the terms and conditions, service targets, responsibilities, closure, renewal, extensions, handling disputes and transfer.
- **Supplier and contract categorization and maintenance of the SCMIS:** A potential supplier will be entered into the SCMIS and all relevant information captured, including the contract. Categorization of the supplier is performed as a method of organizing the supplier based on the services provided or importance of the service. This categorization can be used to indicate about when and how frequent assessments and reassessments of the supplies and contracts should be conducted. Any changes to the supplier information or contract

should be made to the SCMIS and managed through service transition. The SCMIS should be regularly updated and ongoing maintenance performed.

- **Establishment of new suppliers and contracts:** Upon awarding the contract to a supplier, the service and contract should be set up in the SCMIS and other corporate systems. The transition of the service must be conducted to establish the supplier and contract within the current IT environment, including establishing contacts and relationships.

- **Supplier, contract, and performance management:** While the service is being provided by the supplier, some level of management will be performed to ensure SLA criteria is met: this requires monitoring and reporting on the service, its quality, and costs, as well as periodic reviews and improvements. The relationship with the supplier must be managed, with at least one review of the service scope each year to determine any changes in scope or service. Specific times may be indicated where planning is made to close out the contract, renew or extend it.

- **Contract renewal or termination:** most contracts will end. At some point, the IT organization and the supplier will have to review the current contract with the purpose of determining whether the contract should end, be renegotiated, renewed, terminated, and/or transferred to another supplier. If the decision will require the services to be moved in-house or with another supplier, a transition period will be required to migrate the service to the new provider.

Supplier and Contact Management Information System (SCMIS):

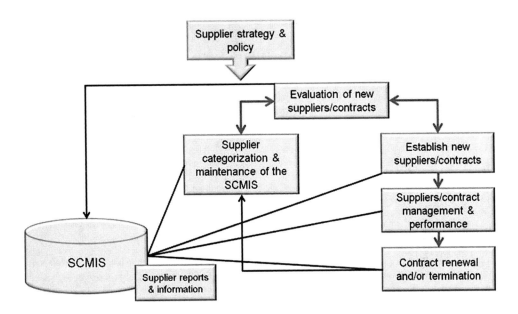

Figure 5.H—The Supplier and Contract Management Information System
© Crown Copyright 2011 Reproduced under license from the
Cabinet Office

ALL SUPPLIER MANAGEMENT PROCESS ACTIVITY should be driven by supplier strategy and policy. In order to achieve consistency and effectiveness in the implementation of the policy, a Supplier and Contract Management Information System (SCMIS) should be established.

Ideally, the SCMIS should form an integrated element of a comprehensive CMS (Configuration Management System) or SKMS (Service Knowledge Management System), recording all supplier and contract details, together with the types of service, products etc. provided by each supplier and all the other information and relationships with other associated CIs (Configuration Items). This will also contribute to the information held in the Service Portfolio and Catalog.

Underpinning Contracts and Agreements (10/11)

THE NATURE AND EXTENT OF an agreement between a service provider and supplier depends on the relationship type and an assessment of the risks involved. A preagreement risk assessment is a vital stage in establishing any external supplier agreement. For each party, it exposes the risks that need to be addressed and must be comprehensive and practical, covering a wide variety of risks, including financial, business reputation, operational, regulatory, and legal.

A comprehensive agreement minimizes the risk of disputes arising from a difference of expectations. A flexible agreement, which adequately caters for its adaptation across the term of the agreement, is maintainable and supports change with a minimum amount of renegotiation.

THE CONTENTS OF A BASIC Underpinning Contract or Service Level Agreement are (Service Design, Page 209):

- **Basic terms and conditions:** *The term (duration) of the contract, the parties, locations, scope, definitions, and commercial basis*
- **Service description and scope:** *The functionality of the services being provided and its extent, along with constraints on the service delivery, such as performance, availability, capacity, technical interface, and security*
- **Service standards:** *The service measures and the minimum levels that constitute acceptable performance and quality—for example, IT may have a performance requirement to respond to a request for a new desktop system in 24 hours, with acceptable service deemed to have occurred where this performance requirement is met in 95% of cases. Service levels must be realistic, measurable, and aligned to the organization's business priorities and underpin the agreed targets within SLRs and SLAs.*
- **Workload ranges:** *The volume ranges within which service standards apply or for which particular pricing regimes apply*
- **Management information:** *The data that must be reported by the supplier on operational performance—take care to ensure that management information is focused on the most important or headline reporting measures on which the relationship will be assessed*
- **Responsibilities and dependencies:** *Description of the obligations of the organization (in supporting the supplier in the service delivery efforts) and of the supplier (in its provision of the service), including communication, contacts, and escalation*

Supplier Categorization $(5-2/8)$

WE'VE ALREADY ESTABLISHED THAT NOT all suppliers are created equally and some need more attention than others. The establishment of a categorization scheme within Supplier Management allows the organization to categorize the importance of the service provider and their products and services to achieving business objectives. While many methods may be used to categorize suppliers, one of the best methods is based on assessing the risk and impact associated with using the supplier and the value and importance of the supplier and its services to the business, as illustrated in figure 5.l.

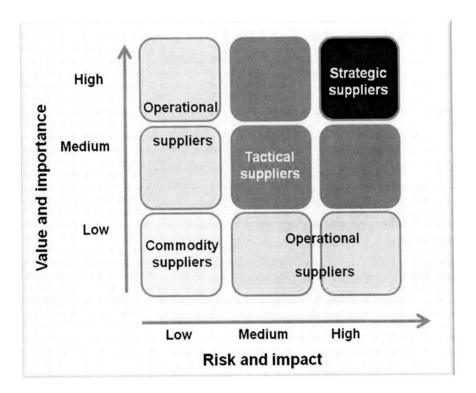

Figure 5.l—Supplier Categorization
© Crown Copyright 2011 Reproduced under license from the Cabinet Office

Categorization of suppliers will allow supplier managers to understand the amount of time and effort needed to manage the supplier and the relationship. ITIL® 2011 explains this correlation (Service Design, page 215):

- **Strategic**: for significant partnering relationships that involve senior managers sharing confidential strategic information to facilitate long-term plans. These relationships would normally be managed and owned at a senior management level within the service provider organization and would involve regular and frequent contact and performance reviews. These relationships would probably require involvement of service strategy and service design resources, and would include ongoing specific improvement programmes (e.g. a network service provider supplying worldwide networks service and their support).
- **Tactical**: for relationships involving significant commercial activity and business interaction. These relationships would normally be managed by middle management and would involve regular contact and performance reviews, often including ongoing improvement programs (e.g., a hardware maintenance organization providing resolution of server hardware failures).
- **Operational**: for suppliers of operational products or services. These relationships would normally be managed by junior operational management and would involve infrequent but regular contact and performance reviews (e.g., an internet hosting service provider supplying hosting space for a low-usage, low-impact website or internally-used IT service).
- **Commodity**: for suppliers providing low-value and/or readily available products and services, which could be alternatively sourced relatively easily (e.g., paper or printer cartridge suppliers)

The suppliers that are strategically important will be given the greatest focus: in these cases, the supplier manager ensures the culture of the service provider organization is extended into the supplier domain so that the relationship works beyond the initial contract. Outsourcing has been the primary driver for diverse types of supplier relationships.

Relationships with other Lifecycle Stages:

THE INFORMATION WITHIN THE SCMIS will provide a complete set of reference information for all Supplier Management procedures and activities needed across the Service Lifecycle. Such activities include:

Lifecycle Stage	Activities
Service Design	Evaluating which components of service provision should/could be provided by an external supplier or partner
	Supplier categorization and maintenance of the SCD
	Evaluation and set-up of new suppliers and contracts
Service Transition	Assessing the transition to new suppliers
	Establishing new suppliers
Service Operation	Ongoing Supplier and Contract Management and performance
	Contract renewal and termination
Continual Service Improvement	Identifying improvement actions involving suppliers
	Collating measurements gathered on supplier arrangements

© **Crown** Copyright 2011 Reproduced under license from the Cabinet Office

This table shows that although Supplier Management is firmly placed within the Service Design Stage of the Lifecycle, many activities are carried out in the other Lifecycle Stages too.

Inputs

THE INPUTS TO SUPPLIER MANAGEMENT are (Service Design, page 223):

- *Business information*: from the organization's business strategy, plans and financial plans, and information on its current and future requirements
- *Supplier and contracts strategy*: this covers the sourcing policy of the service provider and the types of supplier and contract used. It is produced by the service strategy processes.
- *Supplier plans and strategies*: details of the business plans and strategies of suppliers, together with details of their technology developments, plans and statements, and information on their current financial status and projected business viability

- **Supplier contracts, agreements, and targets**: of both existing and new contracts and agreements from suppliers
- **Supplier and contract performance information**: of both existing and new contracts and suppliers
- **IT information: from the IT strategy and plans and current budgets**
- **Performance issues**: the Incident and Problem Management processes, with incidents and problems relating to poor contract or supplier performance
- **Financial information**: from Financial Management for IT services, the cost of supplier service(s) and service provision, the cost of contracts and the resultant business benefit, and the financial plans and budgets, together with the costs associated with service and supplier failure
- **Service information**: from the SLM process, with details of the services from the service portfolio and the service catalog, service level targets within SLAs and SLRs, and possibly from the monitoring of SLAs, service reviews, and breaches of the SLAs—also customer satisfaction data on service quality
- **CMS**: containing information on the relationships between the business, the services, the supporting services, and the technology

Outputs

THE OUTPUTS OF SUPPLIER MANAGEMENT are (Service Design, page 223):

- **SCMIS**: This holds the information needed to execute the activities within Supplier Management—for example, the data monitored and collected as part of Supplier Management. This is then invariably used as an input to all other parts of the Supplier Management process.
- **Supplier and contract performance information and reports**: These are used as input to supplier and contract review meetings to manage the quality of service provided by suppliers and partners. This should include information on shared risk, where appropriate.
- **Supplier and contract review meeting minutes**: These are produced to record the minutes and actions of all review meetings with suppliers.
- **Supplier SIPs**: These are used to record all improvement actions and plans agreed between service providers and their suppliers, wherever they are needed, and should be used to manage the progress of agreed improvement actions, including risk reduction measures.
- **Supplier survey reports**: Often many people within a service provider organization have dealings with suppliers. Feedback from these individuals

should be collated to ensure consistency in the quality of service provided by suppliers in all areas. These can be published as league tables to encourage competition between suppliers.

Service Catalog Management (2/11)

IMAGINE WALKING INTO A RESTAURANT for lunch only to find there is no menu available for you to peruse. How will the staff provide you with information about what options are available to you? How will you know what ingredients and items are included with each meal? What will the price be of those meals? What about drinks or other items? Even if you manage to be served by a very efficient waiter who can recite everything to you flawlessly, how will you manage the large influx of information in such a small time and be able to choose what you want?

While this example may be far removed from the running of an IT organization the principles remain the same. A restaurant is in business to provide dining services to customers and through the use of their menu and the knowledge and skills of staff, customers can understand what is available to them and make effective choices in a simple manner. As an IT service provider, we are in the business of providing IT services to our customers, but what mechanisms do we use to make these transactions simple yet effective for all parties?

For most IT organizations, the Service Catalog provides this mechanism and, in many ways, it serves as the foundation for much of the work involved within the scope of Service Offerings and Agreements. Without some agreed definition of what services we offer, what those services provide, and which customers we provide them to, the development and management of Service Portfolios, Service Level Agreements, IT budgets, and other related items becomes all the more difficult and things only get worse as time progresses.

But it is not enough to simply have some form of Service Catalog. We must also seek to ensure that the Service Catalog is continually maintained and updated to contain correct, appropriate, and relevant information to assist communication and transactions with customers.

Terminology

Term	Definition
service catalog	(*ITIL® Service Design*) (*ITIL® Service Strategy*) A database or structured document with information about all live IT services, including those available for deployment. The service catalog is part of the service portfolio and contains information about two types of IT service: customer-facing services that are visible to the business and supporting services required by the service provider to deliver customer-facing services.

© **Crown** Copyright 2011 Reproduced under license from the Cabinet Office

Purpose

THE SERVICE CATALOG IS A single source of information on all operational services in the IT organization, as well as those services being prepared to be run operationally. The Service Catalog is a large part of the Service Portfolio: however where the portfolio is focused on tracking the business requirements and the investments on a service, the Service Catalog is focused on the service solution and its delivery to the business.

Like Service Portfolio Management, Service Catalog Management does not manage the services contained within – it only manages the information about the services. Within this context of managing information, the objectives of the process is to ensure that the information is accurate and current on all services in the live environment and ensures the catalog is available to those approved to access. The Service Catalog is a vital element to IT Service Management and is utilized by several processes to understand such information as interfaces and dependencies. As these service management processes evolve, the Service Catalog must also evolve.

Scope

THE SCOPE OF THE SERVICE Catalog Management process is to provide and maintain accurate information on all services running in, or being prepared to run in, The Service Catalog can present services individually or, more typically, in the form of service packages The Service Catalog Management process covers (Service Design, Page 97):

- *Contribution to the definition of services and service packages*

- *Development and maintenance of service and service package descriptions appropriate for the Service Catalog*
- *Production and maintenance of an accurate Service Catalog*
- *Interfaces, dependencies, and consistency between the Service Catalog and the overall Service Portfolio*
- *Interfaces and dependencies between all services and supporting services within the Service Catalog and the CMS*
- *Interfaces and dependencies between all services, supporting components, and configuration items (CIs) within the Service Catalog and the CMS*

The Service Catalog Management process does not include:
- *Detailed attention to the capturing, maintenance, and use of service asset and configuration data as performed through the Service Asset and Configuration Management process (see ITIL® Service Transition)*
- *Detailed attention to the capturing, maintenance, and fulfillment of service requests as performed through request fulfillment (see ITIL® Service Operation)*

Depending on the number and complexity of services offered, the size of the customer and end user population, and what objectives have been defined for the process, these activities and items may have little or a great deal of reliance on technology to be effective.

Once the definition of services and their interfaces is finalized, the knowledge and information of the Service Catalog is logically divided into two aspects:

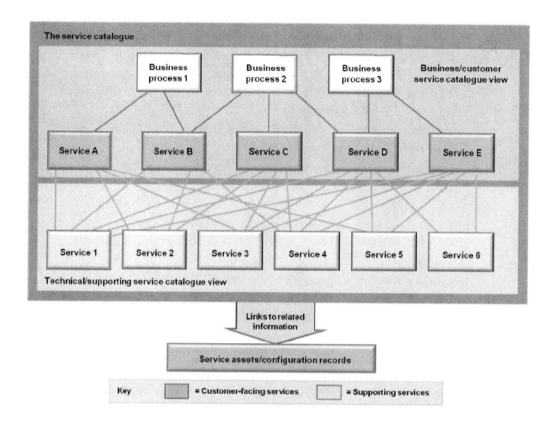

Figure 5.J—The Business and Technical Service Catalogs
© Crown Copyright 2011 Reproduced under license from the
Cabinet Office

Business Service Catalog: the details about IT services are contextually available to the customer, identifying what the services entails, their relationships to the business units and the business process they support. This information creates the customer view of the Service Catalog, using appropriate language and use of business terminology, without being not overly technical, to ensure its effectiveness. In cases where the customer is an IT organization themselves, the technical level of detail provided should be appropriately expanded. Multiple Business Service Catalogs can exist when the service provider provides IT support to multiple customers: each customer will have access to those services they currently are being provided.

Technical Service Catalog: contains the same details about IT services that the customers have access to, but by comparison, the Technical Service Catalog includes records of the relationships that exist with other supporting services, shared services, components, and Configuration Items necessary for the delivery of the service to the business. The Technical Service Catalog supports the Business Service Catalog and is not typically visible to customers and users, unless specifically requested. The Configuration Management System contributes a large portion of the information found in the Technical Service Catalog.

Developing the Service Catalog

WHILE MORE EXTRAVAGANT IMPLEMENTATIONS OF the Service Catalog delivered via extensive internet/intranet solutions will maintain both aspects in an integrated fashion, less mature organizations may choose to maintain these separately. Regardless of the implementation method, the key requirement is that the desired information is easily accessible by the authorized parties and communicated in a form that is appropriate for the audience.

The starting point for any Service Catalog journey is to begin identifying what actual services are being provided and who are the customers of these services. While it sounds simple enough, for an organization with a long history and large amount of customers, there will often be a lack of clarity in this regard, resulting in confusion and debate about what actually constitutes a service.

From an IT perspective, many staff will typically identify IT systems, such as software or applications, as being the service offered to customers. In other cases, the service will be seen to be composed of multiple services (which in turn are formed by one or more IT systems). In short, looking at services from only an IT perspective will lead you down a dangerous path and most likely cause you more headaches and grief in the process.

Instead, the recommended starting point is to look at things from the customer perspective. This is normally performed by asking customers what they perceive to be the IT services they are utilizing and how they map onto and support their business processes. Just like the design of services should be coordinated in a top-down approach, so should the associated definition for inclusion in the Service Catalog. Regardless of exactly how this occurs, each organization needs to develop a policy defining what constitutes a service and how it is defined and agreed within their own organization.

The top-down approach may lead to the creation of a service hierarchy, qualifying types of services such as:

- **Business Services**—what is actually used and seen by the customer
- **Supporting Services**, including further definition as:
  - ‣ Infrastructure Services
  - ‣ Application Services
  - ‣ Network Services
  - ‣ Data Management Services
- **Shared and Commodity Services**
- **Externally provided Service**s—those provided/managed by a 3rd party organization

As the definition of services begins to occur, consideration should be made as to who the actual customers of these services are. Eventually, through a cycle of discussions with customers, a clearer picture will emerge, providing the beginnings of a Business Service Catalog.

Inputs

THE PROCESS INPUTS INTO THE Service Catalog Management process are (Service Design, page 104):

- *Business information from the organization's business and IT strategy, plans and financial plans, and information on their current and future requirements from the Service Portfolio*
- *BIA, providing information on the impact, priority, and risk associated with each service or changes to service requirements*
- *Business requirements, including details of any agreed, new, or changed business requirements from the Service Portfolio*
- *The Service Portfolio and all related data and documents*
- *The CMS*
- *RFCs*
- *Feedback from all other processes*

Outputs

THE PROCESS OUTPUTS OF THE Service Catalog Management process are (Service Design, page 104):

- *The documentation and agreement of a definition of the service*

- *Updates to the service portfolio—should contain the current status of all services and requirements for services*
- *Updates to RFCs*
- *The Service Catalog—should contain the details and the current status of every live service provided by the service provider or service being transitioned into the live environment, together with the interfaces and dependencies*

Capacity Management (6/11)

Terminology

Term	Definition
application sizing	(*ITIL® Service Design*) The activity responsible for understanding the resource requirements needed to support a new application or a major change to an existing application. Application sizing helps to ensure that the IT service can meet its agreed service level targets for capacity and performance.
capacity	(*ITIL® Service Design*) The maximum throughput that a configuration item or IT service can deliver. For some types of CIs, capacity may be the size or volume—for example, a disk drive.
capacity management information system (CMIS)	(*ITIL® Service Design*) A set of tools, data, and information that is used to support capacity management. See *also* service knowledge management system.
capacity planning	(*ITIL® Service Design*) The activity within capacity management responsible for creating a capacity plan.
modeling	A technique that is used to predict the future behavior of a system, process, IT service, configuration item, etc. Modeling is commonly used in financial management, capacity management, and availability management.
service capacity management (SCM)	(*ITIL® Continual Service Improvement*) (*ITIL® Service Design*) The sub-process of capacity management responsible for understanding the performance and capacity of IT services. Information on the resources used by each IT service and the pattern of usage over time are collected, recorded, and analyzed for use in the capacity plan.

| tuning | The activity responsible for planning changes to make the most efficient use of resources. Tuning is most commonly used in the context of IT services and components. Tuning is part of capacity management, which also includes performance monitoring and implementation of the required changes. Tuning is also called optimization, particularly in the context of processes and other nontechnical resources. |

Purpose

CAPACITY MANAGEMENT ENSURES THE AGREED capacity- and performance-related requirements are met through managing the capacity of IT services and IT infrastructure in a cost-effective and timely manner. The concerns for the process are in meeting current and future capacity and performance needs for the business.

Within the domain of capacity management are the following objectives:

- An appropriate and up-to-date capacity plan must be produced and maintained, reflecting the current and future needs of the business
- All other areas of the business and IT are advised and provided guidance on all capacity- and performance-related issues
- Service performance achievements must meet all agreed targets through the management of the performance and capacity for both services and resources
- Proper involvement in the diagnosis and resolution of performance- and capacity-related incidents and problems
- The impact of all changes on the capacity plan and the performance and capacity of all services and resources is adequately assessed
- Proactive measures to improve the performance of services are implemented

Scope

CAPACITY MANAGEMENT PROVIDES THE PREDICTIVE and ongoing capacity indicators needed to align capacity to demand. It is about finding the right balance between resources and capabilities and demand.

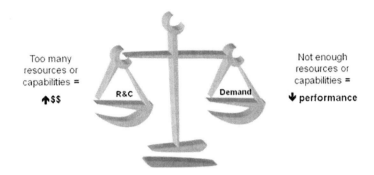

Figure 5.K—The Balancing Act of Capacity Management

IN COORDINATION WITH THE PROCESSES found in the Service Strategy stage, Capacity Management seeks to provide a continual optimal balance between supply against demand and costs against resources needed.

This optimum balance is only achieved both now and in the future by ensuring that Capacity Management is involved in all aspects of the Service Lifecycle. When this doesn't occur, Capacity Management only operates as a reactive process with limited benefits being delivered as a result.

Restaurant management provides a basic analogy for capacity management. The restaurant facility will typically limit the number of seats available to customers and the management of the restaurant requires ensuring that the seats are filled at all times with new customers. When seating in a restaurant is fill, the restaurant has two options, expand the number of seats by expanding the facility which is a long-term proactive action to take, or quickly, but appropriately, improve the performance of the restaurant to move the existing customers through the dining experience, which can be done reactively in the moment.

Like IT, the business of restaurants has peaks and valleys related to the number of customers served at any given time. Management of the restaurant requires that staff, inventory, and other resources are scheduled to appropriately support the number of expected customers at any given time. Since, people are the greatest resource for a restaurant, training is provided to raise the capabilities of the staff so that greater performance can be had. During peaks periods, how resources work together, the speed in which they complete tasks, and the functions they serve all increase the performance of the restaurant and allows more customers to be served in a given time period. If performance is not meeting a specific target, the restaurant manager must identify the problem and resolve, usually by calling in more staff or upgrading equipment. During slow periods, if the restaurant is staffed to support a peak period, the manager is losing money because they are not fully utilizing all their resources.

Capacity Management in IT works in the same manner: plan for peaks and valleys in customer demand. When handling peaks, ensure all the available resources are being used; but cut back in the number of resources available during slow periods. To increase the performance of the IT infrastructure, increase the capabilities of the resources, either through new configurations or new technology, but definitely through improvements. Another way to increase performance is to add more capacity. Capacity Management considers all resources required to deliver the IT service and plans for short-, medium-, and long-term business requirements. The Capacity Management process should be the focal point for all IT performance and capacity issues.

The Capacity Management process should include (Service Design, page 158):

- *Monitoring patterns of business activity through performance, utilization, and throughput of IT services and the supporting infrastructure, environmental, data, and applications components and the production of regular and ad hoc reports on service and component capacity and performance*
- *Undertaking tuning activities to make the most efficient use of existing IT resources*
- *Understanding the agreed current and future demands being made by the customer for IT resources and producing forecasts for future requirements*
- *Influencing demand in conjunction with the Financial Management for IT services and Demand Management processes*
- *Producing a capacity plan that enables the service provider to continue to provide services of the quality defined in SLAs and that covers a sufficient planning timeframe to meet future service levels required as defined in the Service Portfolio and SLRs*
- *Assisting with the identification and resolution of any incidents and problems associated with service or component capacity or performance*
- *The proactive improvement of service or component performance, wherever it is cost-justifiable and meets the needs of the business*

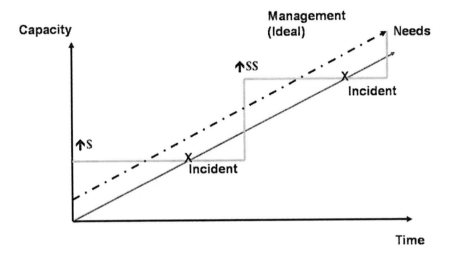

Figure 5.L—Capacity Management When Used Reactively

IN THE ABOVE FIGURE, CAPACITY is only implemented when disruptions begin to occur as demand has exceeded supply. While the implemented capacity does work to resolve the disruptions, there are some consequences to this type of reactive behavior including:

- IT infrastructure components being purchased that do not optimally fit the requirements or architecture
- Budget overruns for the unforeseen and unanticipated purchases
- Periods of time where there are potentially large amounts of excess capacity
- Reduced customer and user satisfaction with the affected IT services
- A general negatively affected perception of the IT organization as a whole

Sub-Processes of Capacity Management:

SOME OF THE ACTIVITIES OF Capacity Management are defined in the context of three sub-processes, consisting of Business, Service, and Component Capacity Management. Besides these, there will also be discussion of the operational activities required as well as the techniques that are utilized in various forms by the three different sub - processes.

Business Capacity Management:
- Manages Capacity to meet future business requirements for IT services
- Identifies changes occurring in the business to assess how they might impact capacity and performance of IT services
- Plans and implements sufficient capacity in an appropriate timescale
- Should be included in Change Management and Project Management activities

Service Capacity Management
- Focuses on managing ongoing service performance as detailed in the Service Level Agreements
- Establishes baselines and profiles of use of services, including all components and sub-services that affect the user experience
- Reports to the Service Level Manager and Service Owner regarding end-to-end service capacity, performance, and utilization

Component Capacity Management
- Identifies and manages each of the individual components of the IT Infrastructure (e.g., CPU, memory, disks, network bandwidth, server load)
- Evaluates new technology and how it might be leveraged to benefit the organization
- Balances loads across resources for optimal performance of services

All three sub-processes collate their data for use by other ITSM processes, primarily Service Level Management and Financial Management.

Activities

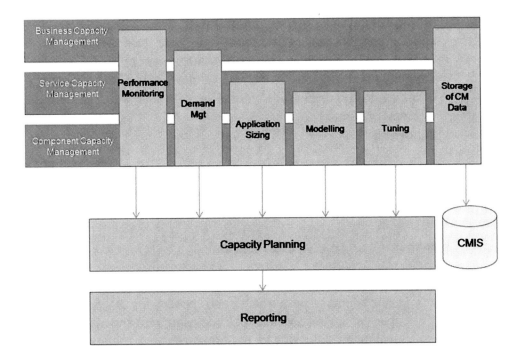

Figure 5.M—Activities of Capacity Management
© Crown Copyright 2011 Reproduced under license from the Cabinet Office

Capacity Management consists of these main activities:

- **Performance Monitoring**: measuring, monitoring, and tuning the performance of IT services and the individual infrastructure components
- **Demand Management**: short term reactive implementation of strategies considered within Service Strategy to manage current demand
- **Application Sizing**: determining the hardware or application capacity required to support new or modified applications and their predicted workload
- **Modeling**: used to forecast the behavior of the infrastructure under *certain conditions* (e.g., *what if the number of users doubled?; what if a network segment fails?*)

- **Tuning**: modifications made under the control of Change Management to enable better utilization of current infrastructure
- **Storage of Capacity Management Data**: storing all business, service, and component capacity data to assist decision-making within the Capacity Management and Financial Management processes
- **Capacity Planning**: forecasting when and where capacity will need to be increased and decreased. A formal Capacity Plan will document these recommendations
- **Reporting**

Roles and Responsibilities

Capacity Manager

- Responsibilities:
  - Ensure adequate performance and capacity for all IT services
  - Capacity Plan (responsible for its development and management)
  - Delegate responsibility for performance and capacity monitoring and alerting tasks
  - Report provision and advice to other areas of IT and the business
- Skills: Strategic business awareness, technical, analytical, consultancy

Capacity Management is critical for ensuring effective and efficient capacity and performance of IT Services and IT components in line with identified business requirements and the overall IT strategic objectives. It is essential that the Capacity Manager ensures that the process is appropriately integrated with all aspects of the Service Lifecycle.

Inputs

A NUMBER OF SOURCES OF information are relevant to the Capacity Management process. Some of these are as follows (Service Design, page 174)

- *Business information*: from the organization's business strategy, plans and financial plans, and information on their current and future requirements
- *Service and IT information*: from Service Strategy, the IT strategy and plans and current budgets, covering all areas of technology and technology

plans, including the infrastructure, environment, data, and applications and the way in which they relate to business strategy and plans

- **Component performance and capacity information**: of both existing and new technology from manufacturers and suppliers
- **Service performance issue information**: the Incident and Problem Management processes, with incidents and problems relating to poor performance
- **Service information**: from the SLM process with details of the services from the Service Portfolio, the Service Catalog, and service level targets within SLAs and SLRs and possibly from the monitoring of SLAs, service reviews, and breaches of the SLAs
- **Financial information**: from Financial Management for IT services, the cost of service provision, the cost of resources, components and upgrades, the resultant business benefit, and the financial plans and budgets, together with the costs associated with service and component failure. Some of the costs of components and upgrades to components will be obtained from procurement, suppliers, and manufacturers
- **Change information**: from the Change Management process, with a change schedule and a need to assess all changes for their impact on the capacity of the technology
- **Performance information**: from the CMIS on the current performance of both all existing services and IT infrastructure components
- **CMS**: containing information on the relationships between the business, the services, the supporting services, and the technology
- **Workload information**: from the IT operations team, with schedules of all the work that needs to be run and information on the dependencies between different services and information and the interdependencies within a service

Outputs
THE OUTPUTS OF CAPACITY MANAGEMENT are (Service Design, page 175):

- **CMIS**: this holds the information needed by all sub-processes within Capacity Management. For example, the data monitored and collected as part of Component and Service Capacity Management is used in Business Capacity Management to determine what infrastructure components or upgrades to components are needed and when.
- **Capacity plan**: this is used by all areas of the business and IT management and is acted on by the IT service provider and senior management of

the organization to plan the capacity of the IT infrastructure. It contains information on the current usage of service and components and plans for the development of IT capacity to meet the needs in the growth of both existing services and any agreed new services. The capacity plan should be actively used as a basis for decision-making.

- **Service performance information and reports**: *This is used by many other processes. For example, the Capacity Management process assists SLM with the reporting and reviewing of service performance and the development of new SLRs or changes to existing SLAs. It also assists the Financial Management for IT services process by identifying when money needs to be budgeted for IT infrastructure upgrades or the purchase of new components.*

- **Workload analysis and reports**: *this is used by IT operations to assess and implement changes in conjunction with Capacity Management to schedule or reschedule when services or workloads are run to ensure that the most effective and efficient use is made of the available resources*

- **Ad hoc capacity and performance reports**: *these are used by all areas of Capacity Management, IT, and the business to analyze and resolve service and performance issues*

- **Forecasts and predictive reports**: *these are used by all areas to analyze, predict, and forecast particular business and IT scenarios and their potential solutions*

- **Thresholds, alerts, and events**

- **Improvement actions**: *for inclusion in an SIP*

Availability Management (3/11)

Terminology

Term	Definition
availability	(*ITIL® Service Design*) Ability of an IT service or other configuration item to perform its agreed function when required. Availability is determined by reliability, maintainability, serviceability, performance, and security. Availability is usually calculated as a percentage. This calculation is often based on agreed service time and downtime. It is best practice to calculate availability of an IT service using measurements of the business output.
availability management information system (AMIS)	(*ITIL® Service Design*) A set of tools, data, and information that is used to support availability management. See *also* service knowledge management system.
downtime	(*ITIL® Service Design*) (*ITIL® Service Operation*) The time when an IT service or other configuration item is not available during its agreed service time. The availability of an IT service is often calculated from agreed service time and downtime.
maintainability	(*ITIL® Service Design*) A measure of how quickly and effectively an IT service or other configuration item can be restored to normal working after a failure. Maintainability is often measured and reported as MTRS. Maintainability is also used in the context of software or IT service development to mean ability to be changed or repaired easily.
reliability	(*ITIL® Continual Service Improvement*) (*ITIL® Service Design*) A measure of how long an IT service or other configuration item can perform its agreed function without interruption. Usually measured as MTBF or MTBSI. The term can also be used to state how likely it is that a process, function, etc. will deliver its required outputs. See *also* availability.
resilience	(*ITIL® Service Design*) The ability of an IT service or other configuration item to resist failure or to recover in a timely manner following a failure. For example, an armored cable will resist failure when put under stress.
response time	A measure of the time taken to complete an operation or transaction. Used in capacity management as a measure of IT infrastructure performance and in incident management as a measure of the time taken to answer the phone or to start diagnosis.

Term	Definition
risk	A possible event that could cause harm or loss or affect the ability to achieve objectives. A risk is measured by the probability of a threat, the vulnerability of the asset to that threat, and the impact it would have if it occurred. Risk can also be defined as uncertainty of outcome and can be used in the context of measuring the probability of positive outcomes as well as negative outcomes.
risk assessment	The initial steps of risk management: analyzing the value of assets to the business, identifying threats to those assets, and evaluating how vulnerable each asset is to those threats. Risk assessment can be quantitative (based on numerical data) or qualitative.
risk management	The process responsible for identifying, assessing, and controlling risks. Risk management is also sometimes used to refer to the second part of the overall process after risks have been identified and assessed, as in 'risk assessment and management'. This process is not described in detail within the core ITIL® publications. See *also* risk assessment.
serviceability	(*ITIL® Continual Service Improvement*) (*ITIL® Service Design*) The ability of a third-party supplier to meet the terms of its contract. This contract will include agreed levels of reliability, maintainability, and availability for a configuration item.
trend analysis	(*ITIL® Continual Service Improvement*) Analysis of data to identify time-related patterns. Trend analysis is used in problem management to identify common failures or fragile configuration items and in capacity management as a modeling tool to predict future behavior. It is also used as a management tool for identifying deficiencies in IT service management processes.
vital business function (VBF)	(*ITIL® Service Design*) Part of a business process that is critical to the success of the business. Vital business functions are an important consideration of business continuity management, IT service continuity management, and availability management.
vulnerability	A weakness that could be exploited by a threat—for example, an open firewall port, a password that is never changed, or a flammable carpet. A missing control is also considered to be a vulnerability.

Purpose

LET'S GO BACK TO OUR restaurant analogy: the restaurant continues to make money for as long as it can serve its customers, in other words, its potential is directly correlated to when and how long it is open usually inside the boundaries of a defined set of business hours. The same is true for a service, its potential is directly correlated to the when the service is available to the customer. For a restaurant, service availability is a simple switch of unlocking the doors, but there are other considerations that can disrupt operations and force the doors to be locked again. Equipment failures, improper handling of food (failed processes), utility disruptions, and such are all components of the restaurant business that if not available can strongly influence keeping the doors open. In technology, the availability of the components used in a service can influence the availability of the service.

In this context, availability is one of the most critical parts of the warranty of a service. In order for the business to experience the value promised by the service, the service must deliver within the required levels of availability. Without availability, the utility of the service cannot be accessed in the same manner that a restaurant customer cannot be fed if the doors are locked.

The goal of the restaurant is to remain open during their defined business hours. The purpose of the Availability Management process is ensure the level of availability delivered to all IT services matches to agreed need for availability or defined service level targets. This must be done in a cost effective and timely manner. Availability Management is concerned with the current and future availability needs of the business.

For Availability Management to fulfil its purpose, the process must define, analyze, plan, measure, and improve all aspects of the availability of IT services and its components in accordance to the agreed availability service level targets. The process is point of focus and management for all availability-related issues..

The objectives of Availability Management are to (Service Design, page 125):

- *Produce and maintain an appropriate and up-to-date availability plan that reflects the current and future needs of the business*
- *Provide advice and guidance to all other areas of the business and IT on all availability-related issues*
- *Ensure that service availability achievements meet all their agreed targets by managing services and resources-related availability performance*

> - *Assist with the diagnosis and resolution of availability-related incidents and problems*
> - *Assess the impact of all changes on the availability plan and the availability of all services and resources*
> - *Ensure that proactive measures to improve the availability of services are implemented wherever it is cost-justifiable to do so.*

Question

WHY COULD USERS BE HAPPY with a 60 minute outage and yet be unhappy with 30 minute outage?

1. 30min outage during peak time, overtime being paid to staff, urgent report required
2. 60min outage on weekend, holiday, off peak, when service not required
3. 30min outage on critical IT Service, 60min outage on non-critical IT Service
4. 30mins unplanned outage, 60min planned outage (e.g., maintenance)

For a consumer/user of an IT service, its availability and reliability can directly influence both the perception and satisfaction of the overall IT service provision. However, when disruptions are properly communicated and managed effectively, the impact on the user population's experience can be significantly reduced.

Scope

THE AVAILABILITY OF A SERVICE is dependent on the capabilities of the components used to deliver the service, and not just a by-product of running the component continuously. For this reason, availability must be designed, implemented, measured, and improved. The Availability Management process is involved in every aspect of availability throughout the service lifecycle and down to the component level of the service solution. The process is initiated when the availability requirements for the IT service are understood and clearly defined and remains active until the service is decommissioned or retired.

The Availability Management process includes two key elements:

- **Reactive activities:** These activities include monitoring, measuring, analysis, and management of all events, incidents, and problems related to unavailability. Typically performed by operational roles in IT, the activities focus on identifying any disruption to the service availability and resolving the disruption sufficiently to make the service available again.
- **Proactive activities:** These activities include any planning, design work, and improvement of availability performed to ensure the service and associated components are available when required by the customer. The activities are performed by individuals or groups involved in the planning and design of the service.

The service and component availability requirements must be understood from the business perspective and can be influenced by current business processes and operations, future business plans, service targets and the current capabilities of IT operations and delivery, and the demand on the service, including its impact and priority in the business.

The Availability Management process is applied to all current services and technology being covered by SLAs, all new IT services or existing services with established SLRs, all supporting services and suppliers, and all aspects of the service and components that may potentially impact availability. , :

The Availability Management process should include (Service Design, page 126):

- *Monitoring of all aspects of availability, reliability, and maintainability of IT services and the supporting components with appropriate events, alarms, and escalation, with automated scripts for recovery*
- *Maintaining a set of methods, techniques, and calculations for all availability measurements, metrics, and reporting*
- *Actively participating in risk assessment and management activities*
- *Collecting measurements and the analysis and production of regular and ad hoc reports on service and component availability*
- *Understanding the agreed current and future demands of the business for IT services and their availability*
- *Influencing the design of services and components to align with business availability needs*

- *Producing an availability plan that enables the service provider to continue to provide and improve services in line with availability targets defined in SLAs and to plan and forecast future availability levels required, as defined in SLRs*
- *Maintaining a schedule of tests for all resilience and fail-over components and mechanisms*
- *Assisting with the identification and resolution of any incidents and problems associated with service or component unavailability*
- *Proactively improving service or component availability wherever it is cost-justifiable and meets the needs of the business.*

While Availability Management may provide substantial information to Business Continuity Management (BCM) and IT Service Continuity Management (ITSCM), the process is not responsible for the resumption of business or IT processes after a major disaster.

Activities

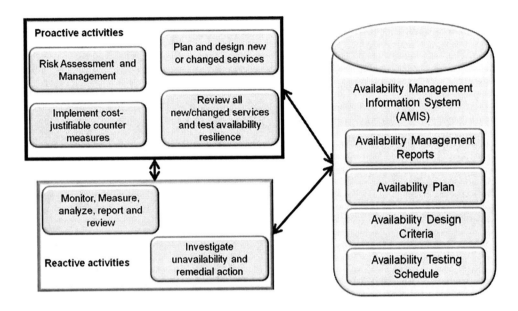

Figure 5.N—The Proactive and Reactive Elements of Availability Management © Crown Copyright 2011 Reproduced under license from the Cabinet Office

- **Proactive Activities (primarily executed in Service Design and Service Transition):**
  - ⊳ The development and maintenance of an availability plan, which documents the current and future requirements for service availability and the methods used to meet these requirements
  - ⊳ Development of a defined set of methods, techniques, and calculations for the assessment and reporting of availability
  - ⊳ Liaison with IT Service Continuity Management and other aligned processes to assist with risk assessment and management activities
  - ⊳ Ensuring consistency in the design of services and components to align with the business requirements for availability

- **Reactive Activities (primarily executed in Service Operation and Continual Service Improvement):**

> ▷ Regular monitoring of all aspects of availability, reliability, and maintainability, including supporting processes such as Event Management for timely disruption detection and escalation
> ▷ Regular and event-based reporting of service and component availability
> ▷ Ensuring regular maintenance is performed according to the levels of risk across the IT infrastructure
> ▷ Assessing the performance of and data gathered by various Service Operation processes, such as Incident and Problem Management, to determine what improvement actions might be made to improve availability levels or the way in which they are met.

Expanded Incident Lifecycle

AN AIM OF AVAILABILITY MANAGEMENT is to ensure the duration and impact from incidents impacting IT services are minimized to enable business operations to resume as quickly as possible.

The expanded incident lifecycle enables the total IT service downtime for any given incident to be broken down and mapped against the major stages that all incidents go through.

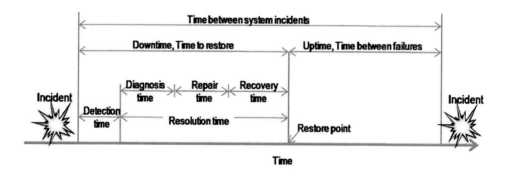

Figure 5.0—The Expanded Incident Lifecycle
© Crown Copyright 2011 Reproduced under license from the Cabinet Office

- **Mean Time Between Failures (MTBF) or Uptime:**
  - ▷ Average time between the recovery from one incident and the occurrence of the next incident, relates to the reliability of the service

- **Mean Time to Restore Service (MTRS) or Downtime:**
  - ▷ Average time taken to restore a CI or IT service after a failure
  - ▷ Measured from when CI or IT service fails until it is fully restored and delivering its normal functionality

- **Mean Time Between System Incidents (MTBSI):**
  - ▷ Average time between the occurrences of two consecutive incidents
  - ▷ Sum of the MTRS and MTBF

- **Relationships of the above terms:**
  - ▷ High ratio of MTBF/MTBSI indicates there are frequently occurring minor faults or disruptions
  - ▷ Low ratio of MTBF/MTBSI indicates there are infrequently occurring major faults or disruptions

Elements making up the Mean Time to Restore Service (MTRS):

- **Detection Time**: Time for the service provider to be informed of the fault (reported)
- **Diagnosis Time**: Time for the service provider to respond after diagnosis completed
- **Repair Time**:
  - ▷ Time for the service provider to restore the components that caused the fault
  - ▷ Calculated from **diagnosis** to **recovery** time
- **Restoration Time (MTRS)**:
  - ▷ The **agreed** level of service is restored to the user
  - ▷ Calculated from **detection** to **restore point**
- **Restore Point**: The point where the agreed level of service has been restored

Roles and Responsibilities

Availability Manager

- **Responsibilities:**
  - ▹ Ensure adequate availability of all IT services
  - ▹ Developing and maintaining an availability plan
  - ▹ Oversee availability monitoring and improvement of the process
  - ▹ Report provision and advice

Skills: Awareness of how IT supports the business, technical, analytical, consultancy, seeks continuous improvement

Note: The Availability Manager does not seek to achieve 100% availability of all services and systems but, instead, seeks to deliver availability that matches or exceeds (within reason) the agreed business requirements.

Availability Management Metrics

TYPICAL METRICS FOR EVALUATING THE effectiveness and efficiency of Availability Management include:

- Percentage reduction in unavailability of services and components
- Percentage increase in the reliability of services and components
- Effective review and follow up of all SLA, OLA, and UC breaches
- Percentage improvement in overall end-to-end availability of service
- Percentage reduction in the number and impact of service breaks
- Improvement of MTBF
- Improvement of MTBSI
- Reduction in MTRS

While the above list does include a number of important measures, the service provider should also seek to demonstrate the impact that availability/unavailability has on the business. Such examples of business-oriented availability reporting include:

- User minutes lost due to disruption
- Transactions lost or delayed due to disruption

- Customer complaints caused by disruption

Inputs

A NUMBER OF SOURCES OF information are relevant to the Availability Management process. Some of these are as follows (Service Design, page 153)

- **Business information**: *from the organization's business strategy, plans and financial plans, and information on their current and future requirements, including the availability requirements for new or enhanced IT services*
- **Business impact information**: *from BIAs and assessment of VBFs underpinned by IT services*
- **Reports and registers:** *previous risk assessment reports and a risk register*
- **Service information**: *from the Service Portfolio and the Service Catalog*
- **Service information**: *from the SLM process, with details of the services from the Service Portfolio and the Service Catalog, service level targets within SLAs and SLRs, service reviews and breaches of the SLAs*
- **Financial information**: *from Financial Management for IT services, the cost of service provision, the cost of resources and components*
- **Change and release information**: *from the Change Management process, with a change schedule, the release schedule from release and deployment management, and a need to assess all changes for their impact on service availability*
- **Service asset and configuration management**: *containing information on the relationships between the business, the services, the supporting services, and the technology*
- **Service targets**: *from SLAs, SLRs, OLAs, and contracts*
- **Component information**: *on the availability, reliability, and maintainability requirements for the technology components that underpin IT service(s)*
- **Technology information**: *from the CMS on the topology and the relationships between the components and the assessment of the capabilities of new technology*
- **Past performance**: *from previous measurements, achievements, and reports and the Availability Management Information System (AMIS)*
- **Unavailability and failure information**: *from incidents and problems*

> • ***Planning information***: *from other processes, such as the capacity plan from Capacity Management*

Outputs

THE OUTPUTS PRODUCED BY AVAILABILITY Management should include (Service Design, page 154):

- *The Availability MIS (AMIS)*
- *The availability plan for the proactive improvement of IT services and technology*
- *Availability and recovery design criteria and proposed service targets for new or changed services*
- *Service availability, reliability, and maintainability reports of achievements against targets, including input for all service reports*
- *Component availability, reliability, and maintainability reports of achievements against targets*
- *Revised risk assessment reviews and reports and an updated risk register*
- *Monitoring, management, and reporting requirements for IT services and components to ensure that deviations in availability, reliability, and maintainability are detected, actioned, recorded, and reported*
- *An availability management test schedule for testing all availability, resilience, and recovery mechanisms*
- *The planned and preventive maintenance schedules*
- *Contributions for the PSO to be created by change in collaboration with Release and Deployment Management*
- *Details of the proactive availability techniques and measures that will be deployed to provide additional resilience to prevent or minimize the impact of component failures on the IT service availability*
- *Improvement actions for inclusion within the SIP*

IT Service Continuity Management

SERVICE CONTINUITY IS AN ESSENTIAL part of the warranty of a service. If a service's continuity cannot be maintained and/or restored in accordance with the requirements of the business, then the business will not experience the value that has been promised. Without continuity the utility of the service cannot be accessed. Service continuity is different from Availability Management, though many of the concepts are the same. Our restaurant analogy fits to describe the difference: with availability management the goal is to keep the doors unlocked for business. With Service Continuity, there is no restaurant to open so the task is to rebuild. This may be dramatic, but it is sufficient to distinguish between the two processes.

Continuity management in IT is often spoken on two levels: Business Continuity Management (BCM) and IT Service Continuity Management (ITSCM). Business Continuity Management is developed by the customer, or business, that the IT organization is providing support. Along the same lines that IT services must support he business operations, it must also support the disruption and recovery of business operations in a continuity event. This is done through the development and implementation of IT Service Continuity Management and its associated process, policies, and technologies. ITSCM is often referred to as Disaster Recovery Planning. The business and IT service provider will agree to minimum service levels and expected service support during these types of events: depending on the conditions of the situation, some services may not be delivered or service levels will be lower than normal operations. To support and align with the BCM process, ITSCM will utilize formal techniques for risk assessment and management to restore the risks to IT services and plan and prepare for recovery of IT services.

The objectives of ITSCM are to (Service Design, page 179):

- *Produce and maintain a set of IT service continuity plans that support the overall business continuity plans of the organization*
- *Complete regular BIA exercises to ensure that all continuity plans are maintained in line with changing business impacts and requirements*
- *Conduct regular risk assessment and management exercises to manage IT services within an agreed level of business risk in conjunction with the business and the Availability Management and Information Security Management processes*
- *Provide advice and guidance to all other areas of the business and IT on all continuity-related issues*
- *Ensure that appropriate continuity mechanisms are put in place to meet or exceed the agreed business continuity targets*
- *Assess the impact of all changes on the IT service continuity plans and supporting methods and procedures*
- *Ensure that proactive measures to improve the availability of services are implemented wherever it is cost-justifiable to do so*

- *Negotiate and agree contracts with suppliers for the provision of the necessary recovery capability to support all continuity plans in conjunction with the Supplier Management process*

Note: ITSCM is often referred to as Disaster Recovery planning.

Terminology

Term	Definition
business continuity plan (BCP)	(ITIL® Service Design) A plan defining the steps required to restore business processes following a disruption. The plan also identifies the triggers for invocation, people to be involved, communications, etc. IT service continuity plans form a significant part of business continuity plans.
business impact analysis (BIA)	(ITIL® Service Strategy) Business impact analysis is the activity in business continuity management that identifies vital business functions and their dependencies. These dependencies may include suppliers, people, other business processes, IT services etc. Business impact analysis defines the recovery requirements for IT services. These requirements include recovery time objectives, recovery point objectives, and minimum service level targets for each IT service.
countermeasure	Can be used to refer to any type of control. The term is most often used when referring to measures that increase resilience, fault tolerance, or reliability of an IT service.
gradual recovery	(ITIL® Service Design) A recovery option that is also known as cold standby. Gradual recovery typically uses a portable or fixed facility that has environmental support and network cabling but no computer systems. The hardware and software are installed as part of the IT service continuity plan. Gradual recovery typically takes more than three days and may take significantly longer.
hot standby	See fast recovery; immediate recovery.
immediate recovery	(ITIL® Service Design) A recovery option that is also known as hot standby. Provision is made to recover the IT service with no significant loss of service to the customer. Immediate recovery typically uses mirroring, load balancing, and split-site technologies.
impact	(ITIL® Service Operation) (ITIL® Service Transition) A measure of the effect of an incident, problem, or change on business processes. Impact is often based on how service levels will be affected. Impact and urgency are used to assign priority.

Term	Definition
intermediate recovery	(ITIL® Service Design) A recovery option that is also known as warm standby. Intermediate recovery usually uses a shared portable or fixed facility that has computer systems and network components. The hardware and software will need to be configured and data will need to be restored as part of the IT service continuity plan. Typical recovery times for intermediate recovery are one to three days.
IT service continuity plan	(ITIL® Service Design) A plan defining the steps required to recover one or more IT services. The plan also identifies the triggers for invocation, people to be involved, communications, etc. The IT service continuity plan should be part of a business continuity plan.
manual workaround	(ITIL® Continual Service Improvement) A workaround that requires manual intervention. Manual workaround is also used as the name of a recovery option in which the business process operates without the use of IT services. This is a temporary measure and is usually combined with another recovery option.
reciprocal arrangement	(ITIL® Service Design) A recovery option. An agreement between two organizations to share resources in an emergency—for example, high-speed printing facilities or computer room space.
risk	A possible event that could cause harm or loss or affect the ability to achieve objectives. A risk is measured by the probability of a threat, the vulnerability of the asset to that threat, and the impact it would have if it occurred. Risk can also be defined as uncertainty of outcome and can be used in the context of measuring the probability of positive outcomes as well as negative outcomes.
risk assessment	The initial steps of risk management: analyzing the value of assets to the business, identifying threats to those assets, and evaluating how vulnerable each asset is to those threats. Risk assessment can be quantitative (based on numerical data) or qualitative.
risk management	The process responsible for identifying, assessing, and controlling risks. Risk management is also sometimes used to refer to the second part of the overall process after risks have been identified and assessed, as in 'risk assessment and management'. This process is not described in detail within the core ITIL® publications. See also risk assessment.
threat	A threat is anything that might exploit a vulnerability. Any potential cause of an incident can be considered a threat. For example, a fire is a threat that could exploit the vulnerability of flammable floor coverings. This term is commonly used in information security management and IT service continuity management but also applies to other areas, such as problem and availability management.

Term	Definition
vital business function (VBF)	(ITIL® Service Design) Part of a business process that is critical to the success of the business. Vital business functions are an important consideration of business continuity management, IT service continuity management, and availability management.
vulnerability	A weakness that could be exploited by a threat—for example, an open firewall port, a password that is never changed, or a flammable carpet. A missing control is also considered to be a vulnerability.
warm standby	See intermediate recovery.

Scope

THE SCOPE OF ITSCM CAN be said to be focused on planning for, managing, and recovering from IT disasters. These disasters are severe enough to have a critical impact on business operations and, as a result, will typically require a separate set of infrastructure and facilities to recover. Less significant events are dealt with as part of the Incident Management process in association with Availability Management.

The disaster does not necessarily need to be a fire, flood, pestilence, or plague; it can any disruption that causes a severe impact to one or more business processes. Accordingly, the scope of ITSCM should be carefully defined according to the organization's needs, which may result in continuity planning and recovery mechanisms for some or all of the IT services being provided to the business.

There are longer-term business risks that are out of the scope of ITSCM, including those arising from changes in business direction, organizational restructures, or emergence of new competitors in the market place. These are more the focus of processes such as Service Portfolio Management and Change Management.

The ITSCM process includes (Service Design, page 180):

- *The agreement of the scope of the ITSCM process and the policies adopted*
- *BIA to quantify the impact loss of IT service would have on the business*
- *Risk assessment and management—the risk identification and risk assessment to identify potential threats to continuity and the likelihood of the threats becoming reality. This also includes taking measures to manage the identified threats where this can be cost-justified. The approach to managing these threats will form the core of the ITSCM strategy and plans.*

- *Production of an overall ITSCM strategy that must be integrated into the BCM strategy. This can be produced following the two steps identified above and is likely to include elements of risk reduction as well as selection of appropriate and comprehensive recovery options.*
- *Production of an ITSCM plan, which again must be integrated with the overall BCM plans*
- *Testing of the plans*
- *Ongoing operation and maintenance of the plans*

Activities of IT Service Continuity Management

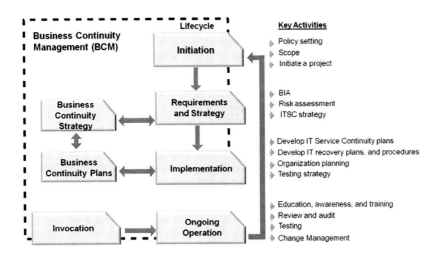

Figure 5.P—Activities of IT Service Continuity Management
© Crown Copyright 2011 Reproduced under license from the Cabinet Office

THE ACTIVITIES SHOWN IN FIGURE 5.P demonstrate what is required to support BCM and maintain a readiness for ITSCM. Two activities are keys to the success of ITSCM: Business Impact Analysis (BIA) and Risk Assessments. A BIA is used to quantify the impact any service loss will have on the business. Tangible losses such as financial loss are often considered "hard" impacts, while loss in morale, health, and safety cannot be clearly quantified and are considered "soft" impacts. The BIA will identify those services that are most important to the business and will need priority attention in the planning of continuity activities. Some of the items identified through a BIA are:

- Critical business processes and Vital Business Functions
- Potential damage or loss caused by disruption
- Possible escalations caused by damage or loss
- Necessary resources required to enable continuity of critical business processes
- Time constraints for minimum recovery of facilities and services
- Time constraints for complete recovery of facilities and services

Risk assessments will focus on the likelihood that a serious service disruption will occur, or threat of disaster. Often used in availability management to proactively ensure the required availability of a service, a risk assessment will identify those potential threats that the business and IT should be aware. Many threats dealt with in ITSCM are geographical, weather related, political, or social issues. Large companies may have several data centers or many third-party suppliers of service, so risk assessments will typically evaluate the threat of one or more data centers or suppliers no longer being in service. The items identified in risk assessments are:

- Gather information on assets (IT infrastructure components)
- Threats from both internal and external sources (the likelihood of occurring)
- Vulnerabilities (the extent of impact or effect on organization)

Ongoing Operation

ITSCM HAS A UNIQUE CHARACTERISTIC that sets it apart from any other service management process: the organization does not want to initiate it but it must be ready to initiate at a moment's notice. For instance, you may not want your house to catch fire, but you and your family should know what to do in case it does. When ITSCM is initiated, it means that a "disaster" has occurred, usually unpredicted and the scope of the impact is typically unknown. Immediate attention is required to assess the damage, respond appropriate and start recovery. The policies and procedures need to be clearly understood and interpretable under the harshest and most emotional conditions.

Because the core of the process is responding to a disaster, many organizations may never use the plans it creates. At the same time, the plans cannot be shelved until they are needed. ITSCM is responsibility for building the awareness and confidence of the organization to be prepared for a continuity event. The activities used for this purpose are done regularly and with full support of management. The activities include:

- Education and awareness
- Involving IT staff, customers, users, suppliers, and other stakeholders
- Training
- Reviews
- Ongoing testing
- At least annually
- Following major changes
- Audits of recovery procedures, risk-reduction measures, and for compliance to procedures.
- Ensuring integration with Change Management so that all changes are assessed as to their requirements for continuity and their potential impact on existing continuity strategies

Roles and Responsibilities

TYPICAL RESPONSIBILITIES FOR ITSCM IN planning and dealing with disasters are similar to how First Aid Officers and Fire Wardens act in planning and operational roles (they may not be full-time roles but are, instead, a 'hat' they wear when required). See the following table for an example of how responsibilities for ITSCM are typically assigned.

Role	Responsibilities
Board	Crisis management Corporate/business decisions External affairs
Senior Management	Co-ordination Direction and arbitration Resource authorization
Management	Invocation of continuity or recovery Team leadership Site management Liaison and reporting

Supervisors and Staff	Task execution
	Team membership
	Team and site liaison

Skill requirements for the ITSCM Manager and other involved staff include:

- Knowledge of the business (help to set priorities for protection and recovery)
- Calm under pressure
- Analytical (problem solving)
- Leadership and team players
- Negotiation and communication

Inputs

THERE ARE MANY SOURCES OF input required by the ITSCM process (Service Design, page 194):

- **Business information**: *from the organization's business strategy, plans and financial plans, and information on their current and future requirements*
- **IT information: from the IT strategy and plans and current budgets**
- **A business continuity strategy** *and a set of business continuity plans: from all areas of the business*
- **Service information**: *from the SLM process, with details of the services from the Service Portfolio and the Service Catalog and service level targets within SLAs and SLRs*
- **Financial information**: *from Financial Management for IT services, the cost of service provision, the cost of resources and components*
- **Change information**: *from the Change Management process, with a change schedule and a need to assess all changes for their impact on all ITSCM plans*
- **CMS**: *containing information on the relationships between the business, the services, the supporting services, and the technology*
- **Business Continuity Management** *and Availability Management testing schedules*

- *Capacity Management information*: identifying the resources required to run the critical services in the event of a continuity event
- **IT service continuity plans and test reports**: from supplier and partners, where appropriate

Outputs

THE OUTPUTS FROM THE ITSCM process include (Service Design, page 194):

- *A revised ITSCM policy and strategy*
- *A set of ITSCM plans*: including all crisis management plans, emergency response plans, and disaster recovery plans, together with a set of supporting plans and contracts with recovery service providers
- **BIA exercises and reports:** in conjunction with BCM and the business
- **Risk assessment and management reviews and reports**: in conjunction with the business, Availability Management, and Information Security Management
- *An ITSCM testing schedule*
- *ITSCM test scenarios*
- *ITSCM test reports and reviews*

Forecasts and predictive reports are used by all areas to analyze, predict, and forecast particular business and IT scenarios and their potential solutions.

Information Security Management (4/1)

Purpose

INFORMATION SECURITY IS PART OF the corporate governance framework, providing strategic direction for security activities and ensures that strategic objectives for the business are achieved. Information Security Management also ensures the management of information security risks and responsible use of information resources. 'Information' in this context is used as a general terms and includes all data stores, databases, and metadata used by the enterprise.

Information security is a critical part of the warranty of a service. The process establishes controls that prevent or mitigate disruptions from security threats impacting the IT environment. This allows IT services to perform as expected and ensures value is generated for the business. Information security also ensures that the users can access the utility of the service. The primary purpose of Information Security Management is to align IT security with business security, ensuring the agreed business needs regarding the confidentiality, integrity, and availability of the organization's assets information, data and IT services are matched. The objective of Information Security Management is to protect the interests of those people and groups from failures of confidentiality, integrity, and availability, specifically when accessing information and systems and communications that deliver the information. For most organizations, the security objective is met when (Service Design, page 197):

- *Information is observed by or disclosed to only those who have a right to know (confidentiality)*
- *Information is complete, accurate, and protected against unauthorized modification (integrity)*
- *Information is available and usable when required, and the systems that provide it can appropriately resist attacks and recover from or prevent failures (availability)*
- *Business transactions, as well as information exchanges between enterprises or with partners, can be trusted (authenticity and non-repudiation)*

Terminology

Term	Definition
confidentiality	(ITIL® Service Design) A security principle that requires that data should only be accessed by authorized people.
information security policy	(ITIL® Service Design) The policy that governs the organization's approach to information security management.
risk	A possible event that could cause harm or loss or affect the ability to achieve objectives. A risk is measured by the probability of a threat, the vulnerability of the asset to that threat, and the impact it would have if it occurred. Risk can also be defined as uncertainty of outcome and can be used in the context of measuring the probability of positive outcomes as well as negative outcomes.
risk assessment	The initial steps of risk management: analyzing the value of assets to the business, identifying threats to those assets, and evaluating how vulnerable each asset is to those threats. Risk assessment can be quantitative (based on numerical data) or qualitative.

risk management	The process responsible for identifying, assessing, and controlling risks. Risk management is also sometimes used to refer to the second part of the overall process after risks have been identified and assessed, as in 'risk assessment and management'. This process is not described in detail within the core ITIL® publications. See also risk assessment.
security	See information security management.
security management information system (SMIS)	(ITIL® Service Design) A set of tools, data, and information that is used to support information security management. The security management information system is part of the information security management system. See also service knowledge management system.
security policy	See information security policy.
threat	A threat is anything that might exploit a vulnerability. Any potential cause of an incident can be considered a threat. For example, a fire is a threat that could exploit the vulnerability of flammable floor coverings. This term is commonly used in information security management and IT service continuity management but also applies to other areas, such as problem and availability management.
vulnerability	A weakness that could be exploited by a threat—for example, an open firewall port, a password that is never changed, or a flammable carpet. A missing control is also considered to be a vulnerability.

© **Crown** Copyright 2011 Reproduced under license from the Cabinet Office

Scope

THE INFORMATION SECURITY MANAGEMENT PROCESS is the focal point for all IT security issues and ensures an information security policy is produced, maintained, and enforced. The information security policy covers the use and misuse of all IT systems and services. The entire IT and business security environment must be understood, specifically (Service Design, page 197):

- *Business security policy and plans*
- *Current business operation and its security requirements*
- *Future business plans and requirements*
- *Legislative and regulatory requirements*
- *Obligations and responsibilities with regard to security contained within SLAs*

- *The business and IT risks and their management*

Understanding all of this will enable Information Security Management to ensure that all the current and future security aspects and risks of the business are cost-effectively managed.

Information Security Management ensures that the **confidentiality**, **integrity**, and **availability** of an organization's assets, information, data, and IT services is maintained. Information Security Management must consider the following four perspectives:

- Organizational—define security policies and staff awareness of these
- Procedural—defined procedures used to control security
- Physical—Controls used to protect any physical sites against security incidents
- Technical—Controls used to protect the IT infrastructure against security incidents

Information Security Management Policy

A CONSISTENT SET OF POLICIES and supporting documents should be developed to define the organization's approach to security, which is supported by all levels of management in the organization.

These policies should be made available to customers and users, and their compliance should be referred to in all SLRs, SLAs, contracts, and agreements. The policies should be authorized by top executive management within the business and IT, and compliance to them should be endorsed on a regular basis. All security policies should be reviewed and, where necessary, revised on at least an annual basis.

The overall Information Security Policy should consist of a number of sub-components or sub-policies, covering:

- The use and misuse of IT assets
- Access control
- Password control
- E-mail
- Internet
- Anti-virus

- Information classification
- Document classification
- Remote access
- Supplier access
- Asset disposal

The Information Security Management System (ISMS)

THE ISMS CONTAINS THE STANDARDS, management procedures, and guidelines that support the Information Security Management policies. Using this in conjunction with an overall framework for managing security will help to ensure that the Four P's of People, Process, Products, and Partners are considered as to the requirements for security and control.

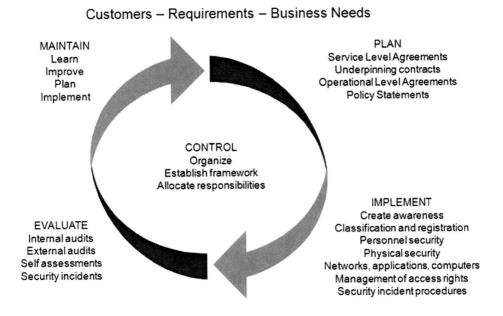

Figure 5.Q—Framework for Managing IT Security
© Crown Copyright 2011 Reproduced under license from Cabinet Office.

AS A GUIDE, STANDARDS SUCH as ISO 27001 provide a formal standard by which to compare or certify their own ISMS, covering the five main elements of:

1. **Plan**

Planning is used to identify and recommend the appropriate security measures that will support the requirements and objectives of the organization. SLAs, OLAs, business and organizational plans and strategies, regulation and compliance requirements (such as Privacy Acts) as well as the legal, moral, and ethical responsibilities for information security will be considered in the development of these measures.

2. **Implement**

The objective of this element is to ensure that the appropriate measures, procedures, tools, and controls are in place to support the Information Security Policy.

3. **Control**

The objectives of the control element of the ISMS are to:

- Ensure the framework is developed to support Information Security Management
- Develop an organizational structure appropriate to support the Information Security Policy
- Allocate responsibilities
- Establish and control documentation

4. **Evaluate**

The evaluate element of the ISMS is focused on ensuring:

- Regular audits and reviews are performed
- Policy and process compliance is evaluated
- Information and audit reports are provided to management and external regulators, if required

5. **Maintain**

As part of Continual Service Improvement, the maintain element seeks to:

- Improve security agreements as documented in SLAs and OLAs
- Improve the implementation and use of security measures and controls

Activities

THE ACTIVITIES OF INFORMATION SECURITY Management are involved in multiple stages of the Service Lifecycle, including the:

- Development and maintenance of the Information Security Policy
- Communication, implementation, and enforcement of the security policies
- Assessment and classification of all information assets and documentation
- Implementation and continual review of appropriate security controls
- Monitoring and management of all security incidents
- Analysis, reporting, and reduction of the volumes and impact of security breaches and incidents
- Scheduling and execution of security reviews, audits, and penetration tests

Training and awareness is particularly vital and is often the weakness in an organization's control of security (particularly at the end-user stage). As part of the maintain element of the ISMS, consideration should be given to methods and techniques that can be improved so that the policies and standards can be more easily followed and implemented.

Inputs

INFORMATION SECURITY MANAGEMENT WILL NEED to obtain input from many areas, including (Service Design, page 204):

- *Business information*: from the organization's business strategy, plans and financial plans, and information on its current and future requirements
- *Governance and security*: from corporate governance and business security policies and guidelines, security plans, risk assessment, and responses
- *IT information*: from the IT strategy and plans and current budgets
- *Service information*: from the SLM process with details of the services from the Service Portfolio and the Service Catalog, service level targets within SLAs and SLRs and possibly from the monitoring of SLAs, service reviews, and breaches of the SLAs
- *Risk assessment processes and reports*: from ISM, Availability Management and ITSCM

- *Details of all security events and breaches*: from all areas of IT and ITSM, especially Incident Management and Problem Management
- *Change information*: from the Change Management process with a change schedule and a need to assess all changes for their impact on all security policies, plans, and controls
- *CMS*: containing information on the relationships between the business, the services, supporting services, and the technology
- *Details of partner and supplier access*: from Supplier Management and Availability Management on external access to services and systems

Outputs

THE OUTPUTS PRODUCED BY THE Information Security Management process are used in all areas and should include (Service Design, page 204):

- An overall information security management policy, together with a set of specific security policies
- A Security Management Information System (SMIS), containing all the information relating to Information Security Management
- Revised security risk assessment processes and reports
- A set of security controls, together with details of the operation and maintenance and their associated risks
- Security audits and audit reports
- Security test schedules and plans, including security penetration tests and other security tests and reports
- A set of security classifications and a set of classified information assets
- Reviews and reports of security breaches and major incidents
- Policies, processes, and procedures for managing partners and suppliers and their access to services and information

Service Design Summary

GOOD SERVICE DESIGN MEANS IT is possible to deliver quality, cost-effective services and to ensure that the business requirements are being met. It also delivers:

- Improved Quality of Service
- Improved Consistency of Service
- Improved Service Alignments
- Standards and Conventions to be followed
- More Effective Service Performance

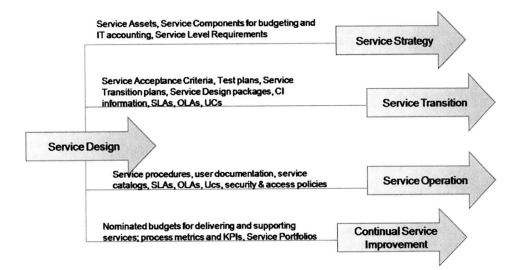

Figure 5.R—Example Service Design Outputs to Other Lifecycle Stages

Service Design Scenario

Design Coordination
- Comprehensive and consistent set of service designs and SDPs
- Revised measurement and metrics methods
- Service portfolio updated

Service Level Management Considerations
- SLR—detailed requirements that constitute the design criteria to be met, e.g., secure, clear uninterrupted voice, real time video, accessible for novice users, etc.
- SLA structure—decision made to develop multi-level structure (based on decision of service level package used, as well as offering greater security and accessibility to various departments/users)

Service Catalog Management Considerations
- Business Service Catalog—will describe HYPE service as business understands it, including levels of service
- Technical Services Catalog—will clearly list technical and supporting service information, e.g., ISP bandwidth, server requirements, etc.

Supplier Management Considerations
- Negotiate UCs with software vendor, ISP, WAN
- Monitor external supplier service—discussions with Availability Management, Service Desk, etc.

Capacity Management Considerations
- Application Sizing—assessing what minimum PC requirements needed to support new HYPE software, as well as type of webcam to best provide service, network bandwidth
- Modeling—how many users can videoconference before quality of service is affected, throughput/bandwidth targets, how may this service impact on other services?
- Demand Management—designing to ensure ability to limit bandwidth/ video access during peak times for certain users/groups

Availability Management Considerations
- To ensure availability targets are met, regular maintenance of components is required, as well as ensuring through Supplier Management that ISP Underpinning Contract is met (serviceability requirements)

Information Security Management Considerations
- Confidentiality—user passwords design (e.g., HYPE service is not controlled locally; all information is stored on the vendor's server. If all users use the same password as their network login, resulting in a clear pattern, then it would be possible for security to be threatened if someone hacked into the vendor's server)
- Integrity—will logs of all conversations/messages/video kept be stored?
- Availability—having those logs available to those who require it, when they require it

ITSCM Considerations
- The business has decided that this is a BCP, so standby arrangements are negotiated with business ($$)
- Decided that the telephone line and/or email will be possible recovery measures until service is restored—included in ITSCM plan

The Service Design processes will ensure that HYPE meets the customer needs, can be developed and deployed by Service Transition, and then maintained and supported within Service Operation.

Service Design Review Questions

Question 1

Which ITIL® process analyzes threats and dependencies to IT services as part of the decision regarding countermeasures to be implemented?

    a) Availability Management
    b) IT Service Continuity Management
    c) Problem Management
    d) Service Asset and Configuration Management

Question 2

What is the name of the activity within the Capacity Management process whose purpose is to predict the future capacity requirements of new and changed services?

    a) Application Sizing
    b) Demand Management
    c) Modeling
    d) Tuning

Question 3

In which ITIL® process are negotiations held with customers about the availability and capacity levels to be provided?

    a) Availability Management
    b) Capacity Management
    c) Financial Management for IT Services
    d) Service Level Management

Question 4

Which of the following statements is false?

a) It is impossible to maintain user and customer satisfaction during a disruption to service
b) When reporting the availability provided for a service, the percentage (%) availability that is calculated takes into account the agreed service hours
c) Availability of services could be improved by changes to the architecture, ITSM processes, or IT staffing levels
d) Reports regarding availability should include more than just uptime, downtime, and frequency of failure and reflect the actual business impact of unavailability

Question 5

Which of the following activities is Service Level Management responsible for?

a) Informing users of available services
b) Identifying customer needs
c) Overseeing service release schedule
d) Keeping accurate records of all configuration items

Question 6

Which process reviews Operational Level Agreements (OLAs) on a regular basis?

a) Supplier Management
b) Service Level Management
c) Service Portfolio Management
d) Contract Management

Question 7
What is another term for Uptime?

   a) Mean Time Between Failures (MTBF)
   b) Mean Time to Restore Service (MTRS)
   c) Mean Time Between System Incidents (MTBSI)
   d) Relationship between MTBF and MTBSI

Question 8
Which of the following is an activity of IT Service Continuity Management?

   a) Advising end users of a system failure
   b) Documenting the recovery procedure for a critical system
   c) Reporting regarding availability
   d) Guaranteeing that the Configuration Items are constantly kept up - to - date

Question 9
Information security must consider the following four perspectives:

   1. Organizational
   2. Physical
   3. Technical?

   a) Process
   b) Security
   c) Procedural
   d) Firewalls

Question 10
The 3 types of Service Level Agreements structures are:

   a) Customer-based, Service-based, Corporate-based
   b) Corporate-level, customer-level, service-level
   c) Service-based, customer-based, user-based
   d) Customer-based, service-based, multi-level

SERVICE TRANSITION

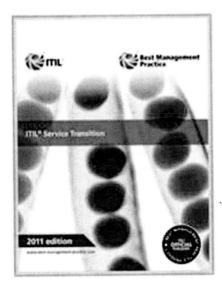

Figure 6.A—Service Transition
"© Crown copyright 2011 Reproduced under licence from the Cabinet Office"

The Service Transition lifecycle stage focuses on the vulnerable transition between the Design stage and the Operation stage of a service. It is particularly critical as functional and technical errors not found during this stage will result in significantly higher impact levels to the business and/or IT infrastructure and will usually cost much more to fix once the service is in operation.

Processes:

* Transition Planning and Support
* Knowledge Management
* Service Asset and Configuration Management
* Change Management
* Release and Deployment Management
* Service Validation and Testing
* Change Evaluation

THE ITIL® FOUNDATION CERTIFICATE IN ITSM syllabus and the corresponding exam requirements only cover five of these Service Transition processes, the other processes are covered in the Intermediate level of study. Therefore, this book and the corresponding eLearning program will cover the following Service Transition processes:

* Transition Planning and Support
* Knowledge Management
* Service Asset and Configuration Management
* Change Management
* Release and Deployment Management

Purpose

THE MAIN GOAL OF THE SERVICE TRANSITION stage of the Service Lifecycle is to make sure that any updates or changes to the live operational environment—that impact either new, modified, retiring, or retired services—are in line with the agreed expectations of all parties involved; being the customers the business, and the users. Meaning that, all changes to operational environments should be managed, planned, and coordinated through Service Transition processes and activities to ensure a smooth transition to live operation is accomplished. This is to make sure that a new, modified, retiring, or retired service accomplishes its operational expectation and has no or limited undesirable impact on the business, its customers or its users.

Successful service transition will not occur until an organization realizes a need for it and its benefits. Business operations and processes are in a constant state of transition making effective service transition a necessary process. The pursuit of a competitive advantage, self-preservation, best-of-breed innovation, and agility are never-ending catalysts for changes that must eventually be delivered.

Service Transition's purpose is also to make sure that the requirements of Service Strategy set in Service Design are in effect fulfilled through to the release of live services within the Service Operation stage of the Service Lifecycle. With the outputs gained from the Service Design stage, Service transition ensures that service solutions are smoothly transferred to live operation, fulfilling the requirements agreed upon by the customer and the business. The transition activity is triggered by the production of a Service Design Package developed by the processes and activities of Service Design. Service Transition uses this new business requirement enclosed within the Service Design Package and, by making use of five aspects of design, creates services and their supporting practices that meet business demands for functionality, security, performance, reliability, and flexibility. The Service Design Package makes possible the build, test, and release and deployment activities of Service Transition and the operation, support, and improvement activities within the Service Operation and Continual Service Improvement stages of the Service Lifecycle.

The objectives of Service Transition are to:

- Plan and manage service changes efficiently and effectively
- Manage risks relating to new, changed, or retired services
- Successfully deploy service releases into supported environments

- Set correct expectations on the performance and use of new or changed services
- Ensure that service changes create the expected business value
- Provide good-quality knowledge and information about services and service assets

In order to achieve these objectives, there are many things that need to happen during the Service Transition Lifecycle stage. These include:

- Planning and managing the capacity and resources required to manage service transitions
- Implementing a rigorous framework for evaluating service capabilities and risk profiles before new or changed services are deployed
- Establishing and maintaining the integrity of service assets
- Providing efficient repeatable mechanisms for building, testing, and deploying services and releases
- Ensuring that services can be managed, operated, and supported in accordance with constraints specified during the Service Design stage of the Service Lifecycle

We have already seen how, In Service Strategy, the business strategy and IT strategy are turned into requirements on IT services at a conceptual level. Within Service Design, the conceptual IT service is made real through ensuring that all aspects of the service is designed to fit within the existing IT environment to create a 'real' service solution. In Service Transition, the 'real' is moved into the 'realized': the components required to ensure the service is delivered as expected by the strategy and as design are put into place, tested, and approved for final use within the operational environment.

Value

THE VALUE OF SERVICE TRANSITION rests squarely on realizing the benefits of the IT service and its particular design. This is done by adopting and implementing standard and consistent approaches for Service Transition. The benefits of these approaches will (Service Transition, page 6):

- *Enable projects to estimate the cost, timing, resource requirement, and risks associated with the Service Transition stage more accurately*

- *Result in higher volumes of successful change*
- *Be easier for people to adopt and follow*
- *Enable Service Transition assets to be shared and re-used across projects and services*
- *Reduce delays from unexpected clashes and dependencies—for example, if multiple projects need to use the same test environment at the same time*
- *Reduce the effort spent on managing the Service Transition test and pilot environments*
- *Improve expectation setting for all stakeholders involved in Service Transition, including customers, users, suppliers, partners, and projects*
- *Increase confidence that the new or changed service can be delivered to specification without unexpectedly affecting other services or stakeholders*
- *Ensure that new or changed services will be maintainable and cost-effective*
- *Improve control of service assets and configurations*

Service Transition Processes

Transition Planning and Support

EFFECTIVE TRANSITION PLANNING AND SUPPORT can greatly increase the ability of a service provider in handling high volumes of change and releases across its customer base. *An integrated approach to planning improves the alignment of the service transition plans with the customer, supplier, and business change project plans* (Service Transition, page 52).

Purpose

THE PURPOSE OF THE TRANSITION planning and support process is ensure proper attention is given to the overall planning for service transitions and to coordinate the resources required to implement the new or changed service.

The objectives of transition planning and support are to (Service Transition, page 51):

- *Plan and coordinate the resources to ensure that the requirements of Service Strategy encoded in Service Design are effectively realized in Service Operation*
- *Coordinate activities across projects, suppliers, and service teams, where required*
- *Establish new or changed services into supported environments within the predicted cost, quality, and time estimates*
- *Establish new or modified management information systems and tools, technology and management architectures, service management processes, and measurement methods and metrics to meet requirements established during the Service Design Stage of the lifecycle*
- *Ensure that all parties adopt the common framework of standard re-usable processes and supporting systems in order to improve the effectiveness and efficiency of the integrated planning and coordination activities*
- *Provide clear and comprehensive plans that enable customer and business change projects to align their activities with the service transition plans*
- *Identify, manage, and control risks to minimize the chance of failure and disruption across transition activities and ensure that service transition issues, risks, and deviations are reported to the appropriate stakeholders and decision-makers*
- *Monitor and improve the performance of the Service Transition Lifecycle stage*

Scope

UNLIKE MANY OF THE OTHER service management processes which are focuses on some aspect of the service delivery, the processes of Service Transition are focused on transitioning the service, not the service itself. During the service transition, some question or issue may arise that will require some attention to be given to the service, its requirements, and its design: at this point, the processes from other Service Lifecycle stages to resolve the situation and allow the transition to move forward. Transition planning and support is not responsible for detailed planning of the build, test, and deployment of individual changes or releases; these activities are carried out as part of Change Management and Release and Deployment Management.

The scope of transition planning and support concentrates on the resources, schedules, and budgets required to move the IT service from a blueprint comprised of the service charter and Service Design Package to a working solution assimilated into the current live environment. Some of the high level activities of transition planning and support include (Service Transition, page 52):

- *Maintaining policies, standards, and models for service transition activities and processes*
- *Guiding each major change or new service through all service transition processes*
- *Coordinating the efforts needed to enable multiple transitions to be managed at the same time*
- *Prioritizing conflicting requirements for service transition resources*
- *Planning the budget and resources needed to fulfill future requirements for service transition*
- *Reviewing and improving the performance of transition planning and support activities*
- *Ensuring that Service Transition is coordinated with program and project management, service design, and service development activities*

The transition planning and support process makes heavy use of the Service Knowledge Management System to provide access to the full range of information needed for short-, medium-, and long-range planning.

In order to create and manage plans, transition and support requires access to information about new or changed services. There are many structured and unstructured documents in which this information may be found, for examples, plans, models, standards and guidelines, as well as documents developed as part of other process e.g. Service Design packages, OLA's (Operational Level Agreements) contracts, and process documentation. It is imperative to the creation and management of service transition plans that access to up-to-date versions of these documents be provided in a timely manner. They should all be managed via Change Management and the CMS, and stored within the Service Knowledge Management System (SKMS).

Inputs

THE MAJORITY OF THE INPUTS to the Transition Planning and Support process will be outputs from the processes of Service Design, including:

- Service Design Package, which includes:
- Release package definition and design specification

- Test plans
- Deployment plans
- Service acceptance criteria (SAC)

During the Service Transition, changes to the operational environment will be made which must be preceded by a change proposal detailing the change, its benefits, and its impact. The change will follow the Change Management process and result in either an authorized changed or rejection of the change. Both the change proposal and authorized change will be deliverables within the transition plan managed by the Transition Planning and Support: therefore, they both will be inputs to the process.

Outputs

THE OUTPUTS OF TRANSITION PLANNING and support are simple. A transition strategy will be constructed to define how all transitions will be managed within the organization based on the type and size of transitions expected in the environment. The purpose of the strategy is to drive consistency across all transition work, no matter what IT service is currently being transition. A transition budget is provided that identifies the funding available to conduct the transitions the next few months.

Lastly, Transition Planning and Support will provide an integrated set of service transition plans that are focuses on the individual transitions of IT services.

Knowledge Management

THE QUALITY OF DECISION-MAKING WITHIN the Service Lifecycle depends on the ability and understanding of those parties involved, the understanding of the benefits and consequences of actions taken, and the analysis of any of the surrounding issues involved. All of this, in turn, depends on the availability of accurate and timely knowledge, information, and data provided in a way that can be easily accessed and interpreted by the appropriate parties.

That knowledge within the Service Transition domain might include (Service Transition, page 181):

- *Identity of stakeholders*
- *Acceptable risk levels and performance expectations*
- *Available resource and timescales*

The quality and relevance of the knowledge rests in turn on the accessibility, quality, and continued relevance of the underpinning data and information available to service staff.

Terminology

Term	Definition
data-to-information-to-knowledge-to-wisdom (DIKW)	(ITIL® Service Transition) A way of understanding the relationships between data, information, knowledge, and wisdom. DIKW shows how each of these builds on the others.
service knowledge management system (SKMS)	(ITIL® Service Transition) A set of tools and databases that is used to manage knowledge, information, and data. The service knowledge management system includes the configuration management system, as well as other databases and information systems. The service knowledge management system includes tools for collecting, storing, managing, updating, analyzing, and presenting all the knowledge, information, and data that an IT service provider will need to manage the full lifecycle of IT services.

Purpose

THE PURPOSE OF THE KNOWLEDGE *Management process is to share perspectives, ideas, experience, and information to ensure that these are available in the right place at the right time to enable informed decisions and to improve efficiency by reducing the need to rediscover knowledge.* (Service Transition, page 181).

The objectives of Knowledge Management are to (Service Transition, page 182):

- *Improve the quality of management decision-making by ensuring that reliable and secure knowledge, information, and data is available throughout the Service Lifecycle*
- *Enable the service provider to be more efficient and improve quality of service, increase satisfaction, and reduce the cost of service by reducing the need to rediscover knowledge*
- *Ensure that staff have a clear and common understanding of the value that their services provide to customers and the ways in which benefits are realized from the use of those services*
- *Maintain a Service Knowledge Management System (SKMS) that provides controlled access to knowledge, information, and data that is appropriate for each audience*
- *Gather, analyze, store, share, use, and maintain knowledge, information, and data throughout the service provider organization*

Scope

WHILE KNOWLEDGE MANAGEMENT IS FOUND and primarily explained within the context of Service Transition, it is a process used by all elements of the Service Lifecycle to improve the decision-making that occurs. Knowledge Management can be potentially utilized by every service management process that generates any form of data, information, or knowledge; though an organization may choose to limit its focus to deal with critical aspects of service delivery. Within Service Transition, knowledge management plays two roles: captures and makes available data, information and knowledge relevant to managing and execution transitions in general, and captures and makes available data, information, and knowledge relevant to the IT service being transitioned.

The Knowledge Management process provides oversight over the management of data, information, and knowledge used in the environment. What is not considered to be within the scope of Knowledge Management is the detailed configuration item information that is captured and maintained by Service Asset and Configuration Management (but is interfaced with the same tools and systems).

Benefits

WITH PARTICULAR FOCUS ON SERVICE Transition, knowledge is one of the important elements that need to be transitioned as part of the service changes and associated releases being managed. Examples where successful transition requires effective Knowledge Management include (Service Transition, page 182):

- *User, service desk, support staff, and supplier understanding of the new or changed service, including knowledge of errors signed off before deployment, to facilitate their roles within that service*
- *Awareness of the use of the service and the discontinuation of previous versions*
- *Establishment of the acceptable risk and confidence levels associated with the transition*

Outside of Service Transition, decision-making at the strategic, tactical, and operational levels all benefit from quality knowledge, information, and data being available. Some benefits include:

- Optimized service portfolios (with appropriate balance of investments, resources, services, and technology)
- Improved feedback loops between the design architects and the support staff for services
- Better real-time information and data for operational staff responding to user requests and incidents, as well as documented procedures for resolving known errors and requests

The Data Information Knowledge Wisdom (DIKW) Structure

KNOWLEDGE MANAGEMENT IS GENERALLY DISPLAYED within the Data-to-Information-to-Knowledge-to-Wisdom (DIKW) structure. The use of these terms is detailed below.

Data is a set of discrete facts. On its own, data has no purpose, understanding, or interpretation. Data is simply numbers on a page or facts in a list. Significant amounts of data are captured every day in most organizations and placed in highly structured databases, such as service management and service asset and configuration management tools/systems and databases. Returning to our restaurant analogy, data would represent the number of customers walking through the door, the number of menu items ordered, and a myriad of other numbers and facts about the restaurant and its operations. In IT, an example of data is the date and time at which an incident was logged.

The key knowledge management activities around data are the ability to (Service Transition, Page 183):

- Capture accurate data
- Analyze, synthesize, and then transform the data into information
- Identify relevant data and concentrate resources on its capture
- Maintain integrity of the data
- Archive and purge data to ensure optimal balance between availability of data and use of resources

Information comes from providing context to data; that is, applying the data to some understanding or interpretation of what the data means. For instance, using the number of customers coming to the restaurant and the menu items ordered will provide information useful in understanding the impact on inventory. Information is always generated by combining two or more sets of related data. An example of information in IT is the average time it takes to close priority 2 incidents. This information is created by combining data from the start time, end time, and priority of many incidents.

Information is typically stored in documents, email, and multimedia, which are all considered semi-structured platforms. Knowledge management must manage the information content in a manner that makes it easy to capture, query, find, re-use, and learn from experiences so that mistakes are not repeated and work is not duplicated.

Knowledge is composed of the implicit experiences, ideas, insights, values, and judgments of individuals. Knowledge is generated through experiences of the person and their peers, as well as the analysis of information and data. Understanding the impact on inventory from the number of customers visiting the restaurant and the menu items ordered, allows the restaurant manager to accurately re-order inventory.

However the data may show an unusual increase in the ordering of one menu item over the last year which does not seem to be permanent. The manager utilizes experience (personal and other people's) and information not provided by the numbers to determine an accurate picture of what to order. An example of knowledge is that the average time it takes to close priority 2 incidents has increased by approximately 10% since the newest version of the service was released.

Knowledge is dynamic and context-based. Knowledge is interpretive because it is generated based on what the knowledge creator perceives at the moment; the person may generate different knowledge the next time the situation with the same conditions occur. The situation must be understood by researchers together. Two people may view the same situation and come to different conclusions (knowledge) based on their viewpoint, biases, and opportunity. To complete the whole picture of the situation, all perspectives must be taken into account.

From a Knowledge Management perspective, knowledge puts information into a format that is easy to use to facilitate decision-making. *In Service Transition, this knowledge is not solely based on the transition in progress but is gathered from experience of previous transitions, awareness of recent and anticipated changes, and other areas, which experienced staff will have been unconsciously collecting for some time* (Service Transition, Page 183).

Wisdom makes use of knowledge to create value through correct and well-informed decisions. After determining the correct order for inventory, the restaurant manager makes the weekly order to ensure inventory is sufficient to support the business the following week. Scientists utilize the knowledge obtained though experimentation to develop a drug to fight cancer. Authorities use eyewitness accounts to determine the cause of a tragedy and decide how best to respond. Wisdom involves having the application and contextual awareness to provide strong common-sense judgment.

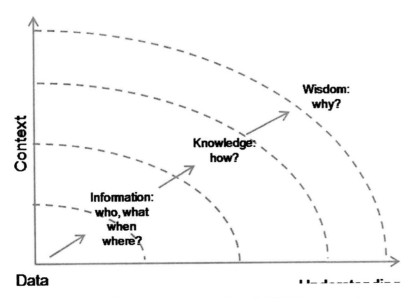

Figure 6.B—Moving from Data to Wisdom (DIKW Structure)
© Crown Copyright 2011 Reproduced under license from the
Cabinet Office

WE CAN USE TOOLS AND databases to capture data, information, and knowledge, but wisdom cannot be captured this way because wisdom is a concept relating to the ability to use knowledge to make correct judgments and decisions.

Service Knowledge Management System (SKMS)

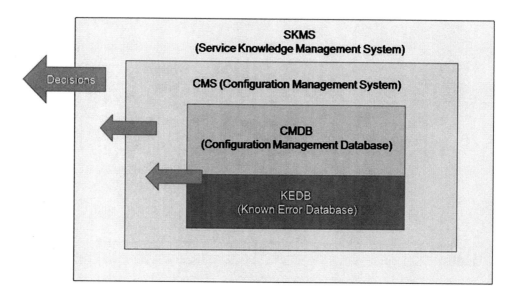

Figure 6.C—Components Making Up the Service Knowledge
Management System

© **Crown** Copyright 2011 Reproduced under license from the Cabinet Office

THE **SKMS** DESCRIBES THE COMPLETE set of tools and databases that are used to manage knowledge and information, including the Configuration Management System as well as other tools and databases. The SKMS stores, manages, updates, and presents all information that an IT service provider needs to manage the full lifecycle of its services. The main purpose of the SKMS is to provide quality information so that informed decisions can be made by the IT service provider.

Whereas the CMS focuses on providing information relating to the configuration of the IT infrastructure, the SKMS has a broader scope (as implied by the diagram), which includes anything pertaining to the needs of service management, including:

- Experience of staff
- Records of peripherals
- Supplier and partner requirements and abilities
- Typical and anticipated user skill levels

Service Asset and Configuration Management

Terminology

Term	Definition
attribute	(ITIL® Service Transition) A piece of information about a configuration item. Examples are name, location, version number, and cost. Attributes of CIs are recorded in a configuration management database (CMDB) and maintained as part of a configuration management system (CMS). See also relationship; configuration management system.
CI type	(ITIL® Service Transition) A category that is used to classify configuration items. The CI type identifies the required attributes and relationships for a configuration record. Common CI types include hardware, document, user, etc.
component	A general term that is used to mean one part of something more complex. For example, a computer system may be a component of an IT service; an application may be a component of a release unit. Components that need to be managed should be configuration items.
configuration	(ITIL® Service Transition) A generic term used to describe a group of configuration items that work together to deliver an IT service or a recognizable part of an IT service. Configuration is also used to describe the parameter settings for one or more configuration items.
configuration baseline	(ITIL® Service Transition) The baseline of a configuration that has been formally agreed and is managed through the change management process. A configuration baseline is used as a basis for future builds, releases, and changes.
configuration item (CI)	(ITIL® Service Transition) Any component or other service asset that needs to be managed in order to deliver an IT service. Information about each configuration item is recorded in a configuration record within the configuration management system and is maintained throughout its lifecycle by service asset and configuration management. Configuration items are under the control of change management. They typically include IT services, hardware, software, buildings, people, and formal documentation, such as process documentation and service level agreements.

Term	Definition
configuration management database (CMDB)	(ITIL® Service Transition) A database used to store configuration records throughout their lifecycle. The configuration management system maintains one or more configuration management databases, and each database stores attributes of configuration items and relationships with other configuration items.
configuration management system (CMS)	(ITIL® Service Transition) A set of tools, data, and information that is used to support service asset and configuration management. The CMS is part of an overall service knowledge management system and includes tools for collecting, storing, managing, updating, analyzing, and presenting data about all configuration items and their relationships. The CMS may also include information about incidents, problems, known errors, changes, and releases. The CMS is maintained by service asset and configuration management and is used by all IT service management processes. See also configuration management database.
configuration record	(ITIL® Service Transition) A record containing the details of a configuration item. Each configuration record documents the lifecycle of a single configuration item. Configuration records are stored in a configuration management database and maintained as part of a configuration management system.
relationship	A connection or interaction between two people or things. In business relationship management, it is the interaction between the IT service provider and the business. In service asset and configuration management, it is a link between two configuration items that identifies a dependency or connection between them. For example, applications may be linked to the servers they run on, and IT services have many links to all the configuration items that contribute to that IT service.
service asset	Any resource or capability of a service provider. See also asset.
status accounting	(ITIL® Service Transition) The activity responsible for recording and reporting the lifecycle of each configuration item.
verification and audit	(ITIL® Service Transition) The activities responsible for ensuring that information in the configuration management system is accurate and that all configuration items have been identified and recorded. Verification includes routine checks that are part of other processes— for example, verifying the serial number of a desktop PC when a user logs an incident. Audit is a periodic, formal check.

Purpose

SERVICES PROVIDE VALUE TO THE business by achieving the objectives and outcomes desired by the business. For services to provide value, its components must be designed to be effective in supporting the service. These components can consist of policies, processes, software, hardware, interfaces, and such. While different organizations may choose to deal with different types of components differently, all components can be considered service assets. If a service asset must be managed in order to ensure the proper delivery of a service, the service asset is considered a configuration item and managed by the Service Asset and Configuration Management (SACM) process.

The purpose of the SACM process is to properly control service assets required to deliver services and ensuring accurate and reliable information about those assets is maintained, including how the assets have been configured and the relationships between assets.

The objectives of SACM are to (Service Transition, page 90):

- *Ensure that assets under the control of the IT organization are identified, controlled, and properly cared for throughout their lifecycle*
- *Identify, control, record, report, audit, and verify services and other configuration items (CIs), including versions, baselines, constituent components, their attributes, and relationships*
- *Account for, manage, and protect the integrity of CIs through the Service Lifecycle by working with Change Management to ensure that only authorized components are used and only authorized changes are made*
- *Ensure the integrity of CIs and configurations required to control the services by establishing and maintaining an accurate and complete Configuration Management System (CMS)*
- *Maintain accurate configuration information on the historical, planned, and current state of services and other CIs*
- *Support efficient and effective service management processes by providing accurate configuration information to enable people to make decisions at the right time—for example, to authorize changes and releases or to resolve incidents and problems*

Scope

SERVICE ASSETS MANAGED BY THE Service Asset and Configuration Management process are known as configuration items (CIs). Some service assets are not configuration items, particularly when they cannot be individually managed: so while all CIs are service assets, not all service assets are CIs. Knowledge is an example of a service asset that is not a configuration item. Service Asset and Configuration Management is focused on the management of the complete lifecycle of every configuration item.

Through Service Asset and Configuration Management, CIs are identified, baselined, and maintained and changes to them are controlled. The process ensures that any release of a new or changed configuration item into operational use or a controlled environment is formally authorized. The relationships between configuration items are captured and presented as a configuration model for the service. The service assets managed by the SACM process do not need to be technology-based and may include work products used in developing services as well as configuration items that would not be considered assets in other parts of the business. SACM also recognizes and managed shared assets between internal and external providers and therefore will manage the interfaces between providers to ensure assets and configuration items are adequately documented and controlled.

Most business will have a process for tracking and reporting the value and ownership of fixed assets: the process is usually called Fixed Asset Management or Financial Asset Management. With this process, the business is covering the financial aspects of the assets in the organization, including IT assets and will maintain an asset register that contains the required financial information. SACM and Fixed Asset Management are not the same process and are typically managed by two different entities in IT and the business, respectively. However, the SACM process must properly care for the fixed assets under the control of IT and have in place a well-defined interface between SACM and Fixed Asset Management. Data from the asset register may be integrated with the Configuration Management System to provide a more complete view of the CIs.

The Configuration Management Database (CDMB)

THE CMDB IS A SET of one or more connected databases and information sources that provide a logical model of the IT infrastructure. It captures Configuration Items (CIs) and the relationships that exist between them. Figure 6.D demonstrates the elements of a CMDB.

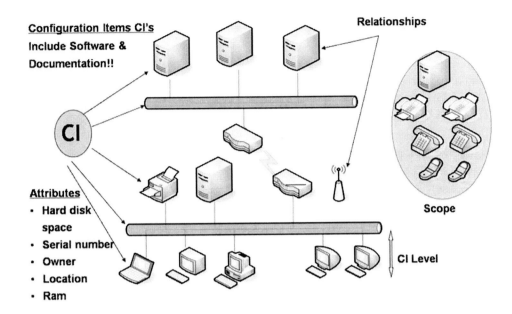

Figure 6.D—The Configuration Management Database (CMDB)

As the above figure shows, it is important to determine the level to which the CMDB will record information about the IT infrastructure and to decide what is not covered within the scope of the CMDB. Components out of scope are those typically not under the control of Change Management (e.g., telecommunication equipment). The CMS is also used for a wide range of purposes, including business processes where information is required for financial, compliance, HR, or other reasons.

At the data level, the CMS may be formed by a combination of physical Configuration Management Databases (CMDBs), as well as other sources they feed and interface information together. Wherever possible, the CMS should provide access to information for other inventories rather than duplicating the data captured. Automation is a factor for success for larger CMS deployments, with discovery, inventory, audit, network management, and other tools being used with interfaces to the CMS.

Activities

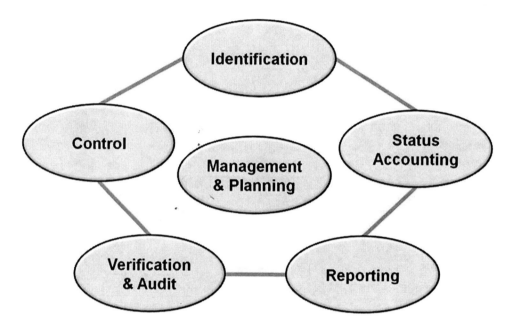

Figure 6.E—Service Asset and Configuration Management Activities

"Based on Cabinet Office ITIL® material. Reproduced under licence from the Cabinet Office"

NOTICE HOW MANAGEMENT AND PLANNING are the central activities. Good, sound Service Asset and Configuration Management requires thorough planning for the operation of the process to work.

Planning:

- Defining the strategy, policy, scope, objectives, processes, and procedures for Service Asset and Configuration Management
- Roles and responsibilities of involved staff and stakeholders
- Location of storage areas and libraries used to hold hardware, software, and documentation
- CMDB design
- CI naming conventions
- Housekeeping, including license management and archiving of CIs

Identification: includes the selection, identification, labeling, and registration of CIs. It is the activity that determines what CIs will be recorded, what their attributes are, and what relationships exist with other CIs. Identification can take place for:
- Hardware and software—including OS
- Business systems—custom built
- Packages—off the shelf
- Physical databases
- Feeds between databases and links
- Configuration baselines
- Software releases
- Documentation

Control: where the CMDB is utilized to store or modify configuration data. Effective control ensures that only authorized and identifiable CIs are recorded from receipt to disposal in order to protect the integrity of the CMDB. Control occurs anytime the CMDB is altered, including:
- Registration of all new CIs and versions
- Updating of CI records and license control
- Updates in connection with RFCs and Change Management
- Updating the CMDB after periodic checking of physical items

Status Accounting: the reporting of all current and historical data concerned with each CI throughout its lifecycle. Provides information on:
- Configuration baselines
- Latest software item versions
- The person responsible for status change
- CI change/incident/problem history

Verification and Audit: reviews and audits verify the existence of CIs, checking that they are correctly recorded in the CMDB and that there is conformity between the documented baselines and the actual environment to which they refer. Configuration audits should occur at the following times:
- Before and after major changes to the IT infrastructure
- Following recovery from disaster
- In response to the detection of an unauthorized CI
- At regular intervals

Benefits

THE MAJORITY OF BENEFITS ENABLED by effective Service Asset and Configuration Management can be seen in improvements of other Service Management processes. By having quality asset and configuration data available, the benefits to other processes include:

- Better forecasting and planning of changes
- Changes and releases to be assessed, planned, and delivered successfully
- Incidents and problems to be resolved within the service level targets
- Changes to be traceable from requirements
- Enhanced ability to identify the costs for a service

Benefits that may be seen to be provided primarily by the process alone include:

- Better adherence to standards
- Greater compliance to legal and regulatory obligations
- Optimum software licensing by ensuring correlation between licenses needed against the number of purchases
- The data about CIs and methods of controlling CIs is consolidated—reduces auditing effort
- Opens opportunities for consolidation in CIs to support services

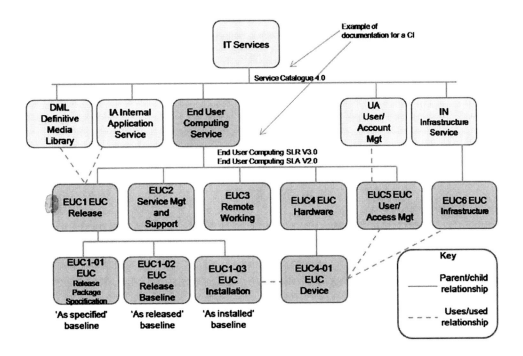

Figure 6.F—Example Configuration Breakdown for an IT Service
© Crown Copyright 2011 Reproduced under license from the
Cabinet Office

Inputs

INPUTS TO SERVICE ASSET AND Configuration Management include (Service Transition, page 112):

- *Designs, plans, and configurations from Service Design Packages*
- *Requests for change and work orders from Change Management*
- *Actual configuration information collected by tools and audits*
- *Information in the organization's fixed asset register*

Outputs

OUTPUTS FROM SERVICE ASSET AND Configuration Management include (Service Transition, page 112):

- *New and updated configuration records*

- *Updated asset information for use in updating the fixed asset register*
- *Information about attributes and relationships of configuration items for use by all other service management processes. This information should be presented in appropriate views for each audience*
- *Configuration snapshots and baselines*
- *Status reports and other consolidated configuration information*
- *Audit reports*

Change Management

THE ABILITY TO CONTROL AND manage changes to defined IT services and their supporting elements is viewed as a fundamental part of quality service management. When reviewing the typical strategic objectives of an IT service provider, most of these are underpinned by the requirement of effective change control. These include strategies focusing on time-to-market, increased market share or high availability, and security platforms, all of which require a controlled process by which to assess, control, and manage changes with varying levels of rigor.

Changes arise for a number of reasons:
- From requests of the business or customers, seeking to improve services, reduce costs, or increase ease and effectiveness of delivery and support
- From internal IT groups looking to proactively improve services or to resolve errors and correct service disruption

The process of Change Management typically exists in order to:
- Optimize risk exposure (defined from both business and IT perspectives)
- Minimize the severity of any impact or disruption
- Deliver successful changes at the first attempt

To deliver these benefits while being careful not to cause excessive delays or bottlenecks as part of a coordinated approach to Service Transition, it is important to consider the diverse types of changes that will be assessed and how a balance can be maintained in regards to the varying needs and potential impacts of changes. In light of this, it is important to interpret the following Change Management guidance with the understanding that is intended to be scaled to suit the organization and the size, complexity, and risk of changes being assessed.

Terminology

Term	Definition
change	(ITIL® Service Transition) The addition, modification, or removal of anything that could have an effect on IT services. The scope should include changes to all architectures, processes, tools, metrics, and documentation, as well as changes to IT services and other configuration items.
change advisory board (CAB)	(ITIL® Service Transition) A group of people that support the assessment, prioritization, authorization, and scheduling of changes. A change advisory board is usually made up of representatives from all areas within the IT service provider, the business, and third parties, such as suppliers.
change model	(ITIL® Service Transition) A repeatable way of dealing with a particular category of change. A change model defines specific agreed steps that will be followed for a change of this category. Change models may be very complex with many steps that require authorization (e.g., major software release) or may be very simple with no requirement for authorization (e.g., password reset). See also change advisory board; standard change.
change proposal	(ITIL® Service Strategy) (ITIL® Service Transition) A document that includes a high level description of a potential service introduction or significant change, along with a corresponding business case and an expected implementation schedule. Change proposals are normally created by the service portfolio management process and are passed to change management for authorization. Change management will review the potential impact on other services, on shared resources, and on the overall change schedule. Once the change proposal has been authorized, service portfolio management will charter the service.
change record	(ITIL® Service Transition) A record containing the details of a change. Each change record documents the lifecycle of a single change. A change record is created for every request for change that is received, even those that are subsequently rejected. Change records should reference the configuration items that are affected by the change. Change records may be stored in the configuration management system or elsewhere in the service knowledge management system.
change request	See request for change.

Term	Definition
change schedule	(ITIL® Service Transition) A document that lists all authorized changes and their planned implementation dates, as well as the estimated dates of longer-term changes. A change schedule is sometimes called a forward schedule of change, even though it also contains information about changes that have already been implemented.
emergency change	(ITIL® Service Transition) A change that must be introduced as soon as possible—for example, to resolve a major incident or implement a security patch. The change management process will normally have a specific procedure for handling emergency changes. See also emergency change advisory board.
emergency change advisory board (ECAB)	(ITIL® Service Transition) A subgroup of the change advisory board that makes decisions about emergency changes. Membership may be decided at the time a meeting is called and depends on the nature of the emergency change.
normal change	(ITIL® Service Transition) A change that is not an emergency change or a standard change. Normal changes follow the defined steps of the change management process.
remediation	(ITIL® Service Transition) Actions taken to recover after a failed change or release. Remediation may include back-out, invocation of service continuity plans, or other actions designed to enable the business process to continue.
request for change (RFC)	(ITIL® Service Transition) A formal proposal for a change to be made. It includes details of the proposed change and may be recorded on paper or electronically. The term is often misused to mean a change record or the change itself.
standard change	(ITIL® Service Transition) A pre-authorized change that is low risk, relatively common, and follows a procedure or work instruction—for example, a password reset or provision of standard equipment to a new employee. Requests for change are not required to implement a standard change, and they are logged and tracked using a different mechanism, such as a service request. See also change model.

Purpose

Like many activities in IT, a change has a beginning and an end. The Change Management process provides a structure for controlling all changes from their initiation to their end and ensures that the benefits of the changes can be realized with minimum disruption to other IT services. If a restaurant owner wanted to change a menu item on the menu, a number of tasks must be considered, such:

- Design layout and publication of new menus
- Ingredients for menu item included in ordering forms
- Possible contracts with new or existing suppliers
- Possible equipment procurement and installation
- Training of staff members
- Marketing of change
- Schedules

All of this must be done without disruption to the business.

The purpose of Change Management is to provide an opportunity and format to ensure that all aspects of the change have been considered. The process will inform potential stakeholders in the change to ensure they have been heard and their support or concerns addressed regarding the change.

The objectives of Change Management are to (Service Transition, page 61):

- *Respond to the customer's changing business requirements, while maximizing value and reducing incidents, disruption, and re-work*
- *Respond to the business and IT requests for change that will align the services with the business needs*
- *Ensure that changes are recorded and evaluated and that authorized changes are prioritized, planned, tested, implemented, documented, and reviewed in a controlled manner*
- *Ensure that all changes to configuration items are recorded in the configuration management system*
- *Optimize overall business risk—it is often correct to minimize business risk, but sometimes it is appropriate to knowingly accept a risk because of the potential benefit.*

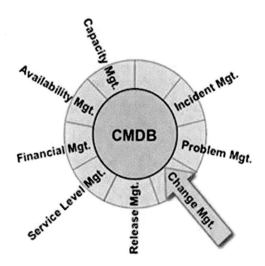

Figure 6.G—Change Management

CHANGE MANAGEMENT ACTS AS the greatest contributor to the CMDB, as changes to the CMDB must be assessed and authorized by Change Management first.

To work effectively, Change Management needs to remain impartial to the needs of any one particular IT group or customer in order to make effective decisions that best support the overall organizational objectives.

Scope

THE TERM 'CHANGE' HAS MANY meanings; however, the best definition of a service change is:

> *"Any alteration in the state of a Configuration Item (CI). This includes the addition, modification, or removal of approved, supported, or baselined hardware, network, software, application, environment, system, desktop build, or associated documentation."*

It is important that every organization defines those changes that lie outside the scope of their service change process (such as operational or business process and policy changes).

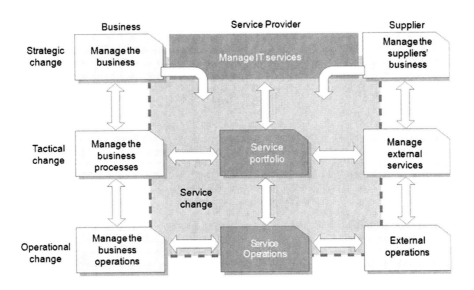

Figure 6.H—Scope of Change Management for IT Services
© Crown Copyright 2011 Reproduced under license from the
Cabinet Office

THIS FIGURE DEMONSTRATES THE TYPICAL scope of the Change Management process for an
IT service provider and how it interfaces with the business and suppliers at strategic,
tactical, and operational levels. As discussed in Service Strategy, Service Portfolios
provide the clear definition of all planned, current, and retired services.

"Remember: Not every change is an improvement, but every improvement is a change!"

Change Models

THE DEFINITION OF DIFFERENT PROCESS models will allow an organization to maintain
a balance between providing an appropriate level of control for changes without
causing bottlenecks or restricting business growth. Change Models define how
various categories of changes are assessed and authorized with different mechanisms
and activities used to process and deliver changes based on the change type. The
defined Change Models should also include:

- What steps should be taken to manage the change
- Roles and responsibilities

- Timescales and thresholds for actions
- Escalation procedures

Change Models defined within ITIL® include the following:

NORMAL Change:	A change that follows all of the steps of the change process. It is assessed by either a Change Manager or Change Advisory Board. Normal changes will often be further defined by the relative impact and complexity, which will escalate the change for assessment to the most appropriate person or group.
STANDARD Change:	A *pre-approved* change that is low risk, relatively common, and follows a procedure or work instruction. E.g., password reset or provision of standard equipment to a new employee. RFCs are not required to implement a standard change, and they are logged and tracked using a different mechanism, such as a **service request**. While standard changes are effectively pre-approved by Change Management, they may still require forms of authorization, such as by other groups like Human Resources (HR) or financial departments.

The main elements of a standard change are that:

- Authority is effectively given ahead of time
- The tasks are well known, documented, and proven
- There is a defined trigger to initiate the Request For Change (RFC)
- Budgetary approval is generally defined or controlled by the requester
- The risk is typically low and always well understood

Over time and as the IT organization matures, the list of standard changes should increase in order to maintain optimum levels of efficiency and effectiveness.

EMERGENCY Change: A change that must be introduced as soon as possible, e.g., to resolve a major incident or implement a security patch.

The Change Management process will normally have a specific procedure for handling emergency changes quickly without sacrificing normal management controls. Organizations should be careful to ensure that the number of emergency changes be kept to a minimum because they are typically more disruptive and prone to failure.

To enable this to occur, methods of assessment and documentation are typically modified with some documentation occurring after the change has occurred.

Activities

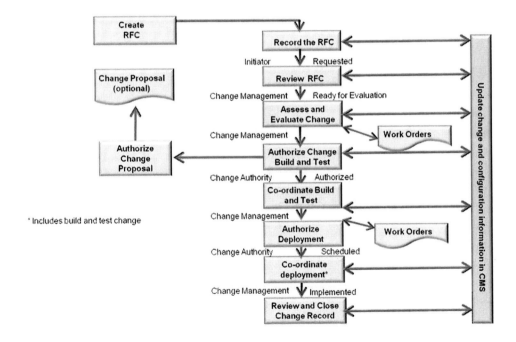

Figure 6.I—The Activities of Change Management
© Crown Copyright 2011 Reproduced under license from the Cabinet Office

Where can RFCs be initiated?
Anywhere (Other ITIL® processes, customers, end-users etc.)

Who does the actual build/test/implement?
- Technical areas
- Project teams
- Release and Deployment Management

Important Steps:
1. The RFC is logged
2. An initial review is performed (to filter RFCs)
3. The RFCs are assessed—may require involvement of CAB or ECAB
4. Authorization of change build and test by the Change Manager
5. Coordination of the build and test, e.g., work orders are issued for the build of the change (carried out by other groups)
6. Change Management authorizes deployment
7. Change Management coordinates the deployment (with multiple checkpoints)
8. The change is reviewed (Post Implementation Review)
9. The change is closed

Change Proposals

CHANGES THAT INVOLVE MAJOR ORGANIZATIONAL impact, risk, or cost will generally be instigated by the Service Portfolio Management process. Before the new or changed service is drawn up, it is important to review the change for its likely impact on other on shared resources, the change schedule and on other services.

In order to identify possible conflicts of resources or other issues change proposals must be submitted to Change Management. Authorizing the change proposal does not imply authorization for the implementation of the change but it will allow the service to be chartered so that service design process can begin.

A change proposal is used to convey a high-level account of the change. This change proposal is generally created by the Service Portfolio Management process and is passed to Change Management to be authorized. In some organizations, change proposals may be created by a program management office or by individual projects. The change proposal should include (Service Transition, Page 67):

- *A high-level description of the new, changed, or retired service, including business outcomes to be supported and utility and warranty to be provided*
- *A full business case including risks, issues, and alternatives, as well as budget and financial expectations*
- *An outline schedule for design and implementation of the change*

Change Management reviews the change proposal and the current change schedule, identifies any potential conflicts or issues, and responds to the change proposal by either authorizing it or documenting the issues that need to be resolved. When the change proposal is authorized, the change schedule is updated to include outline implementation dates for the proposed change.

After the new or changed service is chartered, RFCs will be used in the normal way to request authorization for specific changes. These RFCs will be associated with the change proposal so that Change Management has a view of the overall strategic intent and can prioritize and review these RFCs appropriately (Service Transition, Page 67).

Remediation planning

A CHANGE SHOULD NEVER BE authorized without having addressed what exactly needs to happen if it is not successful. Preferably, back-out plan will be in place, which will return the organization to its original state, often by reloading of a baseline set of CIs, especially data and software. However, not all changes are reversible, in which case an alternative approach to remediation is required.

In the event of a failure, revisiting the change itself may be required, or the situation may be so severe that calling upon the organization's business continuity plan is required. Only by taking in to account what remediation options there are available before bringing about a change and by establishing whether the remediation is feasible (e.g., it successfully passes all tests) can the risk of the proposed change be established and suitable actions taken.

In order for there to be adequate time in the agreed change window for remediation, all change implementation plans should include milestones and other triggers for implementation of the remediation, should it be required.

Assessing and Evaluating Changes

To ensure that the Change Management process does not become a bottleneck, it is important to define what Change Models will be used to ensure effective and efficient control and implementation of RFCs.

Level	Change Authority	Potential Impact/Risk
1	Business Executive Board	High cost/risk change—executive decision
2	The IT Management (Steering) Board	Change impacts multiple services/ organizational divisions
3	Change Advisory Board (CAB) or Emergency CAB (ECAB)	Change impacts only local/service group
4	Change Manager	Change to a specific component of an IT Service
5	Local Authorization	Standard change

Authorization of Changes

While the responsibility for authorization for changes lies with the Change Manager, they in turn will ensure they have the approval of three main areas:

- Financial Approval—what is it going to cost? And what is the cost of not doing it?
- Business Approval—what are the consequences to the business? And what are the consequences of not doing it?
- Technology Approval—what are the consequences to the infrastructure? And what are the consequences of not doing it?

Key Points:
- Change Management should consider the implications of performing the change as well as the impacts of NOT implementing the change
- Importance of empowering Change Manager as their primary role is to protect the integrity of the IT infrastructure

Relationship with Project Management:

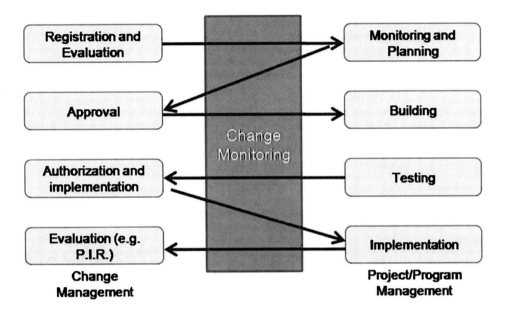

Figure 6.J—Relationship with Project Management
© Crown Copyright 2011 Reproduced under license from Cabinet Office.

How does Change Management work with Project Management?
- Change Management authorizes, controls, and coordinates changes but does not plan, build, test, or implement changes
- Change Management is concerned with Remediation Planning to ensure that each RFC has a fallback/rollback plan

Roles and Responsibilities

- **Change Manager**
  - ▷ Administration of all RFCs
  - ▷ Prepare RFCs for CAB meetings, communicate change schedule for Service Desk
  - ▷ Authorize (or reject) changes
- **Change Advisory Board (CAB)**
- Advises Change Manager on authorization issues for RFCs with significant or major impact

- Typical representatives for a CAB under normal conditions are:
  - ‣ The Change Manager (chairs the CAB)
  - ‣ Customer representatives
  - ‣ User management
  - ‣ Application Developers/Supporters
  - ‣ Technical Experts and Consultants
  - ‣ Other Services Staff
  - ‣ Vendors and Suppliers

Rather than having a static list of members, the CAB should include both static and dynamic members who will attend based on the needs for the changes being discussed.

Inputs

CHANGES MAY BE SUBMITTED AS *an RFC, often with an associated change proposal that provides inputs from the Service Strategy stage of the Service Lifecycle.* (Service Transition, Page 85) *The inputs include:*

- *Policy and strategy for change and release*
- *Request for change*
- *Change proposal*
- *Plans—change, transition, release, test, evaluation, and remediation*
- *Current change schedule and PSO*
- *Evaluation reports and interim evaluation reports*
- *Current assets or configuration items, e.g., baseline, service package, release package*
- *As-planned configuration baseline*
- *Test results, test report, and evaluation report*

Outputs

Outputs from the process will be (Service Transition, Page 85):

- *Rejected and cancelled RFCs*
- *Authorized changes*
- *Authorized change proposals*
- *Change to the services, service, or infrastructure resulting from authorized changes*

- *New, changed, or disposed configuration items, e.g., baseline, service package, release package*
- *Revised change schedule*
- *Revised PSO*
- *Authorized change plans*
- *Change decisions and actions*
- *Change documents and records*
- *Change management reports*

Release and Deployment Management

Often forgotten or ignored in many IT Service Management implementations or initiatives, Release and Deployment can be mistakenly seen as the poor cousin of Change Management—of less importance and priority to both the business and IT organizations.

Much of the confusion and misunderstanding is perpetuated by the idea that Release and Deployment only focuses on the actual distribution of changes to the live environment. While timely and accurate distribution is indeed a goal of the process, the actual scope includes all of the activities, systems, and functions required to build, test, and deploy a release into production and enable effective handover to service operations.

In conjunction with the use of Change Management, Release and Deployment will enhance an organization's capabilities to develop, compile, reuse, distribute, and rollback releases in accordance with defined policies that improve efficiency and reduce business disruption.

Go back to the changing of the menu item on a restaurant manager. The change being made is the addition of a new menu time; however it is likely that a substantial amount of work was already performed before this point. Without going into too much detail about the strategic and design stages of introducing a new menu item, let's assume that a menu item has been under consideration for a couple of months. It may have been a dinner special, or a limited-time offering. Restaurant chains will have focus groups and taste tests. Data would have been collected to determine its popularity and value to the customer. All this activity would have been done before the menu item is formally placed on the menu in a permanent capacity. While Change Management would be responsible for the menu change, most of the other work would be done through Release and Deployment Management.

Terminology

Term	Definition
build	(ITIL® Service Transition) The activity of assembling a number of configuration items to create part of an IT service. The term is also used to refer to a release that is authorized for distribution—for example, server build or laptop build. See also configuration baseline.
definitive media library (DML)	(ITIL® Service Transition) One or more locations in which the definitive and authorized versions of all software configuration items are securely stored. The definitive media library may also contain associated configuration items, such as licenses and documentation. It is a single logical storage area, even if there are multiple locations. The definitive media library is controlled by service asset and configuration management and is recorded in the configuration management system.
deployment	(ITIL® Service Transition) The activity responsible for movement of new or changed hardware, software, documentation, process, etc. to the live environment. Deployment is part of the release and deployment management process.
release	(ITIL® Service Transition) One or more changes to an IT service that are built, tested, and deployed together. A single release may include changes to hardware, software, documentation, processes, and other components.
release package	(ITIL® Service Transition) A set of configuration items that will be built, tested, and deployed together as a single release. Each release package will usually include one or more release units.
release record	(ITIL® Service Transition) A record that defines the content of a release. A release record has relationships with all configuration items that are affected by the release. Release records may be in the configuration management system or elsewhere in the service knowledge management system.
release unit	(ITIL® Service Transition) Components of an IT service that are normally released together. A release unit typically includes sufficient components to perform a useful function. For example, one release unit could be a desktop PC, including hardware, software, licenses, documentation, etc. A different release unit may be the complete payroll application, including IT operations procedures and user training.
release window	See change window.
test	(ITIL® Service Transition) An activity that verifies that a configuration item, IT service, process, etc. meets its specification or agreed requirements.

Purpose

THE RELEASE AND DEPLOYMENT MANAGEMENT process provides the planning, scheduling, and controlling practices applied to the build, test, and deployment of releases, with the intent to deliver new functionality required by the business and protecting the integrity of existing services.

The objectives of Release and Deployment Management are to (Service Transition, Page 114):

- *Define and agree Release and Deployment Management plans with customers and stakeholders*
- *Create and test release packages that consist of related configuration items that are compatible with each other*
- *Ensure that the integrity of a release package and its constituent components is maintained throughout the transition activities and that all release packages are stored in a DML and recorded accurately in the CMS*
- *Deploy release packages from the DML to the live environment following an agreed plan and schedule*
- *Ensure that all release packages can be tracked, installed, tested, verified, and/or uninstalled or backed out if appropriate*
- *Ensure that organization and stakeholder change is managed during release and deployment activities (see Chapter 5)*
- *Ensure that a new or changed service and its enabling systems, technology, and organization are capable of delivering the agreed utility and warranty*
- *Record and manage deviations, risks, and issues related to the new or changed service and take necessary corrective action*
- *Ensure that there is knowledge transfer to enable the customers and users to optimize their use of the service to support their business activities*
- *Ensure that skills and knowledge are transferred to service operation functions to enable them to effectively and efficiently deliver, support, and maintain the service according to required warranties and service levels.*

Scope

THE SCOPE OF RELEASE AND Deployment Management includes the processes, systems, and functions to package, build, test, and deploy a release into live use, establish the service specified in the Service Design Package, and formally hand the service over to the service operation functions. The scope includes all configuration items required to implement a release, for example: (Service Transition, Page 115).

- *Physical assets, such as a server or network*
- *Virtual assets, such as a virtual server or virtual storage*
- *Applications and software*
- *Training for users and IT staff*
- *Services, including all related contracts and agreements*

Release and Deployment Management works with the Service Validation and Testing process to carry out the testing requirements of a new release and Change Management to generate and authorize changes during the various stages of a release. The process will also work with Change Management and the Service Desk to communicate any scheduled deployments of new releases. A well-planned release will significantly but positively impact service costs by reducing the potential risks associated with complexity and preventing any problems from occurring because of poor design. Done effectively, Release and Deployment Management will provide value to IT and the business by (Service Transition, Page 115):

- *Delivering change faster and at optimum cost and minimized risk*
- *Assuring that customers and users can use the new or changed service in a way that supports the business goals*
- *Improving consistency in implementation approach across the business change, service teams, suppliers, and customers*
- *Contributing to meeting auditable requirements for traceability through service transition*

Well-planned and implemented Release and Deployment Management will make a significant difference to an organization's service costs. A poorly designed release or deployment will, at best, force IT personnel to spend significant amounts of time troubleshooting problems and managing complexity. At worst, it can cripple the environment and degrade live services.

Release and Deployment Management also works closely with Change Management and the Service Desk to inform users of scheduled changes/deployments. Tools used to do this can include:

- E-mail notification
- SMS notification
- Verbal communication

Release Policy

A RELEASE POLICY IS THE formal documentation of the overarching strategy for releases and was derived from the Service Design stage of the Service Lifecycle. It is the governing policy document for the process and must accommodate the majority of releases being implemented. Typical contents of a Release Policy include:

- Level of infrastructure to be controlled by releases
- Preferred structure and schedules for release packages
- Definition of major and minor releases, emergency fixes
- Expected deliverables for each type of release
- Policy on the production and execution of back out plans
- How and where releases should be documented
- Blackout windows for releases based on business or IT requirements
- Roles and responsibilities defined for the Release and Deployment process
- Supplier contacts and escalation points

Four phases of Release and Deployment Management

THERE ARE FOUR PHASES TO Release and Deployment Management (see Figure 6.K) (ITIL: Service Transition, Page 122):

- *Release and deployment planning:* This phase focuses on the developing plans for creating and deploying the release. The phase starts with change authorization to plan a release and ends with change authorization to create the release.
- *Release build and test:* This phase will build, test, and check the release package into the Definitive Media Library (DML). The phase starts with change authorization to build the release and ends with change authorization for the baselined release package to be checked into the DML

by *Service Asset and Configuration Management. This phase only happens once for each release.*

- **Deployment:** *This phase ensures the release package in the DML is deployed to the live environment. The phase starts with change authorization to deploy the release package to one or more target environments and ends with handover to the service operation functions and early life support. Several separate deployment phases may exist for each release, depending on the planned deployment options.*
- **Review and close:** *This phase captures and reviews the experience and feedback, performance targets and achievements, and ensures lessons are learned*

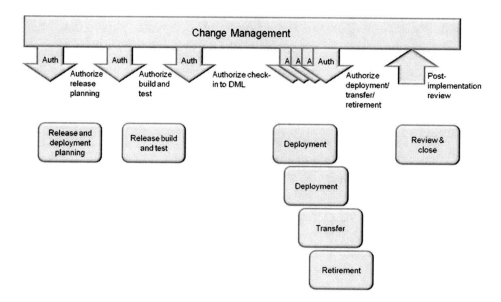

Figure 6.K—Relationship with Project Management
© Crown Copyright 2011 Reproduced under license from the Cabinet Office

FIGURE **6.K** SHOWS MULTIPLE POINTS where an authorized change triggers Release and Deployment Management activity. This does not require a separate RFC at each stage. Some organizations manage a whole release with a single change request and separate authorization at each stage for activities to continue, while other organizations require a separate RFC for each stage. Both of these approaches are acceptable; what is important is that Change Management authorization is received before commencing each stage.

Inputs

The inputs to Release and Deployment management are (Service Transition, Page 146):

- *Authorized change*
- *Service Design Package (SDP) including:*
  - ▷ *A service charter that defines the requirements from the business/ customer for the service, including a description of the expected utility and warranty, as well as outline budgets and timescales*
  - ▷ *Service models that describe the structure and dynamics of how the service is operated and managed*
  - ▷ *Service acceptance criteria*
  - ▷ *IT service continuity plan and related business continuity plan*
  - ▷ *Service management and operations plans and standards*
  - ▷ *Technology and procurement standards and catalogues*
  - ▷ *Acquired service assets and components and their documentation*
  - ▷ *Build models and plans*
  - ▷ *Environment requirements and specifications for build, test, release, training, disaster recovery, pilot, and deployment*
  - ▷ *Release policy and release design from Service Design*
  - ▷ *Release and Deployment models including template plans*
  - ▷ *Exit and entry criteria for each stage of Release and Deployment Management*

Outputs

The outputs from Release and Deployment Management are (Service Transition, Page 147):

- *New, changed, or retired services*
- *Release and deployment plan*
- *Updates to Change Management for the release and deployment activities*
- *Service notification*

- *Notification to Service Catalog Management to update the Service Catalog with the relevant information about the new or changed service*
- *New tested service capability and environment, including SLA, other agreements and contracts, changed organization, competent and motivated people, established business and service management processes, installed applications, converted databases, technology infrastructure, products, and facilities*
- *New or changed service management documentation*
- *SLA, underpinning OLAs, and contracts*
- *New or changed service reports*
- *Tested continuity plans*
- *Complete and accurate configuration item list with an audit trail for the CIs in the release package and also the new or changed service and infrastructure configurations*
- *Updated service capacity plan aligned to the relevant business plans*
- *Baselined release package—checked in to DML and ready for future deployments*
- *Service transition report*

Service Transition Summary

EFFECTIVE SERVICE TRANSITION CAN SIGNIFICANTLY improve a Service Provider's ability to effectively handle high volumes of change and releases across its customer base. Other benefits delivered include:

- Increased success rate of changes and releases
- More accurate estimations of service levels and warranties
- Less variation of costs against those estimated in budgets
- Less variation from resources plans

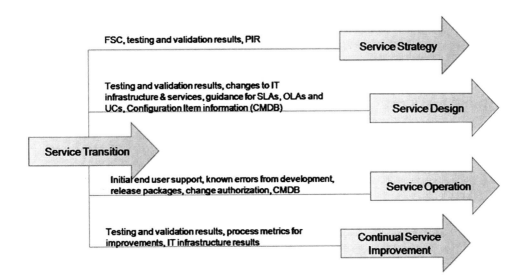

Figure 6.L —Some Service Transition Outputs to Other Lifecycle Stages

Service Transition Scenario

Transition Planning and Support
- Plan and coordinate the resources to ensure that the requirements are met
- Coordinate the activities across projects, suppliers, and service teams

Knowledge Management Considerations
- If your SKMS is established, you would be able to identify if you have the skills required to support videoconferencing, for example
- The SKMS will also help to determine the team required to build, test, and deploy HYPE
- Place to record and transfer user and support documentation

Service Asset and Configuration Management Considerations
- HYPE software is registered as a CI and relationships between it and the other CIs are known if/when an incident occurs. This will assist to speed up resolution times.
- Decision made as to whether webcams are CIs themselves or an attribute of the PC/laptop it is attached to

Change Management Considerations

- Ensure that the introduction of this new service minimizes impact on other services e.g., through testing, it is found that the RAM required slows down the PC, affecting other business critical apps. Change Management will assist with decision-making to determine the best path of action (through CAB).

Release and Deployment Management Considerations

- Builds and tests HYPE—decision here to limit video resolution to minimize bandwidth
- Stores original authorized software in DML
- Ensures that design aspects are adhered to when building (e.g., ensuring that the password policies are adhered to)
- Organizes training on using HYPE—priority given to Service Desk 1st and pilot users

Service Transition Review Questions

Question 1
The key element of a standard change is?
1. Documentation of a pre-approved procedure for implementing the change
2. Low risk to the production environment
3. No requirement for service downtime
4. It can be included in the next monthly or quarterly release

Question 2
The four phases of Release and Deployment are:

1. Release and deployment planning
2. Release build and test
3.
4. Review and close
   ▹ Deployment
   ▹ Change authorization
   ▹ Change coordination
   ▹ Release coordination

Question 3
The 4 spheres of Knowledge Management are:

1. Data, facts, knowledge, wisdom
2. Ideas, facts, knowledge, wisdom
3. Data, information, facts, wisdom
4. Data, information, knowledge, wisdom

Question 4
Which activity in Service Asset and Configuration Management would help to ascertain whether the recorded configuration items conform to the physical environment?

1. Control
2. Verification and audit
3. Identification
4. Status accounting

Question 5

After a change has been implemented, an evaluation is performed. What is this evaluation called?

1. Forward Schedule of Changes (FSC)
2. Post Implementation Review (PIR)
3. Service Improvement Program (SIP)
4. Service Level Requirement (SLR)

Question 6

Which of the following is not a change type?

1. Standard change
2. Normal change
3. Quick change
4. Emergency change

Question 7

Which process is responsible for maintaining software items in the Definitive Media Library (DML)?

1. Release and Deployment Management
2. Service Asset and Configuration Management
3. Service validation and testing
4. Change Management

Question 8

Which process or function is responsible for communicating the change schedule to the users?

1. Change Management
2. Service Desk
3. Release and Deployment Management
4. Service Level Management

Question 9
Which of the following best describes a baseline?

1. Used as a reference point for later comparison
2. The starting point of any project
3. The end point of any project
4. A rollback procedure

Question 10
The main objective of Change Management is to?

1. Ensure that any changes are approved and recorded
2. Ensure that standardized methods and procedures are used for controlled handling of all changes
3. Ensure that any change requests are managed through the CAB
4. Ensure that the CAB takes responsibility for all change implementation

SERVICE OPERATION

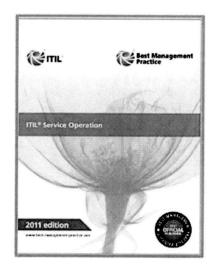

Figure 7.A—Service Operation

"© Crown copyright 2011 Reproduced under licence from the Cabinet Office"

Purpose

The primary purpose of the Service Operation stage of the Service Lifecycle is to coordinate, deliver, and manage services to ensure that the levels agreed with the business, customers, and users are met or exceeded. Service Operation is also responsible for the ongoing management of the technology that is used to deliver and support the services.

Service Operation accepts the new, modified, retiring, or retired services from Service Transition, once the test and acceptance criteria have been met. Service Operation then ensures that those new or modified services will meet all of their agreed operational targets, as well as ensuring that all existing services continue to meet all of their targets. This stage of the lifecycle performs the vital day-to-day activities and processes that collect the data and information that are essential to the activities of Continual Service Improvement, the final stage of the Service Lifecycle.

In the previous sections, the stages of Service Strategy, Service Design, and Service Transition were explored. Through this exploration, the requirements of the business were turned into conceptual services, designed and introduced as real service solutions, and transitioned into a realized state. In Service Operations, the realized is monitored and maintained to ensure that business value and benefits are achieved daily. It does not matter how well the conceptualization, design, or transition of a service is if the service is poorly supported, operated, and managed. Effective processes should be in place with supporting tools to allow an overall view of the service and service operation, which enables operations staff to rapidly detect any threats or failures to the service and service quality.

The objectives of Service Operation are to (Service Operation, Page 4):

- *Maintain business satisfaction and confidence in IT through effective and efficient delivery and support of agreed IT services*
- *Minimize the impact of service outages on day-to-day business activities*
- *Ensure that access to agreed IT services is only provided to those authorized to receive those services*

Value to the business

WHILE MANY OF THE SERVICE management processes will have some responsibilities within Service Operations, the service management processes focused on in Service Operation have one thing in common – they are instance-based. Each of the processes is designed to handle instances decisively and consistently. In request fulfilment and access management, the instances are requests; in incident management, the instances are incidents; problem management; problems; event management; events.

In the restaurant, all the policies, processes, equipment, menu items, and other components are in place to ensure one thing – each customer has an excellent dining experience. Complaints, compliments, and breakdowns must be handled appropriately when they arise. How they are handled must be comply to the pre-defined rules established by the restaurant in the form of policies and they must be consistent to prevent any confusion.

Many of the approaches adopted by Service Operations to deliver IT benefits to the business, customers, and users include (Service Operation, Page 5):

- *Reduce unplanned labor and costs for both the business and IT through optimized handling of service outages and identification of their root causes*
- *Reduce the duration and frequency of service outages, which will allow the business to take full advantage of the value created by the services they are receiving*
- *Provide operational results and data that can be used by other ITIL® processes to improve services continually and provide justification for investing in ongoing service improvement activities and supporting technologies*
- *Meet the goals and objectives of the organization's security policy by ensuring that IT services will be accessed only by those authorized to use them*
- *Provide quick and effective access to standard services, which business staff can use to improve their productivity or the quality of business services and products*
- *Provide a basis for automated operations, thus increasing efficiencies and allowing expensive human resources to be used for more innovative work, such as designing new or improved functionality or defining new ways in which the business can exploit technology for increased competitive advantage*

The processes of Service Operations are performed by every IT staff member in the organization. While the Service Desk may be noted for their extensive involvement in Incident Management or Request Fulfilment, it is also true that any person supporting IT may be involved in resolving incidents or handling requests regardless of their function, role, or assignment. Therefore, every IT staff member must understand when they are working within the scope of these processes and comply to the policies and procedures relevant to the process they are working under. Knowledge Management will play an important role in meeting this need.

Major Concepts

Achieving the Balance

SERVICE OPERATION IS MORE THAN just a repetitive implementation of a standard set of procedures and activities; this stage works in an ever-changing environment. One of Service Operation's key roles is dealing with the conflict between maintaining the status quo, adapting to the changing business and technological environments, and achieving a balance between conflicting sets of priorities.

Internal IT View: Focuses on the way in which IT components and systems are managed to deliver the services. An organization here is out of balance and is in danger of not meeting business requirements.	VS	**External Business View:** Focuses on the way in which services are experienced by users and customers. An organization has business focus, but tends to under-deliver on promises to the business.
Stability: No matter how good the functionality is of an IT service or how well it has been designed, it will be worth far less if the service components are not available or if they perform inconsistently. Service Operation has to ensure that the IT infrastructure is stable and available as required. However an extreme focus on stability means that IT is in danger of ignoring changing business requirements	VS	**Responsiveness:** Service Operation must recognize that the business and IT requirements change. When there is an extreme focus on responsiveness IT may tend to overspend on change and also decrease the stability of the infrastructure.
Cost of Service: An organization with an extreme focus on cost is out of balance and is in danger of losing service quality because of heavy cost cutting. The loss of service quality leads to a loss of customers, which in turn leads to further cost cutting as the negative cycle continues.	VS	**Quality of Service:** An organization with an extreme focus on quality has happy customers but may tend to overspend to deliver higher levels of service than are strictly necessary, resulting in higher costs and effort required. The goal should be to consistently deliver the agreed level of IT service to customer and users, while at the same time keeping costs and resource utilization at an optimal level.

"Based on Cabinet Office ITIL® material. Reproduced under licence from the Cabinet Office"

Reactive:	VS	Proactive:
An organization that is extremely reactive is not able to effectively support the business strategy. Unfortunately a lot of organizations focus on reactive management as the sole means of ensuring that services are highly consistent and stable, actively discouraging proactive behavior from staff. The worst aspect of this approach is that discouraging effort investment in proactive service management can ultimately increase the effort and cost of reactive activities and further risk stability and consistency in services.		An extremely proactive organization tends to fix services that are not broken or introduce services that are not yet needed, resulting in higher levels of change, cost, and effort. This also comes at a cost to the stability of the infrastructure and quality of service already being delivered.

"Based on Cabinet Office ITIL® material. Reproduced under licence from the Cabinet Office"

Service Operation Functions

"Know your role, do your job"

TEAM MOTTO DESCRIBING THE GOAL for every player, coach, and general staff member of the Kansas City Chiefs.

Unique to Service Operations is the introduction of functions. While a defined function does have responsibilities in all stages of the Service Lifecycle, the majority of activities they performed are completed within the scope of Service operations. The functions in Service Operation are:

- Service Desk
- Technical Management
- IT Operations Management
- Application Management

Functions refer to the people (or roles) and automated measures that execute a defined process, an activity, or combination of both. The functions within Service Operation are needed to manage the 'steady state' operation IT environment. Just like in sports where each player will have a specific role to play in the overall team strategy, IT functions define the different roles and responsibilities required for the overall service delivery and support of IT services.

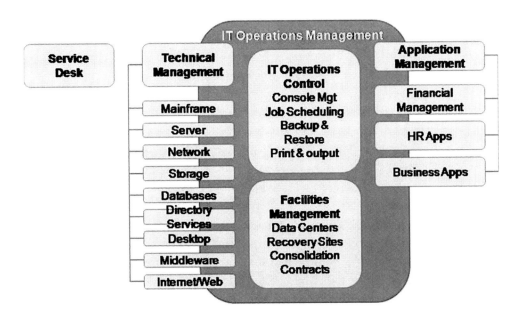

Figure 7.B—The ITIL® Functions from Service Operation

© **Crown** Copyright 2011 Reproduced under license from the Cabinet Office

NOTE: THESE ARE LOGICAL FUNCTIONS and do not necessarily have to be performed by equivalent organizational structure. This means that Technical and Application Management can be organized in any combination and into any number of departments. The lower groupings (e.g., Mainframe, Server) are examples of activities performed by Technical Management and are not a suggested organizational structure.

The Service Desk

Purpose

THE SERVICE DESK PROVIDES A single point of contact between the services being provided and the users. A typical Service Desk will manage incidents and service requests as well as communication with the users: thus the Service Desk staff will execute the Incident Management and Request Fulfillment processes with the intent to restore normal-state service operation to users as quickly as possible. This can involve fixing an error, fulfilling a request, or answering an IT-related question – whatever is needed to allow the users to return to working satisfactorily.

Specific responsibilities will include (Service Operation, Page 158):

- *Logging all relevant incident/service request details, allocating categorization and prioritization codes*
- *Providing first-line investigation and diagnosis*
- *Resolving incidents/service requests when first contacted, whenever possible*
- *Escalating incidents/service requests that they cannot resolve within agreed timescales*
- *Keeping users informed of progress*
- *Closing all resolved incidents, requests, and other calls*
- *Conducting customer/user satisfaction call-backs/surveys as agreed*
- *Communication with users—keeping them informed of incident progress, notifying them of impending changes or agreed outages, etc.*
- *Updating the CMS under the direction and approval of Service Asset and Configuration Management, if so agreed.*

Service Desk Organizational Structures

MANY FACTORS WILL INFLUENCE THE way in which a Service Desk function will be physically structured, such as the location, languages and cultures of end users, diversity in services and technology supported, and the objectives governing the implementation of the Service Desk, such as improved satisfaction or reduced operating costs.

The following are some of the main options chosen when implementing a Service Desk function:

Local Service Desk
A local Service Desk structure is where the Service Desk is co-located within or physically near to the user community it is serving. This may aid in communication and give the Service Desk a visible presence, which some users may like. It may, however, be inefficient and expensive to have multiple Service Desks operating.

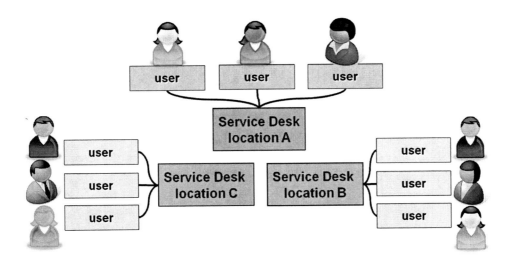

Figure 7.C—The Local Service Desk Structure

"Based on Cabinet Office ITIL® material. Reproduced under licence from the Cabinet Office"

Benefits of a local Service Desk structure	Disadvantages of a local Service Desk structure
• Local and specific user knowledge • Ability to effectively communicate with multiple languages • Appropriate cultural knowledge • Visible (and physical) presence of the Service Desk	• Higher costs for replicated infrastructure and more staff involved • Less knowledge transfer, each Service Desk may spend time rediscovering knowledge • Inconsistency in service levels and reporting • Service Desks may be focused on local issues

Centralized Service Desk

A centralized structure uses a Service Desk in a single location (or smaller number of locations), although some local presence may remain to handle physical support requirements, such as deploying, moving, and disposing of user workstations. This could be more efficient, enabling less staff to manage a higher volume of calls with greater visibility of repeat incidents and requests.

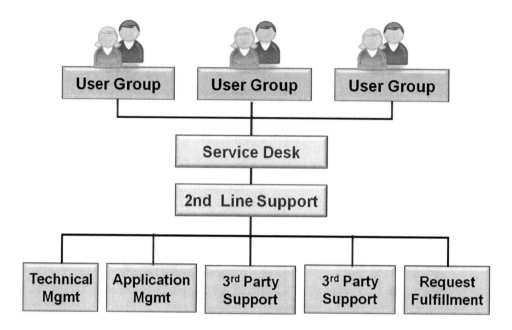

Figure 7.D—The Centralized Service Desk Structure

"Based on Cabinet Office ITIL® material. Reproduced under licence from the Cabinet Office"

Benefits of a centralized Service Desk structure	Disadvantages of a centralized Service Desk structure
• Reduced operational costs • Improved usage of available resources • Consistency of call handling • Improved ability for knowledge sharing • Simplicity for users (call one number) to contact the Service Desk	• Potentially higher costs and challenges in handling 24x7 environment or different time zones • Lack of local knowledge • Possible gaps in language and culture • Higher risk (single point of failure), in case of power loss or other physical threat

Virtual Service Desk

A virtual Service Desk, through the use of technology, particularly the Internet, and the use of corporate support tools, can give users the impression of a single, centralized Service Desk when, in fact, the personnel may be ocated in various geographical or structural locations.

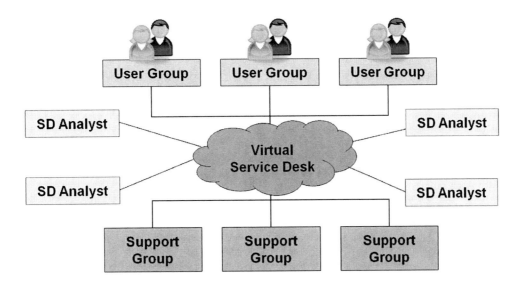

Figure 7.E—A Virtual Service Desk Structure

"Based on Cabinet Office ITIL® material. Reproduced under licence from the Cabinet Office"

Benefits of a virtual Service Desk structure	Disadvantages of a virtual Service Desk structure
• Support for global organizations • 24x7 support in multiple time zones • Reduced operational costs • Improved usage of available resources • Effective matching of appropriate staff for different types of calls	• Initial cost of implementation, requiring diverse and effective voice technology • Lack in the consistency of service and reporting • Less effective for monitoring actions of staff • Staff may feel disconnected from other Service Desk staff

Follow the Sun

Some global and international organizations will choose to combine two or more of their geographically scattered Service Desks to provide their customer with 24-hour follow-the-sun services.

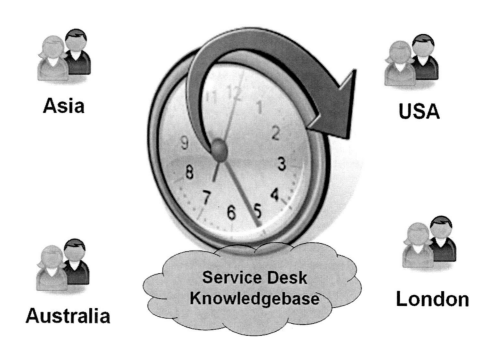

Figure 7.F—A Follow-the-Sun Service Desk structure

"Based on Cabinet Office ITIL® material. Reproduced under licence from the Cabinet Office"

Benefits of a follow-the-sun Service Desk structure	Disadvantages of a follow-the-sun Service Desk structure
• Support for global organizations • 24x7 support in multiple time zones • Improved quality of service • Improved customer/user satisfaction • Effective knowledge sharing and high level visibility of distributed infrastructure	• Typically higher operating costs • Cost of required technology • Challenges in using single language for multiple regions when recording knowledge, workarounds, Known Errors etc.

Skills

DUE TO THE ROLE PLAYED by the Service Desk, staff members need to have (or have the ability to develop):

- Communication Skills
- Technical Skills
- Business Understanding

The most important of these three areas is communication skills, as the primary role of the Service Desk is to provide a Single Point of Contact between the end-users and the IT organization. Because of this, they will need to be able to deal effectively with a wide range of people and situations.

Staff Retention

TO ENSURE A BALANCED MIX of experienced and newer staff, Service Desk managers should use a number of methods and incentives to retain quality staff and to avoid disruption and inconsistency in the quality of support offered.

Some ways in which this can be done include:

- Recognition of staff achievements contributing to service quality
- Rotation of staff onto other activities (projects, second-line support, etc.)
- Team building exercises and celebrations
- Promoting the Service Desk as a potential stepping stone for staff to move into other more technical or supervisory roles (after defined time periods and skills achieved)

Self help

MANY ORGANIZATIONS FIND IT BENEFICIAL to offer self-help capabilities to their users. The technology should, therefore, support this capability, with the web front-end allowing web pages to offer a menu-driven range of self help and service requests—with a direct interface into the back-end process-handling software. This reduces the amount of calls into the Service Desk and is often used as a source for improvements to efficiency. An example of this is the ability for a customer to track the status of their parcels online when shipped through a major courier company.

Aside from this, the Service Desk will use many different tools, systems, and other technology components in order to provide effective and efficient support to end-user calls and requests. To enable this, typical technology components utilized include:

- Computerized Service Desk systems
- Voice services (adv. menu systems, voicemail, SMS)
- Web and email (access, notification, updates)
- Systems that contain linkages to SLAs, CMDB
- Access to availability monitoring tools
- Self help for customers using technology
- Service Desk Metrics

To evaluate the true performance of the Service Desk, a balanced range of metrics should be established and reviewed at regular intervals. Especially dangerous is the tendency to focus on "average call time" or "number of calls answered" metrics, which can mask underlying issues with the quality of support provided.

Some of the typical metrics reviewed when monitoring the performance of the Service Desk include:

- The number of calls to Service Desk (broken down by type and work period)
- First-line resolution rate
- Average Service Desk cost of handling any incident or request
- Number of knowledgebase articles created
- Number or percentage of SLA breaches
- Call resolution time
- Customer satisfaction (surveys)
- Use of self help (where exists)

Outsourcing the Service Desk

ALTHOUGH FAIRLY COMMON, THERE ARE potential risks that can be introduced when outsourcing an organization's Service Desk. When reviewing the potential for this to occur, service managers should consider the following items when developing contracts to reduce these risks:

- Use of your own service management tool, not theirs
- Retain ownership of data
- Ability to maintain required staffing levels
- Agreements on reporting and monitoring needs
- Proven up-to-date procedures
- Agreed and understood support needs
- Engage contract specialists for assistance

Technical Management

TECHNICAL MANAGEMENT COMPRISES THE GROUPS, departments, or teams that provide technical expertise and overall management of the IT infrastructure. These are the people that the Service Desk will typically go to when they do not have the knowledge, access, or capabilities to assist the user. Technical Management has a strong presence in designing the IT infrastructure, transitioning IT service assets, and daily management of configuration items and other service assets. *The objectives of Technical Management are to help plan, implement, and maintain a stable technical infrastructure to support the organization's business processes through*:

- *Well-designed and highly resilient, cost-effective technical topology*
- *The use of adequate technical skills to maintain the technical infrastructure in optimum condition*
- *Swift use of technical skills to speedily diagnose and resolve any technical failures that do occur* (Service Operation, Page 171)

Technical Management plays a dual role (Service Operation, Page 170):

It is the custodian of technical knowledge and expertise related to managing the IT infrastructure. In this role, Technical Management ensures that the knowledge required to design, test, manage, and improve IT services is identified, developed, and refined

It provides the actual resources to support the Service Lifecycle. In this role, Technical Management ensures that resources are effectively trained and deployed to design, build, transition, operate, and improve the technology required to deliver and support IT services

Technical Management ensures the organization has access to human resources to adequately manage technology and meet business objectives. The function must ensure a balance between the skill level, utilization, and cost of these resources. There are many strategies that can be adopted to obtain this balance, including contracting out skills that are used very little or creating pools of resources with specialized skills.

In all but the smallest organizations where a single combined team or department may suffice, separate teams or departments will be needed for each type of infrastructure being used. In many organizations the Technical Management (TM) departments are also responsible for the daily operation of a subset of the IT Infrastructure.

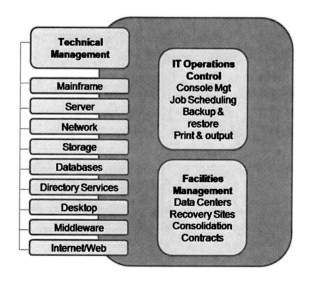

Figure 7.G—Technical Management

© **Crown** Copyright 2011 Reproduced under license from the Cabinet Office

In many organizations, the actual role played by IT Operations Management is carried out by either Technical or Application Management.

Roles and Responsibilities

- Custodian of technical knowledge and expertise related to managing the IT Infrastructure. Provides detailed technical skills and resources needed to support the ongoing operation of the IT Infrastructure.
- Plays an important role in providing the actual resources to support the IT Service Management lifecycle. Ensures resources are effectively trained and deployed to design, build, transition, operate, and improve the technology to deliver and support IT Services.

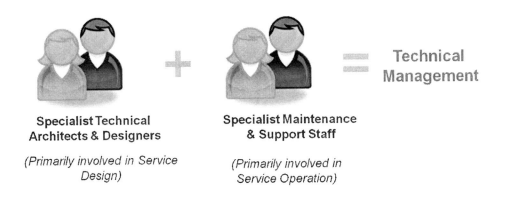

Specialist Technical Architects & Designers

(Primarily involved in Service Design)

Specialist Maintenance & Support Staff

(Primarily involved in Service Operation)

Technical Management

Figure 7.H—Staff making up the Technical Management Function

TO ENABLE QUALITY KNOWLEDGE SHARING and continual improvement of services, technology, processes, and other capabilities, Technical Management staff should develop effective communication channels and meet regularly to discuss issues or potential ideas. History demonstrates that quality design requires involvement from those who will be supporting the product/service, as does quality support require involvement from the designers in turn.

IT Operations Management

THE TERM 'OPERATIONS MANAGEMENT' IS *often used to define the department, group, or team of people responsible for performing the organization's day-to-day operational activities—such as running the production line in a manufacturing environment or managing the distribution centers and fleet movements within a logistics organization* (Service Operation, Page 175).

Operations Management generally has the following characteristics (Service Operation, Page 175):

- *There is work to ensure that a device, system, or process is actually running or working (as opposed to strategy or planning)*
- *This is where plans are turned into actions*
- *The focus is on daily or shorter-term activities; although, it should be noted that these activities will generally be performed and repeated over a relatively long period (as opposed to one-off project-type activities)*
- *These activities are executed by specialized technical staff who often have to undergo technical training to learn how to perform each activity*
- *There is a focus on building repeatable, consistent actions that, if repeated frequently enough at the right level of quality, will ensure the success of the operation*
- *This is where the actual value of the organization is delivered and measured*
- *There is a dependency on investment in equipment or human resources or both*
- *The value generated must exceed the cost of the investment and all other organizational overheads (such as management and marketing costs) if the business is to succeed*

IT Operations Management can be defined in a similar way as the function responsible for the ongoing management and maintenance of an organization's IT infrastructure IT operations is the set of activities used in the day-to-day running of the IT infrastructure to deliver IT services at agreed levels to meet stated business objectives.

In some organizations this is a single, centralized department, while in others some activities and staff are centralized and some are provided by distributed and specialized departments.

In many cases, the role of IT Operations Management is actually performed by the Technical and Application Management functions, where required.

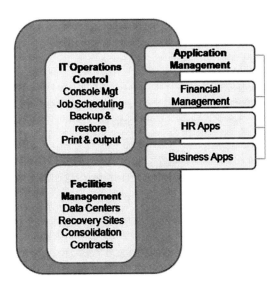

Figure 7.I—IT Operations Management

© **Crown** Copyright 2011 Reproduced under license from the Cabinet Office

IT Operations Control

ONE ROLE PLAYED BY IT Operations Management is that of Operations Control. This role is concerned with the execution and monitoring of the operational activities and events in the IT infrastructure (possibly using an Operations/Network Bridge). In addition to the routine tasks to be performed in accordance with the design specifications of the IT infrastructure, Operations Control is also responsible for the following (Service Operation, Page 176):

- *Console management/operations bridge, which refers to defining central observation and monitoring capability and then using those consoles to exercise event management, monitoring, and control activities*
- *Job scheduling or the management of routine batch jobs or scripts*
- *Backup and restore on behalf of all Technical and Application Management teams and departments and often on behalf of users*

- *Print and output management for the collation and distribution of all centralized printing or electronic output*
- *Performance of maintenance activities on behalf of Technical or Application Management teams or departments*

Facilities Management

FACILITIES MANAGEMENT IS RESPONSIBLE FOR managing all physical IT environments, such as data centers, computer rooms, and recovery sites. Physical components may have been outsourced in some organizations and Facilities Management will manage the outsourcing contracts in cooperation with Supplier Management. Facilities Management should be involved in any large scale project planning to provide advice regarding any physical accommodation of staff or infrastructure required.

Application Management

APPLICATION MANAGEMENT WILL MANAGE APPLICATIONS throughout their lifecycle and performed by any department, group, or team involved in managing and supporting operational applications. Application Management covers the entire ongoing lifecycle of an application, including requirements, design, build, deploy, operate, and optimize. The Application Management function is Application Management plays an important role in the design, testing, and improvement of applications that form part of IT services and may be involved in development projects. Application Management is distinct from application development, where a team of application architects, designers, and programmers are working together to create an application: application management, on the other hand,

will identify functional and manageability requirements for application software and assist in the design and deployment of those applications and the ongoing support and improvement of those applications.

These objectives are achieved through (Service Operation, Page 180):

- *Applications that are well-designed, resilient, and cost-effective*
- *Ensuring that the required functionality is available to achieve the required business outcome*
- *The organization of adequate technical skills to maintain operational applications in optimum condition*

- *Swift use of technical skills to speedily diagnose and resolve any technical failures that do occur*

Roles and Responsibilities

APPLICATION MANAGEMENT IS TO APPLICATIONS *what Technical Management is to the IT infrastructure. Application Management activities are performed in all applications, whether purchased or developed in-house. One of the key decisions that they contribute to is the decision of whether to buy an application or build it (this is discussed in detail in ITIL® Service Design). Once that decision is made, Application Management will have several roles* (Service Operation, Page 179):

- *It is the custodian of technical knowledge and expertise related to managing applications. In this role, Application Management, working together with Technical Management, ensures that the knowledge required to design, test, manage, and improve IT services is identified, developed, and refined.*
- *It provides the actual resources to support the Service Lifecycle. In this role, Application Management ensures that resources are effectively trained and deployed to design, build, transition, operate, and improve the technology required to deliver and support IT services.*

Application Management also performs other specific roles (Service Operation, Page 180):

- *Providing guidance to IT operations about how best to carry out the ongoing operational management of applications. This role is partly carried out during the Service Design process, but it is also a part of everyday communication with IT Operations Management as they seek to achieve stability and optimum performance.*
- *The integration of the Application Management lifecycle into the service ifecycle*

Application Management Lifecycle

APPLICATION DEVELOPMENT PROCESSES SHOULD BE implemented as part of a coordinated approach to IT Service Management, although, in many cases, this fails to happen. When the development of applications is not integrated with the rest of ITSM, it often leads to a breakdown in communication channels between developers and support staff and, ultimately, releasing applications that are not optimal in supporting business processes.

Application development and operations are part of the same overall lifecycle and both should be involved at all stages, although their level of involvement will vary depending on the stage of the lifecycle.

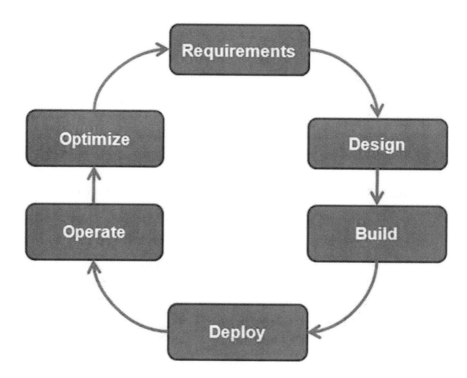

Figure 7.K—The Application Management Lifecycle
© Crown Copyright 2011 Reproduced under license from the Cabinet Office

Service Operation Processes

THE GOAL OF SERVICE OPERATION, as previously mentioned, is to enable effectiveness and efficiency in delivery and support of IT services. The processes that support this goal are:

- Event Management
- Incident Management
- Problem Management
- Request Fulfillment
- Access Management

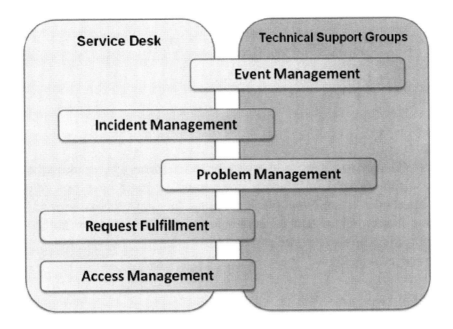

Figure 7.L—Where the Service Operation Processes Get Carried Out

THE FIGURE ABOVE DEMONSTRATES HOW much responsibility the Service Desk and the technical support groups (Technical, IT Operations, and Application Management functions) have in the Service Operation Processes. Incident Management, Request Fulfillment, and Access Management are primarily carried out by the Service Desk, with Event Management and Problem Management as primarily back-of-house processes.

Event Management

Terminology

Term	Definition
alert	(ITIL® Service Operation) A notification that a threshold has been reached, something has changed, or a failure has occurred. Alerts are often created and managed by system management tools and are managed by the event management process.
event	(ITIL® Service Operation) A change of state that has significance for the management of an IT service or other configuration item. The term is also used to mean an alert or notification created by any IT service, configuration item, or monitoring tool. Events typically require IT operations personnel to take actions and often lead to incidents being logged.

© **Crown** Copyright 2011 Reproduced under license from the Cabinet Office

Purpose

THE EVENT MANAGEMENT PROCESS IS designed to manage events throughout their lifecycle, including detecting events, understanding them, and determining the appropriate control action. Event Management is, therefore, the basis for operational monitoring and control. Because events are programmed to communicate operational information, they can also be used as a basis for automating many routine operations management activities.

The objectives of the Event Management process are to (Service Operation, Page 58):

- *Detect all changes of state that have significance for the management of a CI or IT service*
- *Determine the appropriate control action for events and ensure these are communicated to the appropriate functions*
- *Provide the trigger, or entry point, for the execution of many service operation processes and operations management activities*
- *Provide the means to compare actual operating performance and behavior against design standards and SLAs*

- *Provide a basis for service assurance and reporting and service improvement (This is covered in detail in ITIL® Continual Service Improvement)*

Scope

EVENT MANAGEMENT CAN BE APPLIED to any area of service management that needs to be controlled and can be automated. This includes(Service Operation, Page 58-59):

- *Configuration items (CIs):*
  - ⏵ *Some CIs will be included because they need to stay in a constant state (e.g., a switch on a network needs to stay on and event management tools confirm this by monitoring responses to pings)*
- *Some CIs will be included because their status needs to change frequently and Event Management can be used to automate this and update the Configuration Management System (CMS) (e.g., the updating of a file server)*
- *Environmental conditions (e.g., fire and smoke detection)*
- *Software license monitoring for usage to ensure optimum/legal license utilization and allocation*
- *Security (e.g., intrusion detection)*
- *Normal activity (e.g., tracking the use of an application or the performance of a server)*

Types of events

THERE ARE THREE DIFFERENT TYPES of events - informational events, warning events, and exception events

Informational events: provides information that something has occurred, like the completion of a task, the fulfilment of a measured expectation, or simply someone logging onto an application.

Warning events: used to signify unusual but not exceptional operations which may require closer monitoring, such as a threshold being reached. If the situation does not resolve itself or persists, an operator may have to intervene based on the monitoring and control objectives for the service or device.

Exception events: indicates any situation where abnormal operations is clearly present, such as an incorrect password, higher than acceptable utilization rate, unauthorized software, or any situation requiring further investigation.

There is no definitive rule about what constitutes an information, warning, or exception event. Generally speaking, informational events provide data for decision-making, warning events provide information use to predict if some exception might occur, and exception events indicate an abnormal situation that requires action.

Each type of event relies on the sending and receipt of a message of some sort, known as event notifications and they do not just happen without planning.

Event Management requires the correct level of filtering be achieved to focus management and control actions on those events that have significance. Unfortunately, the significance of events will change.

Inputs

INPUTS TO THE EVENT MANAGEMENT process will mostly come from Service Design and Service Transition. Examples of these may include (Service Operation, Page 70):

- *Operational and service level requirements associated with events and their actions*
- *Alarms, alerts, and thresholds for recognizing events*
- *Event correlation tables, rules, event codes, and automated response solutions that will support Event Management activities*
- *Roles and responsibilities for recognizing events and communicating them to those that need to handle them*
- *Operational procedures for recognizing, logging, escalating, and communicating events*

Outputs

EXAMPLES OF OUTPUTS FROM EVENT Management may include (Service Operation, Page 70):

- *Events that have been communicated and escalated to those responsible for further action*

- *Event logs describing what events took place and any escalation and communication activities taken to support forensic, diagnosis, or further CSI activities*
- *Events that indicate an incident has occurred*
- *Events that indicate the potential breach of an SLA or OLA objective*
- *Events and alerts that indicate completion status of deployment, operational, or other support activities*
- *Populated SKMS with event information and history*

Incident Management

INCIDENT MANAGEMENT HAS DEVELOPED OVER time to become one of the most visible and mature ITIL® processes for any organization, largely driven by the need to reduce the business impact of disruptions to IT services. While any effective implementation does balance the efforts towards the various stages of the Service Lifecycle, as Incident Management can be easily demonstrated to have a business benefit, it typically receives more attention and funding than other areas of service management. This section will explain the activities and techniques that represent best practices for Incident Management.

In ITIL® terminology, an incident is defined *as an unplanned interruption to an IT service or reduction in the quality of an IT service or a failure of a CI that has not yet impacted an IT service* (Service Operation, Page 72). Incident Management is responsible for managing the lifecycle of all incidents, Which can be recognized by technical staff, detected and reported by event monitoring tools, communicated by users, or reported by third-party suppliers and partners.

Terminology

Term	Definition
escalation	(ITIL® Service Operation) An activity that obtains additional resources when these are needed to meet service level targets or customer expectations. Escalation may be needed within any IT service management process but is most commonly associated with incident management, problem management, and the management of customer complaints. There are two types of escalation: functional escalation and hierarchic escalation.
functional escalation	(ITIL® Service Operation) Transferring an incident, problem, or change to a technical team with a higher level of expertise to assist in an escalation.
hierarchic escalation	(ITIL® Service Operation) Informing or involving more senior levels of management to assist in an escalation.
impact	(ITIL® Service Operation) (ITIL® Service Transition) A measure of the effect of an incident, problem, or change on business processes. Impact is often based on how service levels will be affected. Impact and urgency are used to assign priority.

Term	Definition
incident	(ITIL® Service Operation) An unplanned interruption to an IT service or reduction in the quality of an IT service. Failure of a configuration item that has not yet affected service is also an incident—for example, failure of one disk from a mirror set.
incident record	(ITIL® Service Operation) A record containing the details of an incident. Each incident record documents the lifecycle of a single incident.
major incident	(ITIL® Service Operation) The highest category of impact for an incident. A major incident results in significant disruption to the business.
resolution	(ITIL® Service Operation) Action taken to repair the root cause of an incident or problem or to implement a workaround. In ISO/IEC 20000, resolution processes is the process group that includes incident and problem management.
restore	(ITIL® Service Operation) Taking action to return an IT service to the users after repair and recovery from an incident. This is the primary objective of incident management.
urgency	(ITIL® Service Design) (ITIL® Service Transition) A measure of how long it will be until an incident, problem, or change has a significant impact on the business. For example, a high-impact incident may have low urgency if the impact will not affect the business until the end of the financial year. Impact and urgency are used to assign priority.
workaround	(ITIL® Service Operation) Reducing or eliminating the impact of an incident or problem for which a full resolution is not yet available—for example, by restarting a failed configuration item. Workarounds for problems are documented in known error records. Workarounds for incidents that do not have associated problem records are documented in the incident record.

Purpose

REMEMBER THAT EVERY IT SERVICE designed to support the business has service level agreements, usually to define the desired availability, performance, or security of that service. Enabling and enhancing services will have operational level agreements. If IT services and their components are operating within the agreed SLA limits. An incident is a disruption in service that threatens the achievement of SLAs and OLAs based on the severity of the incident and how long it persists. The purpose of Incident Management is not to prevent an incident, but to reduce its impact by restoring normal service operation as quickly as possible.

The objectives of the Incident Management process are to (Service Operation, Page 73):

- *Ensure that standardized methods and procedures are used for efficient and prompt response, analysis, documentation, ongoing management, and reporting of incidents*
- *Increase visibility and communication of incidents to business and IT support staff*
- *Enhance business perception of IT through use of a professional approach in quickly resolving and communicating incidents when they occur*
- *Align Incident Management activities and priorities with those of the business*
- *Maintain user satisfaction with the quality of IT services*

What is the difference between Incident Management and Problem Management?

If our garden had weeds, how would we address the situation?

Incident Management: Use techniques that address the symptoms but still allow the weeds to grow back (e.g., pull them out, mow over them, use a hedge-trimmer, or buy a goat)

Problem Management: Use techniques that address the root-cause of the symptoms so that weeds will no longer grow (e.g., use poison, dig roots out, re-lawn, concrete over, etc.)

Incident Management is not concerned with the root cause; it is instead focused on addressing the symptoms as quickly as possible.

Scope

INCIDENT MANAGEMENT CAN BE UTILIZED to manage any event that disrupts or has the potential to disrupt an IT service and associated business processes. Careful distinction needs to be made between the role of Event Management and Incident Management, as only events that indicate exception to normal service operation and are determined by the Event Correlation engine to be significant are escalated to Incident Management. This means that incident records may be generated as a result of:

- End users calling the Service Desk to notify of a disruption to their normal use of IT services
- Events representing an exception that are resolved using automated means with an associated incident record also being generated for informational purposes
- An IT staff member noticing that a component of the IT infrastructure is behaving abnormally, despite no current impact on the end user community
- An end user logging an incident using self help means, which is then resolved by IT operations staff
- An external supplier observing that a portion of the IT infrastructure under their control is experiencing issues and logs an incident ticket via email

While the process of Request Fulfillment does typically operate in a similar fashion to Incident Management, a service request does not involve any (potential) disruption to an IT service.

Incident Models

INCIDENT MODELS PROVIDE A PRE-DEFINED set of steps and procedures that should be used to manage previously seen and documented incidents. They are used to help provide efficient resolution to the most frequently occurring or specialized incidents. Incident Models should define (Service Operation, Page 75):

- *The steps that should be taken to handle the incident*
- *The chronological order these steps should be taken in, with any dependencies or co-processing defined*
- *Responsibilities—who should do what*
- *Timescales and thresholds for completion of actions*

> - *Escalation procedures—who should be contacted and when*
> - *Any necessary evidence-preservation activities*

Any service management tools that are used for Event and Incident Management should be utilized with the defined incident models that can automate the handling, management, and escalation of the process.

Specialized incidents include those that need routing to particular groups or ITIL® processes. An example of this is for capacity related incidents, in which the model would define what impact reduction measures could be performed before routing the incident to Capacity Management.

Major incidents

FOR THOSE INCIDENTS THAT RESULT in significant or organization-wide business impact, planning needs to consider how separate procedures should be used with shorter timescales and greater urgency to provide appropriate response and resolution. The first requirement is to define what constitutes a major incident for the organization and customers, with reference to the incident prioritization mechanisms that are used.

The key role of separate major incident procedures is to establish a fast and coordinated response that can manage and resolve the issues at hand. This may require the establishment of a team with the immediate focus of resolving the incident and reducing the associated business impact. The Service Desk maintains responsibility throughout the process so that users are kept fully informed of the incident status and progress for resolution.

Problem Management will typically be involved when major incidents occur, though the focus is not the resolution of the incident. Instead Problem Management seeks to identify the root cause of the incident, how this can be removed, and if there are any other areas of the infrastructure where this could occur (e.g., replicated infrastructure across multiple locations).

Incident Status Tracking

INCIDENTS HAVE A BEGINNING AND an end. The beginning typically coincides with the opening of an incident in the Incident Management system and the end of an incident occurs when the incident record closes. In between these two events, an incident has its own lifecycle with several states it can be in. The state of the incident is represented by a status code and allows better management over all incidents.. Typical examples of these status codes might include (Service Operation, Page 75):

- *Open: An incident has been recognized but not yet assigned to a support resource for resolution*
- *In progress: The incident is in the process of being investigated and resolved*
- *Resolved: A resolution has been put in place for the incident but normal state service operation has not yet been validated by the business or end user*
- *Closed: The user or business has agreed that the incident has been resolved and that normal state operations have been restored*

Activities

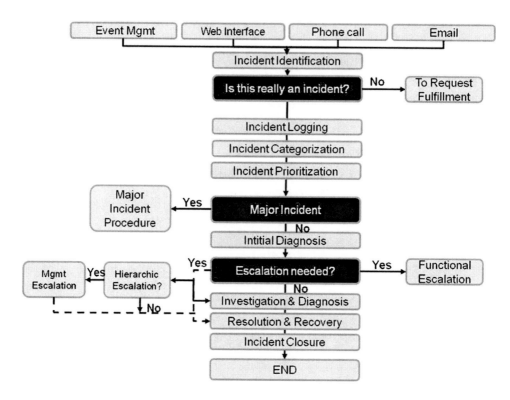

Figure 7.M—Typical Activities for Incident Management
"Based on Cabinet Office ITIL® material. Reproduced under licence from the Cabinet Office"

Overview of steps

1. Incident identification
2. Incident logging
3. Incident categorization
4. Incident prioritization
5. Initial diagnosis
6. Incident escalation
7. Investigation and diagnosis
8. Resolution and recovery
9. Incident closure

1. **Incident identification**

The implementation of Incident Management should consider the range of sources where incidents can be identified. These typically include:

- Customers and end users
- External customers (of the business)
- IT staff members
- Automated mechanisms, including those governed by Event Management
- External suppliers

2. **Incident logging**

All incidents, regardless of source, must be recorded with a unique reference number and be date/time stamped. While this can be easily managed for automated mechanisms, positive behaviors need to be developed for IT staff and end users to ensure the consistent recording of identified incidents. It may also be necessary to record more than one incident for any given call/discussion so that a historical record is kept and that time/work tracking can be performed.

3. **Incident categorization**

During the initial logging of the incident, a category is assigned so that the exact type of incident is recorded. This information is important to allow effective escalation, trend analysis of incidents, and future infrastructure improvements. Multi-level categorization is typically used for Incident Management, where the service management tool is populated with up to three of four levels of category details.

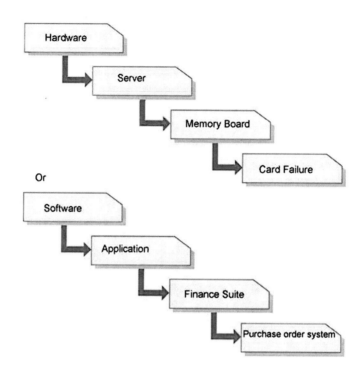

4. **Incident prioritization**

An agreed prioritization matrix should be used to determine the appropriate timescales and effort applied for response and resolution to identified incidents. The general formula by which to calculate incident priority is:

IMPACT + URGENCY = PRIORITY

- **Impact**: Degree to which the **user/business** is affected by the incident(s)
- **Urgency**: Degree to which the **resolution** of the incident can be delayed

The following factors are usually taken into account for determining the impact of an incident:

- The number of users being affected
  - ▷ (e.g., single user, multiple users, entire business unit, organization wide)
- Possible risk of injury or death

- The number of services affected
- The level of financial loss
- Effect on credibility and reputation of business
- Regulatory or legislative breaches

Urgency is calculated by assessing when the potential impact of the incident will be felt. In some cases the incident resolution can be delayed when the disruption to an IT service (e.g., payroll) has not yet affected business operations (but will if the service is not available in three days time).

Urgency

Impact	High	Med	Low
High	1	2	3
Med	2	3	4
Low	3	4	5

Priority

Figure 7.0—Example Incident Prioritization Matrix
"Based on Cabinet Office ITIL® material. Reproduced under licence from the Cabinet Office"

The prioritization matrix above would be accompanied by agreed timelines for resolution.

E.g.   Priority 1 =   Critical   = 1 hour target resolution time

Priority 2 =   High   = 8 hours

Priority 3 =   Medium   = 24 hours

Priority 4 =   Low   = 48 hours

5. **Initial diagnosis**

For calls forwarded to the Service Desk, the staff member will use pre-defined questioning techniques to assist in the collection of useful information for the incident record. At this point, the Service Desk analyst can begin to provide some initial support by referencing known errors and simple diagnostic tools. Where possible, the incident will be resolved using these sources of information, closing the incident after verifying the resolution was successful.

For incidents that cannot be resolved at this stage and the user is still on the phone, the Service Desk analyst should inform the user of the next steps that will be taken, give the unique incident reference number, and confirm user contact details for follow-ups.

6. **Incident escalation**

If the Service Desk analyst requires assistance from other groups due to an inability to resolve the incident or because of specialized circumstances (e.g., VIP user), escalation will be utilized to transfer the incident to the appropriate party or group. Rules for escalation should be defined when implementing Incident Management and agreed upon by all involved groups and stakeholders.

The two forms of escalation that are typically used are functional (horizontal) and hierarchical (vertical) escalation. Escalations can also be combined.

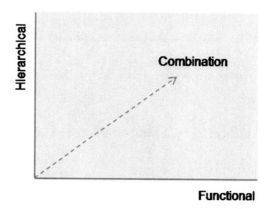

Figure 7.P—Example Incident Prioritization Matrix

Functional:
- Based on *knowledge* or *expertise*
- Also known as Horizontal Escalation, through level 1, 2, and 3 support

Hierarchical:
- For corrective actions by authorized *line management*
- Also known as Vertical Escalation
- When resolution of an incident will not be in time or satisfactory

7. **Investigation and diagnosis**

The incident investigation is likely to include such actions as:

- Identifying the error or determining what is being sought by the user
- Recognizing the chronological order of events
- Confirming the outcome and consequences of the detected incident, including the number and range of users affected
- Distinguish any events that could have triggered the incident
- Knowledge searches looking for any noticeable previous occurrences performed by searching previous incident or problem records and/or known error databases etc.
- Seeking knowledge from system developers as to possible guidance for resolution

8. **Resolution and recovery**

When a potential resolution of an incident has been identified, it should be applied and tested in a controlled manner. The specific requirements for performing this will vary depending on the elements required for resolution, but could involve:

- Guiding the user to perform specific actions on their own equipment
- Specialist support groups performing specific actions on the infrastructure (such as rebooting a server)
- External suppliers performing updates on their infrastructure in order to resolve the incident
- The Service Desk or other specialist staff controlling a user's desktop remotely in order to resolve the incident

9. **Incident closure**

Depending on the nature of the incident (level of impact, users affected, etc.), the Service Desk may be required to call the affected users and confirm that the users are satisfied that the resolution was successful and that the incident can be closed. For other incidents, closure mechanisms may be automated and communicated via email. Closure mechanisms, whether automated or manual, should also check for the following:

- Closure categorization, with comparison to the initial categorization to ensure accurate historical tracking
- User satisfaction survey, usually be email or web-forms for an agreed percentage of random incidents
- Incident documentation, ensuring all required fields are completed satisfactorily
- Potential problem identification, assisting Problem Management in the decision of whether any preventative action is necessary to avoid this in the future

When the requirements for incident documentation are complete, the incident should be closed via agreed methods.

Roles and Responsibilities

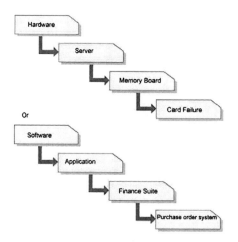

Figure 7.N—Multi-Level Incident Categorization
© Crown Copyright 2011 Reproduced under license from the Cabinet Office

- **Incident Manager:**
  - ▹ Drive effectiveness and efficiency of process
  - ▹ Manage incident management team
  - ▹ Ensure SLA targets for incident resolution are met

Skills: Analytical, technical, business understanding, communication, calm under pressure

- **Service Desk:**
  - ▹ Log/record incidents
  - ▹ Incident classification and categorization
  - ▹ Provide initial support
  - ▹ Match to existing incident or problem records
  - ▹ Manage communication with end users

- **1st, 2nd, 3rd line support groups (including Technical and Application Management):**
  - ▹ Incident classification
  - ▹ Investigation and resolution of incidents

Inputs

EXAMPLES OF INPUTS TO THE Incident Management process may include (Service Operation, Page 83):

- *Information about CIs and their status*
- *Information about known errors and their workarounds*
- *Communication and feedback about incidents and their symptoms*
- *Communication and feedback about RFCs and releases that have been implemented or planned for implementation*
- *Communication of events that were triggered from Event Management*
- *Operational and service level objectives*
- *Customer feedback on success of incident resolution activities and overall quality of incident management activities*
- *Agreed criteria for prioritizing and escalating incidents*

Outputs

EXAMPLES OF OUTPUTS FROM THE Incident Management process may include (Service Operation, Page 83):

- *Resolved incidents and actions taken to achieve their resolution*
- *Updated Incident Management records with accurate incident detail and history*
- *Updated classification of incidents to be used to support proactive Problem Management activities*
- *Raising of problem records for incidents where an underlying cause has not been identified*
- *Validation that incidents have not recurred for problems that have been resolved*
- *Feedback on incidents related to changes and releases*
- *Identification of CIs associated with or impacted by incidents*
- *Satisfaction feedback from customers who have experienced incidents*
- *Feedback on level and quality of monitoring technologies and Event Management activities*
- *Communications about incident and resolution history detail to assist with identification of overall service quality*

"Based on Cabinet Office ITIL® material. Reproduced under licence from the Cabinet Office"

Problem Management

Terminology

Term	Definition
escalation	(ITIL® Service Operation) An activity that obtains additional resources when these are needed to meet service level targets or customer expectations. Escalation may be needed within any IT service management process but is most commonly associated with incident management, problem management, and the management of customer complaints. There are two types of escalation: functional escalation and hierarchic escalation.
functional escalation	(ITIL® Service Operation) Transferring an incident, problem, or change to a technical team with a higher level of expertise to assist in an escalation.
hierarchic escalation	(ITIL® Service Operation) Informing or involving more senior levels of management to assist in an escalation.

Term	Definition
impact	(ITIL® Service Operation) (ITIL® Service Transition) A measure of the effect of an incident, problem, or change on business processes. Impact is often based on how service levels will be affected. Impact and urgency are used to assign priority.
incident	(ITIL® Service Operation) An unplanned interruption to an IT service or reduction in the quality of an IT service. Failure of a configuration item that has not yet affected service is also an incident—for example, failure of one disk from a mirror set.
known error	(ITIL® Service Operation) A problem that has a documented root cause and a workaround. Known errors are created and managed throughout their lifecycle by problem management. Known errors may also be identified by development or suppliers.
known error database (KEDB)	(ITIL® Service Operation) A database containing all known error records. This database is created by problem management and used by incident and problem management. The known error database may be part of the configuration management system or may be stored elsewhere in the service knowledge management system.
known error record	(ITIL® Service Operation) A record containing the details of a known error. Each known error record documents the lifecycle of a known error, including the status, root cause, and workaround. In some implementations, a known error is documented using additional fields in a problem record.
proactive problem management	(ITIL® Service Operation) Part of the problem management process. The objective of proactive problem management is to identify problems that might otherwise be missed. Proactive problem management analyzes incident records and uses data collected by other IT service management processes to identify trends or significant problems.
problem	(ITIL® Service Operation) A cause of one or more incidents. The cause is not usually known at the time a problem record is created, and the problem management process is responsible for further investigation.
problem record	(ITIL® Service Operation) A record containing the details of a problem. Each problem record documents the lifecycle of a single problem.
resolution	(ITIL® Service Operation) Action taken to repair the root cause of an incident or problem or to implement a workaround. In ISO/IEC 20000, resolution processes is the process group that includes incident and problem management.
root cause	(ITIL® Service Operation) The underlying or original cause of an incident or problem.

Term	Definition
threat	A threat is anything that might exploit a vulnerability. Any potential cause of an incident can be considered a threat. For example, a fire is a threat that could exploit the vulnerability of flammable floor coverings. This term is commonly used in information security management and IT service continuity management but also applies to other areas, such as problem and availability management.
trend analysis	(ITIL® Continual Service Improvement) Analysis of data to identify time-related patterns. Trend analysis is used in problem management to identify common failures or fragile configuration items and in capacity management as a modeling tool to predict future behavior. It is also used as a management tool for identifying deficiencies in IT service management processes.
urgency	(ITIL® Service Design) (ITIL® Service Transition) A measure of how long it will be until an incident, problem, or change has a significant impact on the business. For example, a high-impact incident may have low urgency if the impact will not affect the business until the end of the financial year. Impact and urgency are used to assign priority.

© **Crown** Copyright 2011 Reproduced under license from the Cabinet Office

Purpose

PROBLEM MANAGEMENT HAS TWO PURPOSES: *to manage all problems through their lifecycle and to minimize the impact of or prevent the occurrence of incidents and problems. Problems are often confused with incidents, but they are distinct: the most simplistic method for making the distinction is to say incidents are the symptoms while problems are the cause. ITIL® defines a problem as the underlying cause of one or more incidents*

A problem also has a beginning and an end, characterized by the opening of a problem record in the Problem Management system and the closing of the problem record. During the lifecycle of the problem, it will be identified, investigated, documented, and eventually removed. Because incidents are an indication that problems exist, many organization will tightly integrate the systems for incident and problem management. Problem management will manage the lifecycle of the problem.

The Problem Management process will also attempt to affect the problem to minimize any adverse effect on the organization caused by underlying errors and proactively prevent the recurrence of incidents related to the problem. Within this context of its purpose, Problem Management works to identify the root cause of incidents, document and communicate known errors, and initiate actions to improve or correct the situation.

The objectives of the Problem Management process are to (Service Operation, Page 97):

- *Prevent problems and resulting incidents from happening*
- *Eliminate recurring incidents*
- *Minimize the impact of incidents that cannot be prevented*

Scope

THE ACTIVITIES OF PROBLEM MANAGEMENT concentrate on diagnosing the root cause of incidents and determine any resolution to those problems. When a resolution is found, Problem Management will engage the appropriate service management processes, particularly Change Management and Release and Deployment Management to ensure the resolution is implemented into the environment.

Problem Management will maintain information about problems and the appropriate alternatives and resolutions. This information can be used to reduce the number and impact of incidents over time. The Known Error Database is a likely repository for this information and because of this, Problem Management must have a strong interface with Knowledge Management. Although Incident and Problem Management are separate processes, they are closely related and will typically use the same tools and may use similar categorization, impact, and priority coding systems.

This will ensure effective communication when dealing with related incidents and problems.

The Problem Management process has both reactive and proactive aspects (Service Operation, Page 97):

- *Reactive Problem Management is concerned with solving problems in response to one or more incidents*
- *Proactive Problem Management is concerned with identifying and solving problems and known errors before further incidents related to them can occur again*
- *While reactive Problem Management activities are performed in reaction to specific incident situations, proactive Problem Management activities take place as ongoing activities targeted to improve the overall availability and end user satisfaction with IT services. Examples of proactive Problem Management activities might include conducting periodic scheduled reviews of incident records to find patterns and trends in reported symptoms that may indicate the presence of underlying errors in the infrastructure.*
- *Conducting major incident reviews where review of 'How can we prevent the recurrence?' can provide identification of an underlying cause or error*
- *Conducting periodic scheduled reviews of operational logs and maintenance records identifying patterns and trends of activities that may indicate that an underlying problem might exist*
- *Conducting periodic scheduled reviews of event logs targeting patterns and trends of warning and exception events that may indicate the presence of an underlying problem*
- *Conducting brainstorming sessions to identify trends that could indicate the existence of underlying problems*
- *Using check sheets to proactively collect data on service or operational quality issues that may help to detect underlying problems*

While proactive Problem Management is conducted within the scope of Service Operation, it has some strong ties to Continual Service Improvement. Resolutions to identified problems may find themselves in the CSI register as an improvement opportunity.

Remember the weeding analogy used for Incident Management? Problem Management seeks to identify and remove the root cause of incidents in the IT Infrastructure.

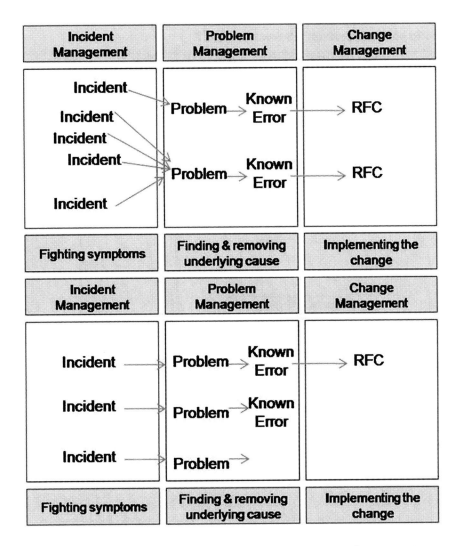

Figure 7.Q—Relationships Between Incidents, Problems and Known Errors

As SHOWN ABOVE, PROBLEMS ARE identified and corrected in multiple ways. For most organizations, the primary benefit of Problem Management is demonstrated in the many-to-one relationship between incidents and problems. This enables an IT service provider to resolve many incidents in an efficient manner by correcting the underlying root cause. Change Management is still required so that the actions being performed to correct and remove the error are done so in a controlled and efficient manner.

Why do some Problems not get diagnosed?
- Because the root cause is not always found

Why do some Known Errors not get fixed?
- Because we may decide that the costs exceed the benefits of fixing the error
- Because it may be fixed in an upcoming patch from development teams or suppliers

Reactive and Proactive Problem Management Activities

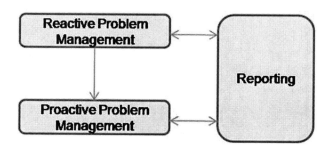

Figure 7.R—Reactive and Proactive Problem Management Activities

Both reactive and proactive Problem Management activities seek to raise problems, manage them through the Problem Management process, find the underlying causes of the incidents they are associated with, and prevent future recurrences of those incidents. The difference between reactive and proactive Problem Management lies in how the Problem Management process is triggered (**Service Operation, Page 98**):

- With reactive Problem Management, process activities will typically be triggered in reaction to an incident that has taken place. Reactive Problem Management complements Incident Management activities by focusing on the underlying cause of an incident to prevent its recurrence and identifying workarounds when necessary.
- With proactive Problem Management, process activities are triggered by activities seeking to improve services. One example might be trend analysis activities to find common underlying causes of historical incidents that took place to prevent their recurrence. Proactive Problem Management complements CSI activities by helping to identify workarounds and improvement actions that can improve the quality of a service.

By redirecting the efforts of an organization from reacting to large numbers of incidents to preventing incidents, an organization provides a better service to its customers and makes more effective use of the available resources within the IT support organization.

Problem Models

PROBLEMS MAY BE SIMILAR TO each other from a high level perspective, but in truth they are all unique. Because of similarities, it is possible to handle different problems in a consistent way based on identified characteristics. Problem Models allow this consistency to be maintained across multiple problems. Problem Management supports the creation of a known error record in the KEDB. These records will ensure quicker diagnosis of the problem and resolution if one exists. Problem Models are used primarily when a problem is present and no solution is currently available, such as when a third party application has a design flaw.

Problem models are similar in concept to incident models and request models..

Incidents versus problems

MANY ORGANIZATIONS HAVE DIFFICULTY UNDERSTANDING the difference between incidents and problems and think they are the same. This is not the case. A single event may indicate an incident and a problem simultaneously: which is most of the time. The event is an incident if its results in an unplanned interruption to a service or the quality of the service decreases. The goal when dealing with an incident is to restore the services to a normal state to ensure the service is providing business value as soon as possible after event.

Incident management does not deal with the underlying issue causing the disruption or loss in quality. The underlying issue, or problem, is handled by problem management. By dealing with the underlying problem, Problem Management hopes to prevent any future incidents from occurring.

Problem Management and Incident Management are not invoked simultaneously: Incident Management is invoked first. If the situation warrants that Problem Management be invoked, a problem is initiated out of the incident and typically a problem record can be created based on the incident record. Organizations must define when a problem record will be invoked: some situations the ITIL® identifies are (Service Operation, Page 99):

- *Incident Management cannot match an incident to existing problems and known errors*
- *Trend analysis of logged incidents reveals that an underlying problem might exist*
- *A major incident has occurred where Problem Management activities need to be undertaken to identify the root cause*
- *Other IT functions identify that a problem condition exists*
- *The Service Desk may have resolved an incident but has not determined a definitive cause and suspects that it is likely to recur*
- *Analysis of an incident by a support group, which reveals that an underlying problem exists or is likely to exist*
- *A notification from a supplier that a problem exists that has to be resolved* (Service Operations, page 99)

Reactive Problem Management

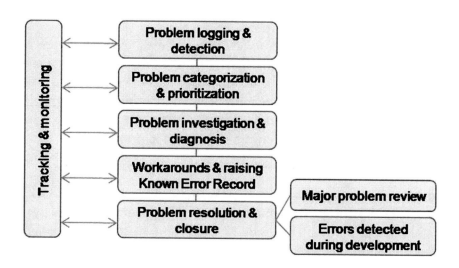

Figure 7.S—The Activities of Reactive Problem Management
"Based on Cabinet Office ITIL® material. Reproduced under licence from the Cabinet Office"

THE ACTIVITIES OF REACTIVE PROBLEM Management are similar to those of Incident Management for the logging, categorization, and classification for problems. The subsequent activities are different as this is where the actual root-cause analysis is performed and the Known Error corrected.

Overview of reactive Problem Management activities:

1. Problem detection
2. Problem logging
3. Problem categorization
4. Problem investigation and diagnosis
5. Workarounds (attached to the Problem or Known Error record)
6. Raising a Known Error record
7. Problem resolution
8. Problem closure
9. Major problem reviews

Major problem review:

After every major problem a review should be conducted to learn any lessons necessary for the future. Specifically, the review should examine (Service Operation, Page 105):

- *Those things that were done correctly*
- *Those things that were done wrong*
- *What could be done better in the future?*
- *How to prevent recurrence*
- *Whether there has been any third-party responsibility and whether follow-up actions are needed*

Such reviews can be used as part of training and awareness activities for staff—any lessons learned should be documented in appropriate procedures, working instructions, diagnostic scripts, or Known Error Records.

Proactive Problem Management

THE TWO MAIN ACTIVITIES OF proactive Problem Management are:

Trend analysis
- Review reports from other processes (e.g., trends in incidents, availability levels, relationships with changes and releases)
- Identify recurring problems or training opportunities for IT staff, customers, and end users.

Targeting preventative action
- Perform a cost-benefit analysis of all costs associated with prevention
- Target specific areas taking up the most support attention
- Coordinate preventative action with Availability and Capacity Management, focusing on vulnerable areas of the infrastructure (e.g., single points of failure, components reaching full capacity/utilization)

Inputs

EXAMPLES OF INPUTS TO THE Problem Management process may include (Service Operation, Page 106):

- *Incident records for incidents that have triggered Problem Management activities*
- *Incident reports and histories that will be used to support proactive problem trending*
- *Information about CIs and their status*
- *Communication and feedback about incidents and their symptoms*
- *Communication and feedback about RFCs and releases that have been implemented or planned for implementation*
- *Communication of events that were triggered from Event Management*
- *Operational and service level objectives*
- *Customer feedback on success of problem resolution activities and overall quality of Problem Management activities*
- *Agreed criteria for prioritizing and escalating problems*
- *Output from risk management and risk assessment activities*

Outputs

EXAMPLES OF OUTPUTS FROM THE Problem Management process may include (Service Operation, Page 106):

- *Resolved problems and actions taken to achieve their resolution*
- *Updated Problem Management records with accurate problem detail and history*
- *RFCs to remove infrastructure errors*
- *Workarounds for incidents*
- *Known error records*
- *Problem Management reports*

- *Output and improvement recommendations from major problem review activity*

Request Fulfillment

Terminology

Term	Definition
request model	(ITIL® Service Operation) A repeatable way of dealing with a particular category of service request. A request model defines specific agreed steps that will be followed for a service request of this category. Request models may be very simple with no requirement for authorization (e.g., password reset) or may be more complex with many steps that require authorization (e.g., provision of an existing IT service). See also request fulfillment.
service request	(ITIL® Service Operation) A formal request from a user for something to be provided—for example, a request for information or advice, to reset a password, or to install a workstation for a new user. Service requests are managed by the request fulfillment process, usually in conjunction with the service desk. Service requests may be linked to a request for change as part of fulfilling the request.

"Service request" is a generic term encompassing several types of demands from users on the IT organization, usually in the form of changes that are small in nature, low risk, and low cost in its execution, and frequently performed. Many of these requests are related to hardware moves, application installations, new user add to a directory structure, or password resets. The Request Fulfilment is dedicated to handling these requests to ensure they do not interfere or congest other service management processes, such as Change Management or Incident Management.

Purpose

REQUEST FULFILLMENT IS THE PROCESS *responsible for managing the lifecycle of all service requests from the users* (Service Operation, Page 87).

The objectives of the Request Fulfillment process are to (Service Operation, Page 87):

- *Maintain user and customer satisfaction through efficient and professional handling of all service requests*
- *Provide a channel for users to request and receive standard services for which a predefined authorization and qualification process exists*
- *Provide information to users and customers about the availability of services and the procedure for obtaining them*
- *Source and deliver the components of requested standard services (e.g., licenses and software media)*
- *Assist with general information, complaints, or comments*

Scope

THE BENEFIT OF THE REQUEST Fulfilment process is that supported "service request" has already been pre-defined, its activities are to be performed and broken down and assigned to resources, and documented as a request model and stored in the SKMS. Service requests do not need to be restricted to IT-specifci requests, but can also include and request from the business, such as servicing a photocopier, repairing a hole in the wall, or fixing a squeak in the door. Service requests are known and planned, though their frequency or volume may be unknown. Some organizations will treat service requests as another type of incident, but incidents are typically characterized as unplanned events. The organization must decide what constitutes a service request.

Resolving a service request will generally require varied types of activities or a level of specialization in the activity. In large organizations, the number of service requests to be handled may be extremely large. A requirement may be in place to track requests significantly different from incidents, problems, or changes. For these reasons, it may be appropriate to handle service requests separate from other processes.

Note that ultimately it will be up to each organization to decide and document which service requests it will handle through the request fulfillment process and which will have to go through other processes. (Service Operation, Page 87).

Request Models

As MANY SERVICE REQUESTS ARE frequently recurring, predefined Request Models should be defined that document:

- What activities are required to fulfill the request
- The roles and responsibilities involved
- Target timescales and escalation paths
- Other policies or requirements that apply

Similar to Change Models, this will enable the IT department (and the Service Desk in particular) to have a clear definition of the appropriate types of service requests and repeatable actions describing how requests should be fulfilled.

Activities

1. Menu selection

Where practical, some mechanism of self help should be utilized so that users can generate service requests using technology that interfaces with existing service management tools. This might be via a website that offers users a menu-driven interface where they can select common services and provide input details. In some instances, the fulfillment of the service request can be entirely automated using workflow, ERP, software deployment, and other tools. For others, manual activities will be required to fulfill the request using resources from the IT department, suppliers, or other parties involved in the provision of IT services.

2. Financial Approval

While the service request may already have approval from Change Management, there may be some form of financial approval that is required when there are financial implications (usually those above a defined dollar amount). It may be possible to agree upon fixed prices for standard requests, otherwise the cost must be estimated and submitted to the user/customer for financial approval (who may in turn require their own line management/financial approval).

3. Other Approval

Where there may be compliance and regulatory implications for the service request, wider business approval may be needed. These approval mechanisms should be built into the request models as appropriate. Change Management should establish that there are mechanisms in place to check for and safeguard these conditions in order for the standard change to be qualified for preapproval.

4. **Fulfillment**

The tasks required for Fulfillment will vary depending on the characteristics of the service request at hand. Some requests can be fulfilled using only automated mechanisms. Others may be fulfilled by the Service Desk at the first-line or escalated, where necessary, to internal or external specialist groups. To ensure compatibility, Request Fulfillment should be interfaced with existing procurement and supplier processes; however, the Service Desk should maintain control and visibility for all requests regardless of where it is fulfilled.

5. **Closure**

When the Service Request has been fulfilled, it should be referred back to the Service Desk to initiate closure. This should include some verification that the request has been satisfied using either confirmation with the end user or other automated means.

Inputs

EXAMPLES OF INPUTS TO THE Request Fulfillment process can include (Service Operation, Page 94):

- *Work requests*
- *Authorization forms*
- *Service requests*
- *RFCs*
- *Requests from various sources, such as phone calls, web interfaces, or email*
- *Request for information*

Outputs

EXAMPLES OF OUTPUTS FROM THE Request Fulfillment process may include (Service Operation, Page 94):

- *Authorized/rejected service requests*
- *Request fulfillment status reports*
- *Fulfilled service requests*
- *Incidents (rerouted)*

- *RFCs/standard changes*
- *Asset/CI updates*
- *Updated request records*
- *Closed service requests*
- *Cancelled service requests*

Access Management

WHEN AN IT SERVICE IS available for use by the customer and end-users, specified components of the service will typically be accessed. Without this access, the service holds no value for the business. Access Management is a process designed to manage the access to the different components of a service. The process serves two roles: ensure those individuals who are allowed to access the service are granted authority to do so and those individuals who do not have authorization are denied access. Different organization know access management as identity management or rights management.

Terminology

Term	Definition
rights	(ITIL® Service Operation) Entitlements or permissions granted to a user or role—for example, the right to modify particular data or to authorize a change.

© **Crown** Copyright 2011 Reproduced under license from the Cabinet Office

Purpose

THE PURPOSE OF ACCESS MANAGEMENT is to execute the policies and actions defined in the Information Security Management process by providing users the rights to use a service or group of services. The objectives of the Access Management process are to (Service Operation, Page 110):

- *Manage access to services based on policies and actions defined in Information Security Management (see ITIL® Service Design)*
- *Efficiently respond to requests for granting access to services, changing access rights, or restricting access, ensuring that the rights being provided or changed are properly granted*

- *Oversee access to services and ensure rights being provided are not improperly used*

Scope

THE SCOPE ACCESS MANAGEMENT IS to effectively execute of the policies in Information Security Management, enabling the organization to manage the confidentiality, availability and integrity of the organization's data and intellectual property. With Access Management, users are given the right to use a service, and works in cooperation with Availability Management to ensure access is available at all agreed times. Access Management is executed by all Technical and Application Management functions and is usually not considered a separate function; though, a single control point of coordination may exist, usually in IT Operations Management or on the Service Desk. Access Management can be initiated by a service request.

Relationship with Other Processes

AS DESCRIBED ABOVE, ACCESS MANAGEMENT is often centrally coordinated by the Service Desk (being the single point of contact with the end user community) but can involve the Technical and Application Management functions. Where access is controlled by external suppliers, interfaces need to be developed to coordinate requests for/ modifications to access levels.

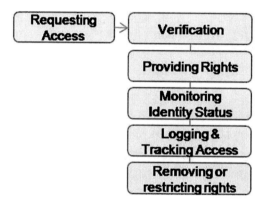

Figure 7.T—Access Management Activities

"Based on Cabinet Office ITIL® material. Reproduced under licence from the Cabinet Office"

FIGURE 7.T DEMONSTRATES THE LIFECYCLE for managing access to services, information, and facilities. In many implementations, these activities relate to the lifecycle of a user as they join the organization, change roles (possibly many times), and finally leave the organization. There should be integration with existing business processes for human resources so that access levels can be continually checked for accuracy against defined job roles.

Request access

Any number of mechanisms can be used to request access or restrict access. The most common mechanisms are:

- A service request from human resources, typically in conjunction with a new hire, promotion, transfer, or termination of employment
- A Request for Change
- A service request submitted via the Request Fulfilment system
- As part of a pre-authorized script or option, such as when an application is downloaded from a staging server.

The guidelines or rules for requesting access are usually documented as part of the Request Fulfillment model associated with requests for access and described in the Service Catalog.

Verification

Every request for access to an IT service must be verified to ensure the user requesting access is who they say they are and they have a legitimate requirements to access the service.

Verifying a person's identity is usually achieved by the user providing their user name and password, but this is contingent on the organization's security policies. Sometimes, further authentication may be required, such as biometric readings, use of an electronic access key, encryption device, database of secret questions and answers known only to the user, or other such methods.

Establishing a legitimate requirement for access will require some independent verification, other than the user's request. This can be done through a notification from human resources communicating the change in employment status, authorization from an appropriate manager, submission of a service request of RFC with supporting evidence, or a policy stating users can have access to optional services if needed.:

When new services are introduced to the environment, the change record should reflect which users or groups of users will have access to the service, which Access Management will determine if all the users are still authorized and automatically provide access as specified in the RFC.

Provide rights

Once a request for access has been submitted and the user and access permissions verified, the appropriate rights are provided. Access Management does not decide who has access to which IT services; it simply executes the policies and regulations defined during Service Strategy and Service Design. Access Management will enforce decisions to restrict or provide access, not make the decision.

To provide a user with the rights to use a requested service, a request is sent to every team or department involved in supporting that service to take the necessary action. For some organizations, these tasks are automated..

As the number of roles and groups used to provide access to users grows, the probability that a role conflict will occur also grows. A role conflict is a situation where two specific roles or groups, if assigned to a single user, will create issues with separation of duties or conflict of interest.

Careful planning of roles and groups will prevent role conflicts; however, most role conflicts are caused by policies and decisions made outside of service operation—either by the business or by different project teams working during Service Design. When a role conflict is identified, the conflict must be documented and escalated to the stakeholders to resolve.

The definitions of roles and groups can also be too broad or too narrow to be effective. Using only predefined roles precludes that some users may need a little more or less access than the generic offering provides. These 'exceptions' require specific rights to be added or subtracted from the standard roles. Each exception must be coordinated and implemented by Access Management and approved through the originating process.

A regular review of the roles and groups will be performed by Access Management to verify the roles created and ensure that they are appropriate for the services that IT delivers and supports. Any obsolete or unwanted roles/groups should be removed.

Check and monitor identity status

During the lifecycle of an employee, their status may change as they are promoted, transferred, assigned to projects, or their employment ends. As their status changes, so does their access and this change has to be monitored. This monitoring is usually done in cooperation with the human resources department of the organization, but can also be performed through periodic audits of users. ITITL provides the following examples of changes include (Service Operation, Page 113):

- *Job changes: In this case, the user will possibly need access to different or additional services.*
- *Promotions or demotions: The user will probably use the same set of services but will need access to different levels of functionality or data.*
- *Transfers: In this situation, the user may need access to exactly the same set of services but in a different region with different working practices and different sets of data.*
- *Resignation or death: Access needs to be completely removed to prevent the user name being used as a security loophole.*
- *Retirement: In many organizations, an employee who retires may still have access to a limited set of services, including benefits systems or systems that allow them to purchase company products at a reduced rate.*
- *Disciplinary action: In some cases, the organization will require a temporary restriction to prevent the user from accessing some or all of the services that they would normally have access to. There should be a feature in the process and tools to do this, rather than having to delete and reinstate the user's access rights.*
- *Dismissals: Where an employee or contractor is dismissed or where legal action is taken against a customer (for example, for defaulting on payment for products purchased on the internet), access should be revoked immediately. In addition, Access Management, working together with Information Security Management, should take active measures to prevent and detect malicious action against the organization from that user.*

The process can also be automated after clearly understanding and documenting the typical user lifecycle in the organization. The more Access Management understands about specific status changes, the more efficiency they can achieve through the process. All changes in access must leave an audit trail.

Log and track access

Access Management also has a proactive element in its process to ensure users are properly using the rights they were provided through access monitoring and control. This activity is usually included in the monitoring activities of all Technical and Application Management functions and all service operation processes and exceptions found are handled by incident Management. Abuse of access rights must be handled carefully and confidentiality because any information related to these situations can expose vulnerabilities in the organization's security.

Information Security Management has an important role in detecting unauthorized access. Any suspicious access will be compared to the rights provided by Access Management. Access Management will, in turn, define the parameters to be used in intrusion detection. Access Management may be asked to provide a record of access for specific services for use in forensic investigations where a user is suspected of breaches of policy, inappropriate use of resources, or fraudulent use of data. Through access monitoring, Access Management may acquire evidence of dates, times, and even content of that user's access to specific services.

Remove or restrict rights

Access Management is also responsible for revoking rights to use a service. This revocation is not arbitrarily performed but based on a request, usually in conjunction with a change in employment status for a user.

Removing access is usually done in the event of death, resignation, termination, change in responsibilities, or transfers or traveling between countries.

In some cases, access should be restricted, not removed. A restriction of access can be for the level of access, the times when access is permitted or not permitted, or how longer access is permitted or not permitted. Restricting access is usually done in the event of changes in responsibilities, demotions, user is under investigation, user is away from company temporarily.

Inputs
EXAMPLES OF INPUTS TO ACCESS Management may include (Service Operation, Page 115):

- *Information security policies (from Service Design)*
- *Operational and service level requirements for granting access to services, performing Access Management administrative activities and responding to Access Management related events*
- *Authorized RFCs to access rights*
- *Authorized requests to grant or terminate access rights*

Outputs
EXAMPLES OF OUTPUTS FROM ACCESS Management may include (Service Operation, Page 115):

- *Provision of access to IT services in accordance with information security policies*
- *Access Management records and history of access granted to services*
- *Access Management records and history where access has been denied and the reasons for the denial*
- *Timely communications concerning inappropriate access or abuse of services*

Service Operation Summary

FROM A CUSTOMER VIEWPOINT, SERVICE Operation is where actual value is seen. This is because it is the execution of strategies, designs and plans, and improvements from the Service Lifecycle stages.

Key benefits delivered as a result of Service Operation are:

- Effectiveness and efficiency in IT service delivery and support
- Increased return on investment
- More productive and positive users of IT services

Other benefits can be defined as:

1. **Long term**: Over a period of time, the Service Operation processes, functions, performance, and output are evaluated. These reports will be analyzed and decisions made about whether the improvement is needed and how best to implement it through Service Design and Transition, e.g., deployment of new tools, changes to process designs, reconfiguration of the infrastructure.
2. **Short term**: Improvement of working practices within the Service Operations processes, functions, and technology itself. Generally they involve smaller improvements that do not mean changes to the fundamental nature of a process or technology, e.g., tuning, training, personnel redeployment, etc.

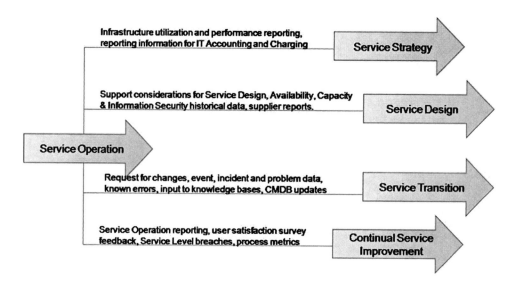

Figure 7.U—Some Outputs to Other Lifecycle Stages

Service Operation Scenario

- **Functions**

Service Desk

> ▷ Service Desk has been trained in HYPE and can support users
> ▷ Has access to known errors and workarounds to resolve incidents

Technical Management

> ▷ Designed, built, tested, and rolled HYPE out into live environment
> ▷ Supports HYPE service

Application Management

> ▷ Made modifications to HYPE application to ensure effectively interfaced with XY app
> ▷ Provided training on HYPE to users and Service Desk

IT Operations Management

> ▷ Creates backups of logs, monitors component events

- **Processes**

Event Management

- Sends alerts to IT Ops when HYPE logs backups pass/fail
- Monitors thresholds for triggers on bandwidth (set up in Availability Management)

Request Fulfillment Management

- Users use this process to request copy of logs

Access Management

- Password reset of HYPE account—provide authorized users access

Incident Management and Problem Management are not discussed in this example.

Service Operation Review Questions

Question 1
What is the best definition of an Incident Model?

    a)   Predicting the impact of incidents on the network
    b)   A type of incident that is used as a best practice model
    c)   A set of pre-defined steps to be followed when dealing with a known type of incident
    d)   An incident that requires a separate system

Question 2
What is the difference between a known error and a problem?

    a)   The underlying cause of a known error is known. The underlying cause of a problem is not known
    b)   A known error involves an error in the IT infrastructure. A problem does not involve such an error.
    c)   A known error always originates from an incident. This is not always the case with a problem.
    d)   With a problem, the relevant configuration items have been identified. This is not the case with a known error.

Question 3
Information is regularly exchanged between Problem Management and Change Management. What information is this?

    a)   Known errors from Problem Management on the basis of which Change Management can generate Requests for Change (RFCs)
    b)   RFCs resulting from known errors
    c)   RFCs from the users that Problem Management passes on to Change Management
    d)   RFCs from the Service Desk that Problem Management passes on to Change Management

Question 4

Incident Management has a value to the business by?

a) Helping to control cost of fixing technology
b) Enabling customers to resolve problems
c) Helping to maximize business impact
d) Helping to reduce the business impact

Question 5

Which of the following is NOT an example of a service request?

a) A user calls the Service Desk to order a new mouse
b) A user calls the Service Desk because they would like to change the functionality of an application
c) A user calls the Service Desk to reset their password
d) A user logs onto an internal website to download a licensed copy of software from a list of approved options

Question 6

The BEST definition of an event is?

a) A situation where a capacity threshold has been exceeded and an agreed service level has already been impacted
b) An occurrence that is significant for the management of the IT infrastructure or delivery of services
c) A problem that requires immediate attention
d) A social gathering of IT staff to celebrate the release of a service

Question 7

Technical Management is NOT responsible for?

a) Maintenance of the local network
b) Identifying technical skills required to manage and support the IT infrastructure
c) Defining the service agreements for the technical infrastructure
d) Response to the disruption to the technical infrastructure

Question 8

Which of the following is NOT an objective of Service Operation?

a) Thorough testing to ensure that services are designed to meet business needs
b) To deliver and support IT Services
c) To manage the technology used to deliver services
d) To monitor the performance of technology and processes

Question 9

Which of the following BEST describes the purpose of Event Management?

a) The ability to detect events, analyze them, and determine the appropriate control action
b) The ability to coordinate changes in events
c) The ability to monitor and control projected service outages
d) The ability to report on success of all batch processing jobs

Question 10

Which process or function is responsible for management of the Data Center facility?

a) IT Operations Control
b) Supplier Management
c) Facilities Management
d) Technical Function

CONTINUAL SERVICE IMPROVEMENT

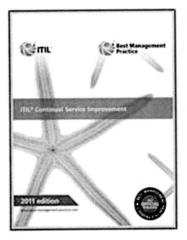

Figure 8.A—Continual
Service Improvement
*"© Crown copyright 2011
Reproduced under licence from the
Cabinet Office"*

Processes:

• The Seven-Step Improvement process

The main areas of focus for Continual Service Improvement (CSI) to address are (Continual Service Improvement, Page 4):

• *The overall health of ITSM as a discipline*
• *Continual alignment of the portfolio of IT services with the current and future business needs*
• *Maturity of the enabling IT processes for each service in a continual service lifecycle approach*

Purpose

The purpose of the CSI stage of the lifecycle is to align IT services with changing business needs by identifying and implementing improvements to IT services that support business processes. These improvement activities support the lifecycle approach through Service Strategy, Service Design, Service Transition and Service Operation. CSI is always seeking ways to improve service effectiveness, process effectiveness, and cost effectiveness. (Continual Service Improvement, Page 4)

If we lived in a world where market places, business strategies, management practices, innovation, and technology were stagnant, we would be complete with the Service Lifecycle and focus on providing value to the business. Unfortunately, the world is not stagnant and is always changing. These changes will impact how IT services are provided to the business, including how the value of these services is interpreted and accepted. While some changes will require a major overhaul of an IT service, the majority of changes will be minor.

In addition to the inevitable influences of change on IT, there is always the drive to improve how the service perform, goals to reduce cost, or commitment to provide greater value to business leading to finding ways to improve the IT service. An important part of determining opportunities for improvement is the measurement of current performance. Consider the following sayings about measurements and management (Continual Service Improvement, Page 4):

- ***You cannot manage what you cannot control.***
- ***You cannot control what you cannot measure.***
- ***You cannot measure what you cannot define.***

Continuous Service Improvement (CSI) is a Service Lifecycle stage designed to address influencing changes on the environment and seek out opportunities for improving services.

The objectives of CSI are to (Continual Service Improvement, Page 4):

- *Review, analyze, prioritize, and make recommendations on improvement opportunities in each lifecycle stage: Service Strategy, Service Design, Service Transition, Service Operation and CSI itself*
- *Review and analyze service level achievement*
- *Identify and implement specific activities to improve IT service quality and improve the efficiency and effectiveness of the enabling processes*
- *Improve cost effectiveness of delivering IT services without sacrificing customer satisfaction*
- *Ensure applicable quality management methods are used to support continual improvement activities*
- *Ensure that processes have clearly defined objectives and measurements that lead to actionable improvements*
- *Understand what to measure, why it is being measured, and what the successful outcome should be*

Scope

ITIL® CONTINUAL SERVICE IMPROVEMENT PROVIDES guidance in four main areas (Continual Service Improvement, Page 4):

- *The overall health of ITSM as a discipline*
- *The continual alignment of the Service Portfolio with the current and future business needs*
- *The maturity and capability of the organization, management, processes, and people utilized by the services*
- *Continual improvement of all aspects of the IT service and the service assets that support them*

To implement CSI successfully, it is important to understand the different activities that need to be applied. The following activities support CSI (Continual Service Improvement, Page 4):

- *Reviewing management information and trends to ensure that services are meeting agreed service levels*
- *Reviewing management information and trends to ensure that the output of the enabling processes are achieving the desired results*
- *Periodically conducting maturity assessments against the process activities and associated roles to demonstrate areas of improvement or, conversely, areas of concern*
- *Periodically conducting internal audits verifying employee and process compliance*
- *Reviewing existing deliverables for appropriateness*
- *Periodically proposing recommendations for improvement opportunities*
- *Periodically conducting customer satisfaction surveys*
- *Reviewing business trends and changed priorities and keeping abreast of business projections*
- *Conducting external and internal service reviews to identify CSI opportunities*
- *Measuring and identifying the value created by CSI improvements*

Improvement activities need structure within an IT environment. Some companies, such as financial, are heavily regulated and some control must be in place to limit unplanned changed in the environment, even down to small changes in the configuration of some systems. Improvements do not happen automatically either, and opportunities must be identified, evaluated, and prioritized. Continuous improvement is a process within ITSM with defined activities, inputs, outputs, roles and reporting. The responsibility of CSI is to ensure ITSM processes are developed and deployed to support business customers. Each of the ITSM processes and associated services must have an continuous improvement strategy in place to ensure value is always provided to the business customer.

Indicators and metrics within the environment must be monitored to identify improvement opportunities. Improvements to the environment will bring about change which must be controlled using Change Management. Deliverables from CSI must be reviewed regularly to ensure they are complete, functional, reachable, and relevant to the current environment. The CSI stage of the Service Lifecycle is designed to ensure all of these requirements are met.

Value to the Business

ADOPTING AND IMPLEMENTING STANDARD AND consistent approaches for CSI will (Continual Service Improvement, Page 5):

- *Lead to a gradual and continual improvement in service quality, where justified*
- *Ensure that IT services remain continuously aligned to business requirements*
- *Result in gradual improvements in cost effectiveness through a reduction in costs and/or the capability to handle more work at the same cost*
- *Use monitoring and reporting to identify opportunities for improvement in all lifecycle stages and in all processes*
- *Identify opportunities for improvements in organizational structures, resourcing capabilities, partners, technology, staff skills and training, and communications*

Major Concepts

The Continual Service Improvement Approach

THE CSI APPROACH PROVIDES THE basis by which improvements to IT Service Management processes can be made. They are questions to ask in order to ensure all the required elements are identified to achieve the improvements desired.

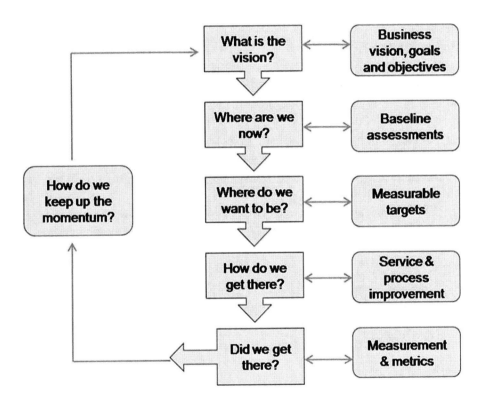

Figure 8.B—Continual Service Improvement Approach
© Crown Copyright 2011 Reproduced under license from the Cabinet Office

THE CONTINUAL SERVICE IMPROVEMENT APPROACH summarizes the constant cycle for improvement. While there may be a focus on a particular lifecycle stage, the questions require close interactions with all the other ITIL® processes in order to achieve Continual Service Improvement.

Example improvement initiative for Service Operation:

- **What is the Vision?** Defining what wants to be achieved by improving Service Operation. Is the focus on service quality, compliance, security, costs, or customer satisfaction? What is the broad approach that we should take?
- **Where are we now?** Baselines taken by performing maturity assessments and by identifying what practices are currently being used (including informal and ad-hoc processes). What information can be provided by the Service Portfolio regarding strengths, weaknesses, risks, and priorities of the service provider?
- **Where do we want to be?** Defining key goals and objectives that wish to be achieved by the formalization of Service Operation processes, including both short-term and long-term targets.
- **How do we get there?** Perform a gap analysis between the current practices and defined targets to begin developing plans to overcome these gaps. Typically, the process owners and Service Operation manager will oversee the design/improvement of the processes, making sure they are fit for purpose and interface as needed with other service management processes.
- **Did we get there?** At agreed time schedules, checks should be made as to how the improvement initiatives have progressed. Which objectives have been achieved? Which haven't? What went well and what went wrong?
- **How do we keep the momentum going?** Now that the targets and objectives have been met, what is the next course of improvements that can be made? This should feed back into re-examining the vision and following the CSI approach steps again.

Since Continual Service Improvement involves ongoing change, it is important to develop an effective communication strategy to support CSI activities and ensure people remain appropriately informed. This communication must include aspects of:

- What the service implications are
- What the impact on personnel will be
- Approach/process used to reach the objective

If this communication does not exist, staff will fill the gaps with their own perceptions. Proper reporting should assist in addressing any misconceptions about improvements.

To aid in understanding the differences in perception between the service provider and the customer, a Service Gap Model can be used. This identifies the most obvious potential gaps in the Service Lifecycle from both a business and IT perspective.

SLM will produce Service Improvement Plans (SIPs) to meet the identified gaps.

Relationships within the Service Lifecycle:

- **What is the Vision?** Service Strategy, Service Portfolio
- **Where are we now?** Baselines taken using Service Portfolios, Service Level Management, and Financial Management for IT, etc.
- **Where do we want to be?** Service Portfolio, Service Measurement and Reporting
- **How do we get there?** CSI and all ITIL® processes
- **Did we get there?** Service Measurement and Reporting
- **How do we keep the momentum going?** Continual Service Improvement

The Deming Cycle

IN THE 1950s, W. EDWARDS Deming proposed that business processes should be analyzed and measured to identify sources of variations that cause products to deviate from customer requirements. He recommended that business processes be placed in a continuous feedback loop so that managers and supporting staff can identify and change the parts of the process that need improvements. As a theorist, Deming created a simplified model to illustrate this continuous process, commonly known as the PDCA cycle for Plan, Do, Check, Act:

- **Plan**: Design or revise business process components to improve results
- **Do**: Implement the plan and measure its performance
- Check: Assess the measurements and report the results to decision-makers
- **Act**: Decide on changes needed to improve the process

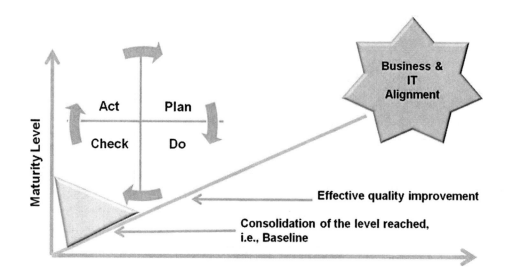

Figure 8.C—Plan-Do-Check-Act Cycle
© Crown Copyright 2011 Reproduced under license from the
Cabinet Office

TOO OFTEN ORGANIZATIONS ARE LOOKING for a big-bang approach to improvements. It is important to understand that a succession or series of small, planned increments of improvements will not stress the infrastructure as much and they will eventually amount to a large amount of improvement over time.

So in relation to Continual Service Improvement, the PDCA model can be applied with the following steps.

1. Plan—scope, establishing goals, objectives and requirements, interfaces, process activities, framework of roles and responsibilities, appropriate tools, methods and techniques for measuring, assessing, analyzing, and reporting
2. Do (implement)—funding and budgets, documenting and allocation roles and responsibilities, documentation and maintaining CSI policies, plans and procedures, communication and training, ensuring monitoring, analysis and trend evaluating, and reporting tools are in place, integration with the other lifecycle stages
3. Check (monitor, measure, review)—reporting against plans, documentation review, conducting process assessments and audits. The key here is identifying and recommending CSI process improvement opportunities.

4. Act—implementing actual CSI enhancements (e.g., updating CSI policies, procedures, roles, and responsibilities)

CSI Register

THE CORE TOOL OF CSI is the CSI record, where all improvement opportunities are recorded and organized to show small, medium, and large endeavours. The size of an improvement can be based on several factors, including scope, impact, risk, cost, time, and benefit. Knowing this information will also allow the organization to prioritize improvement opportunities accordingly. One possible drawback to identifying and prioritizing improvement opportunities is lower priority improvements may never get the attention they need, so it is advisable to review the CSI register regularly and raise the priority of long-standing improvements in the list. Some organizations adopt policies to address this issue and other similar issues related to aging improvements.

The CSI register is part of the Service Knowledge Management System (SKMS) and provides important information to the service provider. Usually, there are no restrictions on who in the IT organization has access to the CSI register and can submit a potential improvement. The production and maintenance of the CSI register is the accountability and responsibility of the CSI manager.

The CSI register provides a structure for capturing and recording improvement opportunities, their initiatives, and the realized benefits (predicted and actual). The CSI register must have a defined interface with strategic initiatives and several service management processes, such as Problem Management, Change Management, and Capacity Management. Many of the improvement opportunities captured in the CSI will be the result of regular service review meetings.

IT Governance

GOVERNANCE RELATES TO DECISIONS THAT define expectations, grant power, or verify performance. It consists either of a separate process or of a specific part of management or leadership processes. In the case of a business or of a non-profit organization, governance relates to consistent management, cohesive policies, processes, and decision-rights for a given area of responsibility. For example, managing at a corporate level might involve evolving policies on privacy, on internal investment, and on the use of data.

There are 3 main areas of governance:

- **Enterprise governance**: describes a framework that covers both corporate governance and the business management aspects of the organization. This achieves good corporate governance that is linked strategically with performance metrics and enables companies to focus all their energy on the key drivers that move their business forward.
- **Corporate governance**: concerned with promoting corporate fairness, transparency, and accountability. One example is the SOX act (2002) in the United States that was created in the aftermath of fraudulent behavior by corporate giants and states accountability provisions, such as criminal charges and incarceration for non-compliance.
- **IT governance**: Consisting of leadership, organizational structures, and processes, IT governance plays a major role in enterprise governance and ensures that the IT of an organization sustains and extends their strategies and objectives.. The board of directors and executive management are responsible for IT governance.

Service Measurement

Baselines

IMPROVEMENTS CAN BE SEEN AS movement within a service, process, or component: a move from point A to point B. For an improvement to be described and understood, one must be able to describe and understand both point A and point B. At the beginning, point B may be conceptual and defined as a prediction for where the improvement should lead; but when the improvement is complete, point B will be actual and clearly described.

To fully understand the improvement before, during, and after its implementation, point A must be marked or highlights. This is done by establishing a baseline – an initial data point for the improvement. Baselines are documented and accepted throughout the organization: they establish where the organization is in relation to a particular service or process. Baselines can be created at every level of the organization – strategic, tactical, and operational.

Baselines are created though measurements. If a baseline is not formally established, the first measurement efforts for a service are automatically used as the baseline. Throughout the improvement initiative and after, the service is monitored and measured. The data captured will be compared to baseline to understand the extent of the improvement, if any exists.

Why do we measure?

THERE ARE FOUR REASONS TO monitor and measure (Continual Service Improvement, Page 39):

- *To validate*: monitoring and measuring to validate previous decisions
- *To direct*: monitoring and measuring to set the direction for activities in order to meet set targets—it is the most prevalent reason for monitoring and measuring
- *To justify*: monitoring and measuring to justify with factual evidence or proof that a course of action is required
- *To intervene*: monitoring and measuring to identify a point of intervention, including subsequent changes and corrective actions

Types of Metrics

THERE ARE 3 TYPES OF metrics that an organization will need to collect to support CSI activities, as well as other process activities:

- **Technology metrics**: often associated with component and application-based metrics, such as performance, availability, etc. The various design architects and technical specialists are responsible for defining the technology metrics.
- **Process metrics**: captured in the form of Key Performance Indicators (KPIs) and activity metrics for the service management processes that determine the overall health of a process. Four key questions that KPIs can help to answer are centered on quality, performance, value, and compliance. CSI uses these metrics to identify improvement opportunities for each process. The various process owners are responsible for defining the metrics for the process that they are responsible for coordinating and managing.
- **Service metrics**: the results of the end-to-end service. Component metrics are used to calculate the service metrics. The service level manager(s) and service owners are responsible for defining appropriate service metrics.

Tension Metrics

ALL SERVICE PROVIDERS ARE FACED with the challenge of a balancing act between three main elements:

- Resources—people, IT infrastructure, consumables, and money
- Features—the product or service and its quality
- Time schedule—the timeframes within which various stages and the final delivery of a service or product are required to be achieved

Delivering a product or service is then a result of a balanced trade-off between the resources, the features, and the time schedule. Tension metrics can help find an equilibrium between the three elements by preventing a focus on one particular element. If an initiative is primarily focused towards on-time delivery of a product to the omission of other factors, it will be achieved by reducing the service features and resources in order to meet the delivery timeframe. This lack of focus will either lead to an increased budget or to a lower quality of product. Tension metrics assist in creating a balance between shared goals and delivering a product or service in line with the business requirements within a fixed time and budget.

Seven-Step Improvement Process

FUNDAMENTAL TO CSI IS THE concept of measurement. CSI uses the seven-step improvement process shown in Figure 8.D.

The value of the seven-step improvement process is that, by monitoring and analyzing the delivery of services, it will ensure that the current and future business outcome requirements can be met. The seven-step improvement process enables continual evaluation of the situation against current business needs and identifies opportunities to improve service provision for customers.

Terminology

Term	Definition
seven-step improvement process	(ITIL® Continual Service Improvement) The process responsible for defining and managing the steps needed to identify, define, gather, process, analyze, present, and implement improvements. The performance of the IT service provider is continually measured by this process and improvements are made to processes, IT services, and IT infrastructure in order to increase efficiency, effectiveness, and cost effectiveness. Opportunities for improvement are recorded and managed in the CSI register.

© **Crown** Copyright 2011 Reproduced under license from the Cabinet Office

Purpose

AS WITH EVERYTHING IN IT Service Management, activities must be measurable and controlled to ensure that services to the business generate value. This holds true for CSI. The seven-step improvement process ensures a consistent approach is established to make meaningful improvements to IT and increase the value of the services to the business. The process is used to identify, define, gather, process, analyze, present, and implement improvements.

The objectives of the seven-step improvement process are to (Continual Service Improvement, Page 47):

- *Identify opportunities for improving services, processes, tools, etc.*
- *Reduce the cost of providing services and ensuring that IT services enable the required business outcomes to be achieved. A clear objective will be cost reduction, but this is not the only criterion. If service delivery or quality reduces as a result, the overall impact may be neutral or even negative.*
- *Identify what needs to be measured, analyzed, and reported to establish improvement opportunities*
- *Continually review service achievements to ensure they remain matched to business requirements, continually align and re-align service provision with outcome requirements*
- *Understand what to measure, why it is being measured, and carefully define the successful outcome*
- *The value of the seven-step improvement process is that by monitoring and analyzing the delivery of services, it will ensure the current and future business outcome requirements can be met. The seven-step improvement*

process enables continual assessment of the current situation against business needs and identifies opportunities to improve service provision for customers.

Scope

THE SEVEN-STEP IMPROVEMENT PROCESS CONSISTS of a number of activities and responsibilities relevant to ensuring improvements are properly identified, defined, developed, and implemented, including:

- Analysis of the performance and capabilities of services, processes throughout the lifecycle, partners, and technology.
- Continual alignment with the service portfolio of IT services and current and future business needs
- Maturing enabling IT processes for each service
- Using technology effectively and efficiently, including exploring and exploiting new technologies
- Increasing and appropriately utilizing the capabilities of the personnel

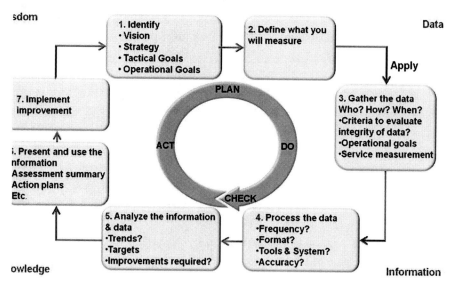

Figure 8.D—Seven Step Improvement Process
        © Crown Copyright 2011 Reproduced under license from the Cabinet Office

THE SEVEN-STEP IMPROVEMENT PROCESS IS a integral part of CSI. All the activities of the improvement process assist with CSI in some form. It is relatively easy to identify what happens but more challenging to understand how this will take place. The improvement process spans not only the management organization but the entire Service Lifecycle. This is a cornerstone of CSI, the main steps of which are as follows (Continual Service Improvement, Page 39):

1. *Identify the strategy for improvement*: *Identify the overall vision, business need, the strategy, and the tactical and operational goals*

2. *Define what you will measure:* *Service Strategy and Service Design should have identified this information early in the lifecycle. CSI can then start its cycle all over again at 'Where are we now?' and 'Where do we want to be?' This identifies the ideal situation for both the business and IT. CSI can conduct a gap analysis to identify the opportunities for improvement as well as answering the question 'How do we get there?'*

3. *Gather the data*: *In order to properly answer the question 'Did we get there?', data must first be gathered (usually through service operations). Data can be gathered from many different sources based on goals and objectives identified. At this point the data is raw and no conclusions are drawn.*

4. *Process the data*: *Here the data is processed in alignment with the critical success factors (CSFs) and KPIs specified. This means that timeframes are coordinated, unaligned data is rationalized and made consistent, and gaps in the data are identified. The simple goal of this step is to process data from multiple disparate sources to give it context that can be compared. Once we have rationalized the data we can begin analysis.*

5. *Analyze the information and data*: *As we bring the data more and more into context, it evolves from raw data into information where we can start to answer questions about who, what, when, where, and how, as well as trends and the impact on the business. It is the analyzing step that is most often overlooked or forgotten in the rush to present data to management.*

6. *Present and use the information*: *Here the answer to 'Did we get there?' is formatted and communicated in whatever way necessary to present to the various stakeholders an accurate picture of the results of the improvement efforts. Knowledge is presented to the business in a form and manner that reflects their needs and assists them in determining the next steps.*

7. *Implement improvement*: *The knowledge gained is used to optimize, improve, and correct services and processes. Issues have been identified and now solutions are implemented—wisdom is applied to the knowledge. The improvements that need to be taken to improve the service or process are*

communicated and explained to the organization. Following this step the organization establishes a new baseline and the cycle begins anew.

Inputs and Outputs

MONITORING TO IDENTIFY IMPROVEMENT OPPORTUNITIES is and must be an ongoing process. New incentives may trigger additional measurement activities, such as changing business requirements, poor performance with a process, or spiraling costs.

Many inputs and outputs to the process are documented within the steps discussed earlier, but examples of key inputs include (Continual Service Improvement, Page 64):

- *Service Catalog*
- *SLRs*
- *The service review meeting*
- *Vision and mission statements*
- *Corporate, divisional, and departmental goals and objectives*
- *Legislative requirements*
- *Governance requirements*
- *Budget cycle*
- *Customer satisfaction surveys*
- *The overall IT strategy*
- *Market expectations (especially in relation to competitive IT service providers)*
- *New technology drivers (e.g., cloud-based delivery and external hosting)*
- *Flexible commercial models (e.g., low capital expenditure and high operational expenditure commercial models and rental models)*

Continual Service Improvement Summary

THERE IS GREAT VALUE TO the business when service improvement takes a holistic approach throughout the entire lifecycle. Continual Service Improvement enables this holistic approach to be taken.

- Some key benefits of the Continual Service Improvement stage:
- Increased growth
- Competitive Advantage
- Increased Return On Investment
- Increased Value On Investment

ROI: Return on investment—difference between the benefit (saving) achieved and the amount expended to achieve that benefit, expressed as percentage. Logically we would like to spend a little to save a lot.

VOI: Value on investment—extra value created by establishment of benefits that include non-monetary or long-term outcomes. ROI is a subcomponent of VOI.

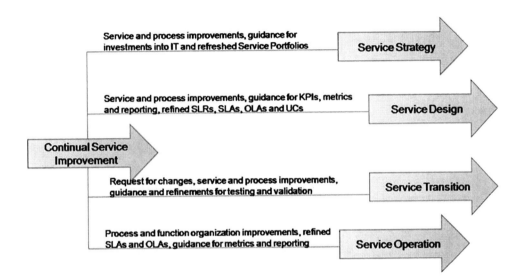

Figure 8.E—Some Outputs to Other Lifecycle Stages

Continual Service Improvement Scenario

To do this effectively, it was necessary to take metrics and data and analyze this against targets.

The CSI improvement approach was used as a roadmap for this SIP (Service Improvement Scenario). As the business needs changed, so did the perceived value of HYPE. HYPE had become an integral part of the business communication plan. As a result, new business plans/goals were established and new targets set with an action plan for improvement.

This will identify:

- Technology improvements
- Process improvements
- Document improvements
- Training, etc.

As plans were formalized and accepted by the business, Request for Changes to technology, process, and documentation were submitted to Change Management.

And so it continues!

Continual Service Improvement Review Questions

Question 1
Why should monitoring and measuring be used when trying to improve services?

    a)   To validate, justify, monitor, and improve
    b)   To validate, direct, justify, and intervene
    c)   To validate, check, act, and improve
    d)   To validate, analyze, direct, and improve

Question 2
Which is the first activity of the Continual Service Improvement (CSI) approach?

    a)   Assess the customer's requirements
    b)   Understand the vision of the business
    c)   Identify what can be measured
    d)   Develop a plan for improvement

Question 3
The four stages of the Deming Cycle are?

    a)   Plan, Assess, Check, Report
    b)   Plan, Do, Check, Act
    c)   Plan, Check, Revise, Improve
    d)   Plan, Do, Act, Assess

Question 4
Which of the following is NOT a step in the Continual Service Improvement (CSI) approach?

    a)   What is the vision?
    b)   Did we get there?
    c)   Who will help us get there?
    d)   Where are we now?

Question 5

Which of the following provides the correct set of governance levels managed by an organization?

    a)   Technology, Service, Business
    b)   Financial, Legal, Security
    c)   Process, Service, Technology
    d)   IT, Corporate, Enterprise

ITIL® FOUNDATION EXAM TIPS

Exam Details:
- 40 questions
- The correct answer is only one of the four
- 60 minutes duration
- 26 out of 40 is a pass (65%)
- Closed book
- No notes

Practical Suggestions:
- Read the question **CAREFULLY**
- At this exam level, the obvious answer is often the correct answer (*if you have read the question carefully!*)
- Beware of being misled by the preliminary text for the question
- If you think there should be another choice that would be the right answer, then you have to choose the most right answer
- Use strategies such as *"What comes first?"* or *"What doesn't belong?"* to help with the more difficult questions
- Where there are questions that involve multiple statements (i.e., 1, 2, 3, 4), then try to eliminate combinations that are immediately incorrect (based on something you can remember) so that the question is broken into smaller and more manageable pieces.

Make sure that you prepare adequately in the lead up to your exam by reviewing your notes, reading any available material, and attempting the sample exams.

We hope this book has been of value and wish you luck in your exam and future IT Service Management career!

ANSWERS FOR REVIEW QUESTIONS

The following section provides example reasoning for each answer. This is only a guide, however, and does not cover every possible reason why an answer is correct or incorrect.

Service Strategy

ANSWERS

1c, 2a, 3b, 4c, 5b, 6a, 7d, 8b, 9b, 10d

Question 1

Which ITIL® process is responsible for developing a charging system?

- a) Availability Management
- b) Capacity Management
- c) **Financial Management for IT Services—this is an element of IT accounting and chargeback**
- d) Service Level Management

Question 2

What is the RACI model used for?

- a) **Documenting the roles and relationships of stakeholders in a process or activity—this is the primary purpose of RACI, i.e., mapping processes to functions and roles**
- b) Defining requirements for a new service or process
- c) Analyzing the business impact of an incident
- d) Creating a balanced scorecard showing the overall status of Service Management

Question 3

Which of the following identifies two Service Portfolio components within the Service Lifecycle?

a) Catalog Service Knowledge Management System and Requirements Portfolio
b) **Service Catalog and Service Pipeline—correct, the three areas are Pipeline, Catalog, and Retired Services**
c) Service Knowledge Management System and Service Catalog
d) Service Pipeline and Configuration Management System

Question 4
Which of the following is NOT one of the ITIL® core publications?

a) Service Operation
b) Service Transition
c) **Service Derivation**
d) Service Strategy

Question 5
A Service Level Package is best described as?

a) A description of customer requirements used to negotiate a Service Level Agreement
b) **A defined level of utility and warranty associated with a core service package—correct, a combination of utility and warranty that meets the customer's needs**
c) A description of the value that the customer wants and for which they are willing to pay
d) A document showing the service levels achieved during an agreed reporting period

Question 6

Setting policies and objectives is the primary concern of which of the following elements of the Service Lifecycle?

a) **Service Strategy—see objectives of Service Strategy**
b) Service Strategy and Continual Service Improvement
c) Service Strategy, Service Transition, and Service Operation
d) Service Strategy, Service Design, Service Transition, Service Operation, and Continual Service Improvement

Question 7

A service owner is responsible for which of the following?

a) Designing and documenting a service
b) Carrying out the service operations activities needed to support a service
c) Producing a balanced scorecard showing the overall status of all services
d) **Recommending improvements—correct, the service owner is responsible for continually improving their service**

Question 8

The utility of a service is best described as:

a) Fit for design
b) **Fit for purpose**
c) Fit for function
d) Fit for use

Question 9

The warranty of a service is best described as:

a) Fit for design
b) **Fit for use**
c) Fit for purpose
d) Fit for function

Question 10

The contents of a service package includes:

a) Base Service Package, Supporting Service Package, Service Level Package

b) Core Service Package, Supporting Process Package, Service Level Package

c) Core Service Package, Base Service Package, Service Support Package

Core Service Package, Supporting Services Package, Service Level Package—correct, see Service Packages

Service Design

ANSWERS

1b, 2a, 3d, 4d, 5b, 6b, 7a, 8b, 9c, 10d

Question 1
Which ITIL® process analyzes threats and dependencies to IT services as part of the decision regarding countermeasures to be implemented?

   a) Availability Management
   b) **IT Service Continuity Management**
   c) Problem Management
   d) Service Asset and Configuration Management

Question 2
What is the name of the activity within the Capacity Management process whose purpose is to predict the future capacity requirements of new and changed services?

   a) **Application Sizing**
   b) Demand Management
   c) Modeling
   d) Tuning

Question 3
In which ITIL® process are negotiations held with customers about the availability and capacity levels to be provided?

   a) Availability Management
   b) Capacity Management
   c) Financial Management for IT Services
   d) **Service Level Management—SLM is always the process that negotiates with customers about any aspect of service quality**

Question 4

Which of the following statements is false?

a) It is impossible to maintain user and customer satisfaction during a disruption to service
b) When reporting the availability provided for a service, the percentage (%) availability that is calculated takes into account the agreed service hours
c) Availability of services could be improved by changes to the architecture, ITSM processes, or IT staffing levels
d) **Reports regarding availability should include more than just uptime, downtime, and frequency of failure and reflect the actual business impact of unavailability—correct, this is called business-oriented availability reporting**

Question 5
Which of the following activities is Service Level Management responsible for?

a) Informing users of available services
b) **Identifying customer needs**
c) Overseeing service release schedule
d) Keeping accurate records of all configuration items

Question 6

Which process reviews Operational Level Agreements (OLAs) on a regular basis?

    a)   Supplier Management
    b)   **Service Level Management**
    c)   Service Portfolio Management
    d)   Contract Management

Question 7

What is another term for Uptime?

    a)   **Mean Time Between Failures (MTBF)**
    b)   Mean Time to Restore Service (MTRS)
    c)   Mean Time Between System Incidents (MTBSI)
    d)   Relationship between MTBF and MTBSI

Question 8

Which of the following is an activity of IT Service Continuity Management?

    a)   Advising end users of a system failure
    b)   **Documenting the recovery procedure for a critical system—correct, this is an activity of the ITSCM process**
    c)   Reporting regarding availability
    d)   Guaranteeing that the Configuration Items are constantly kept up - to - date

Question 9
Information security must consider the following four perspectives:

1. Organizational
2. Physical
3. Technical
4. ?

a) Process
b) Security
c) **Procedural—see scope of Information Security Management**
d) Firewalls

Question 10
The 3 types of Service Level Agreements structures are:

a) Customer-based, Service-based, Corporate-based
b) Corporate-level, customer-level, service-level
c) Service-based, customer-based, user-based
Customer-based, service-based, multi-level

Service Transition

ANSWERS

1a, 2a, 3d, 4b, 5b, 6c, 7a, 8b, 9a, 10b

Question 1
The key element of a standard change is _____?

a) **Documentation of a pre-approved procedure for implementing the change**
b) Low risk to the production environment—this in itself does not guarantee a standard change
c) No requirement for service downtime—the risk of unplanned disruption may still be high
d) It can be included in the next monthly or quarterly release—this relates to the packaging of releases, not the classification of changes

Question 2
The four phases of Release and Deployment are:

1. Release and deployment planning
2. Release build and test
3. ?
4. Review and close
a) **Deployment**
b) Change authorization
c) Change coordination
d) Release coordination

Question 3

The 4 spheres of Knowledge Management are:

a) Data, facts, knowledge, wisdom
b) Ideas, facts, knowledge, wisdom
c) Data, information, facts, wisdom
d) **Data, information, knowledge, wisdom—easier to remember as DIKW**

Question 4

Which activity in Service Asset and Configuration Management would help to ascertain whether the recorded configuration items conform to the physical environment?

a) Control—this is the modification of CIs themselves
b) **Verification and audit**
c) Identification—this collects all the information to be stored for a CI
d) Status accounting—this does not itself include validation procedures

Question 5

After a change has been implemented, an evaluation is performed. What is this evaluation called?

a) Forward Schedule of Changes (FSC)
b) **Post Implementation Review (PIR)**
c) Service Improvement Program (SIP)
d) Service Level Requirement (SLR)

Question 6
Which of the following is not a change type?

    a) Standard change
    b) Normal change
    c) **Quick change**
    d) Emergency change

Question 7
Which process is responsible for maintaining software items in the Definitive Media Library (DML)?

    a) **Release and Deployment Management—as R&D will be responsible for storing and deploying all software items in the DML**
    b) Service Asset and Configuration Management—only responsible for maintaining the records associated with the DML
    c) Service validation and testing
    d) Change Management

Question 8
Which process or function is responsible for communicating the change schedule to the users?

    a) Change Management—responsible for maintaining the change schedule but provides this to the Service Desk for communicating to users
    b) **Service Desk—should be the single point of contact for ALL user** communication
    c) Release and Deployment Management
    d) Service Level Management

Question 9

Which of the following best describes a baseline?

   a) **Used as a reference point for later comparison**
   b) The starting point of any project—only one example of a baseline
   c) The end point of any project – only one example of a baseline
   d) A rollback procedure

Question 10

The main objective of Change Management is to?

   a) Ensure that any changes are approved and recorded—not all changes are approved
   b) **Ensure that standardized methods and procedures are used for controlled handling of all changes**
   c) Ensure that any change requests are managed through the CAB—this is not true for standard changes
Ensure that the CAB takes responsibility for all change implementation—CAB only coordinates implementation, the work is performed within the Release and Deployment process

Service Operation

ANSWERS

1c, 2a, 3b, 4d, 5b, 6b, 7c, 8a, 9a, 10c

Question 1
What is the best definition of an Incident Model?

    a) Predicting the impact of incidents on the network
    b) A type of incident that is used as a best practice model
    c) **A set of pre-defined steps to be followed when dealing with a known type of incident**
    d) An incident that requires a separate system

Question 2
What is the difference between a known error and a problem?

    a) **The underlying cause of a known error is known. The underlying cause of a problem is not known.**
    b) A known error involves an error in the IT infrastructure. A problem does not involve such an error.
    c) A known error always originates from an incident. This is not always the case with a problem.
    d) With a problem, the relevant configuration items have been identified. This is not the case with a known error—explanation is reversed.

Question 3
Information is regularly exchanged between Problem Management and Change Management. What information is this?

    a) Known Errors from Problem Management on the basis of which Change Management can generate Requests for Change (RFCs)—Change Management accepts the RFC, does not create it itself
    b) **RFCs resulting from Known Errors**

c) RFCs from the users that Problem Management passes on to Change Management

d) RFCs from the Service Desk that Problem Management passes on to Change Management

Question 4

Incident Management has a value to the business by?

a) Helping to control cost of fixing technology

b) Enabling customers to resolve Problems—this is problem management

c) Helping to maximize business impact

d) **Helping to reduce the business impact**

Question 5

Which of the following is NOT an example of a service request?

a) A user calls the Service Desk to order a new mouse

b) **A user calls the Service Desk because they would like to change the functionality of an application—this would be a normal change, due to the potential risk and implications of the change**

c) A user calls the Service Desk to reset their password

d) A user logs onto an internal website to download a licensed copy of software from a list of approved options—this is an example of a service request workflow that has been automated

Question 6

The BEST definition of an event is?

a) A situation where a capacity threshold has been exceeded and an agreed service level has already been impacted—only one type of event (exception)

b) **An occurrence that is significant for the management of the IT Infrastructure or delivery of services**

c) A problem that requires immediate attention

d) A social gathering of IT staff to celebrate the release of a service

Question 7

Technical Management is NOT responsible for?

a) Maintenance of the local network
b) Identifying technical skills required to manage and support the IT Infrastructure
c) **Defining the service agreements for the technical infrastructure— this is the role of Service Level Management**
d) Response to the disruption to the technical infrastructure

Question 8

Which of the following is NOT an objective of Service Operation?

a) **Thorough testing to ensure that services are designed to meet business needs—this is an objective of Service Transition**
b) To deliver and support IT Services
c) To manage the technology used to deliver services
d) To monitor the performance of technology and processes

Question 9

Which of the following BEST describes the purpose of Event Management?

a) **The ability to detect events, analyze them, and determine the appropriate control action**
b) The ability to coordinate changes in events
c) The ability to monitor and control projected service outages—this is only one role of Event Management
d) The ability to report on success of all batch processing jobs—this is only one role of Event Management

Question 10
Which process or function is responsible for management of the Data Center facility?

    a)   IT Operations Control
    b)   Supplier Management
    c)   **Facilities Management**
    d)   Technical Function

Continual Service Improvement

ANSWERS

1b, 2b, 3b, 4c, 5d

Question 1
Why should monitoring and measuring be used when trying to improve services?

    a) To validate, justify, monitor, and improve
    b) **To validate, direct, justify, and intervene—see Service Measurement and Reporting**
    c) To validate, check, act, and improve
    d) To validate, analyze, direct, and improve

Question 2
Which is the first activity of the Continual Service Improvement (CSI) approach?

    a) Assess the customer's requirements
    b) **Understand the vision of the business**
    c) Identify what can be measured
    d) Develop a plan for improvement

Question 3
The four stages of the Deming Cycle are?

    a) Plan, Assess, Check, Report
    b) **Plan, Do, Check, Act**
    c) Plan, Check, Revise, Improve
    d) Plan, Do, Act, Assess

Question 4

Which of the following is NOT a step in the Continual Service Improvement (CSI) approach?

- a)   What is the vision?
- b)   Did we get there?
- c)   **Who will help us get there?**
- d)   Where are we now?

Question 5

Which of the following provides the correct set of governance levels managed by an organization?

- a)   Technology, Service, Business
- b)   Financial, Legal, Security
- c)   Process, Service, Technology
- d)   **IT, Corporate, Enterprise**

GLOSSARY

Term	Definition
accounting	(ITIL® Service Strategy) The process responsible for identifying the actual costs of delivering IT services, comparing these with budgeted costs, and managing variance from the budget.
activity	A set of actions designed to achieve a particular result. Activities are usually defined as part of processes or plans and are documented in procedures.
alert	(ITIL® Service Operation) A notification that a threshold has been reached, something has changed, or a failure has occurred. Alerts are often created and managed by system management tools and are managed by the event management process.
application	Software that provides functions that are required by an IT service. Each application may be part of more than one IT service. An application runs on one or more servers or clients.
application sizing	(ITIL® Service Design) The activity responsible for understanding the resource requirements needed to support a new application or a major change to an existing application. Application sizing helps to ensure that the IT service can meet its agreed service level targets for capacity and performance.
asset	(ITIL® Service Strategy) Any resource or capability. The assets of a service provider include anything that could contribute to the delivery of a service. Assets can be one of the following types: management, organization, process, knowledge, people, information, applications, infrastructure, or financial capital. See also customer asset; service asset; strategic asset.
attribute	(ITIL® Service Transition) A piece of information about a configuration item. Examples are name, location, version number, and cost. Attributes of CIs are recorded in a configuration management database (CMDB) and maintained as part of a configuration management system (CMS). See also relationship; configuration management system.

Term	Definition
availability	(ITIL® Service Design) Ability of an IT service or other configuration item to perform its agreed function when required. Availability is determined by reliability, maintainability, serviceability, performance, and security. Availability is usually calculated as a percentage. This calculation is often based on agreed service time and downtime. It is best practice to calculate availability of an IT service using measurements of the business output.
availability management information system (AMIS)	(ITIL® Service Design) A set of tools, data, and information that is used to support availability management. See also service knowledge management system.
baseline	(ITIL® Continual Service Improvement) (ITIL® Service Transition) A snapshot that is used as a reference point. Many snapshots may be taken and recorded over time but only some will be used as baselines. For example: An ITSM baseline can be used as a starting point to measure the effect of a service improvement plan A performance baseline can be used to measure changes in performance over the lifetime of an IT service A configuration baseline can be used as part of a back-out plan to enable the IT infrastructure to be restored to a known configuration if a change or release fails. See also benchmark.
benchmark	(ITIL® Continual Service Improvement) (ITIL® Service Transition) A baseline that is used to compare related data sets as part of a benchmarking exercise. For example, a recent snapshot of a process can be compared to a previous baseline of that process, or a current baseline can be compared to industry data or best practice. See also benchmarking; baseline.
benchmarking	(ITIL® Continual Service Improvement) The process responsible for comparing a benchmark with related data sets, such as a more recent snapshot, industry data, or best practice. The term is also used to mean creating a series of benchmarks over time and comparing the results to measure progress or improvement. This process is not described in detail within the core ITIL® publications.

Term	Definition
Best Management Practice (BMP)	The Best Management Practice portfolio is owned by the Cabinet Office, part of HM Government. Formerly owned by CCTA and then OGC, the BMP functions moved to the Cabinet Office in June 2010. The BMP portfolio includes guidance on IT service management and project, program, risk, portfolio, and value management. There is also a management maturity model as well as related glossaries of terms.
best practice	Proven activities or processes that have been successfully used by multiple organizations. ITIL® is an example of best practice.
budget	A list of all the money an organization or business unit plans to receive and plans to pay out over a specified period of time. See also budgeting.
budgeting	The activity of predicting and controlling the spending of money. Budgeting consists of a periodic negotiation cycle to set future budgets (usually annual) and the day-to-day monitoring and adjusting of current budgets.
build	(ITIL® Service Transition) The activity of assembling a number of configuration items to create part of an IT service. The term is also used to refer to a release that is authorized for distribution—for example, server build or laptop build. See also configuration baseline.
business case	(ITIL® Service Strategy) Justification for a significant item of expenditure. The business case includes information about costs, benefits, options, issues, risks, and possible problems.
business continuity plan (BCP)	(ITIL® Service Design) A plan defining the steps required to restore business processes following a disruption. The plan also identifies the triggers for invocation, people to be involved, communications, etc. IT service continuity plans form a significant part of business continuity plans.
business impact analysis (BIA)	(ITIL® Service Strategy) Business impact analysis is the activity in business continuity management that identifies vital business functions and their dependencies. These dependencies may include suppliers, people, other business processes, IT services etc. Business impact analysis defines the recovery requirements for IT services. These requirements include recovery time objectives, recovery point objectives, and minimum service level targets for each IT service.

Term	Definition
business relationship management	(ITIL® Service Strategy) The process responsible for maintaining a positive relationship with customers. Business relationship management identifies customer needs and ensures that the service provider is able to meet these needs with an appropriate catalog of services. This process has strong links with service level management.
capability	(ITIL® Service Strategy) The ability of an organization, person, process, application, IT service, or other configuration item to carry out an activity. Capabilities are intangible assets of an organization. See also resource.
capacity	(ITIL® Service Design) The maximum throughput that a configuration item or IT service can deliver. For some types of CIs, capacity may be the size or volume—for example, a disk drive.
capacity management information system (CMIS)	(ITIL® Service Design) A set of tools, data, and information that is used to support capacity management. See also service knowledge management system.
capacity planning	(ITIL® Service Design) The activity within capacity management responsible for creating a capacity plan.
change	(ITIL® Service Transition) The addition, modification, or removal of anything that could have an effect on IT services. The scope should include changes to all architectures, processes, tools, metrics, and documentation, as well as changes to IT services and other configuration items.
change advisory board (CAB)	(ITIL® Service Transition) A group of people that support the assessment, prioritization, authorization, and scheduling of changes. A change advisory board is usually made up of representatives from all areas within the IT service provider, the business, and third parties, such as suppliers.
change model	(ITIL® Service Transition) A repeatable way of dealing with a particular category of change. A change model defines specific agreed steps that will be followed for a change of this category. Change models may be very complex with many steps that require authorization (e.g., major software release) or may be very simple with no requirement for authorization (e.g., password reset). See also change advisory board; standard change.

Term	Definition
change proposal	(ITIL® Service Strategy) (ITIL® Service Transition) A document that includes a high level description of a potential service introduction or significant change, along with a corresponding business case and an expected implementation schedule. Change proposals are normally created by the service portfolio management process and are passed to change management for authorization. Change management will review the potential impact on other services, on shared resources, and on the overall change schedule. Once the change proposal has been authorized, service portfolio management will charter the service.
change record	(ITIL® Service Transition) A record containing the details of a change. Each change record documents the lifecycle of a single change. A change record is created for every request for change that is received, even those that are subsequently rejected. Change records should reference the configuration items that are affected by the change. Change records may be stored in the configuration management system or elsewhere in the service knowledge management system.
change request	See request for change.
change schedule	(ITIL® Service Transition) A document that lists all authorized changes and their planned implementation dates, as well as the estimated dates of longer-term changes. A change schedule is sometimes called a forward schedule of change, even though it also contains information about changes that have already been implemented.
change window	(ITIL® Service Transition) A regular, agreed time when changes or releases may be implemented with minimal impact on services. Change windows are usually documented in service level agreements.
charging	(ITIL® Service Strategy) Requiring payment for IT services. Charging for IT services is optional and many organizations choose to treat their IT service provider as a cost centre.
CI type	(ITIL® Service Transition) A category that is used to classify configuration items. The CI type identifies the required attributes and relationships for a configuration record. Common CI types include hardware, document, user, etc.
classification	The act of assigning a category to something. Classification is used to ensure consistent management and reporting. Configuration items, incidents, problems, changes, etc. are usually classified.

Term	Definition
component	A general term that is used to mean one part of something more complex. For example, a computer system may be a component of an IT service; an application may be a component of a release unit. Components that need to be managed should be configuration items.
confidentiality	(ITIL® Service Design) A security principle that requires that data should only be accessed by authorized people.
configuration	(ITIL® Service Transition) A generic term used to describe a group of configuration items that work together to deliver an IT service or a recognizable part of an IT service. Configuration is also used to describe the parameter settings for one or more configuration items.
configuration baseline	(ITIL® Service Transition) The baseline of a configuration that has been formally agreed and is managed through the change management process. A configuration baseline is used as a basis for future builds, releases, and changes.
configuration item (CI)	(ITIL® Service Transition) Any component or other service asset that needs to be managed in order to deliver an IT service. Information about each configuration item is recorded in a configuration record within the configuration management system and is maintained throughout its lifecycle by service asset and configuration management. Configuration items are under the control of change management. They typically include IT services, hardware, software, buildings, people, and formal documentation, such as process documentation and service level agreements.
configuration management database (CMDB)	(ITIL® Service Transition) A database used to store configuration records throughout their lifecycle. The configuration management system maintains one or more configuration management databases, and each database stores attributes of configuration items and relationships with other configuration items.

Term	Definition
configuration management system (CMS)	(ITIL® Service Transition) A set of tools, data, and information that is used to support service asset and configuration management. The CMS is part of an overall service knowledge management system and includes tools for collecting, storing, managing, updating, analyzing, and presenting data about all configuration items and their relationships. The CMS may also include information about incidents, problems, known errors, changes, and releases. The CMS is maintained by service asset and configuration management and is used by all IT service management processes. See also configuration management database.
configuration record	(ITIL® Service Transition) A record containing the details of a configuration item. Each configuration record documents the lifecycle of a single configuration item. Configuration records are stored in a configuration management database and maintained as part of a configuration management system.
countermeasure	Can be used to refer to any type of control. The term is most often used when referring to measures that increase resilience, fault tolerance, or reliability of an IT service.
critical success factor (CSF)	Something that must happen if an IT service, process, plan, project, or other activity is to succeed. Key performance indicators are used to measure the achievement of each critical success factor. For example, a critical success factor of 'protect IT services when making changes' could be measured by key performance indicators such as 'percentage reduction of unsuccessful changes', 'percentage reduction in changes causing incidents', etc.
CSI register	(ITIL® Continual Service Improvement) A database or structured document used to record and manage improvement opportunities throughout their lifecycle.
customer asset	Any resource or capability of a customer. See also asset.
customer portfolio	(ITIL® Service Strategy) A database or structured document used to record all customers of the IT service provider. The customer portfolio is the business relationship manager's view of the customers who receive services from the IT service provider. See also service catalog; service portfolio.
Data-to-Information-to-Knowledge-to-Wisdom (DIKW)	(ITIL® Service Transition) A way of understanding the relationships between data, information, knowledge, and wisdom. DIKW shows how each of these builds on the others.

Term	Definition
definitive media library (DML)	(ITIL® Service Transition) One or more locations in which the definitive and authorized versions of all software configuration items are securely stored. The definitive media library may also contain associated configuration items, such as licenses and documentation. It is a single logical storage area, even if there are multiple locations. The definitive media library is controlled by service asset and configuration management and is recorded in the configuration management system.
Deming Cycle	See Plan-Do-Check-Act.
deployment	(ITIL® Service Transition) The activity responsible for movement of new or changed hardware, software, documentation, process, etc. to the live environment. Deployment is part of the release and deployment management process.
design coordination	(ITIL® Service Design) The process responsible for coordinating all service design activities, processes, and resources. Design coordination ensures the consistent and effective design of new or changed IT services, service management information systems, architectures, technology, processes, information, and metrics.
document	Information in readable form. A document may be paper or electronic—for example, a policy statement, service level agreement, incident record, or diagram of a computer room layout. See also record.
downtime	(ITIL® Service Design) (ITIL® Service Operation) The time when an IT service or other configuration item is not available during its agreed service time. The availability of an IT service is often calculated from agreed service time and downtime.
emergency change	(ITIL® Service Transition) A change that must be introduced as soon as possible—for example, to resolve a major incident or implement a security patch. The change management process will normally have a specific procedure for handling emergency changes. See also emergency change advisory board.
emergency change advisory board (ECAB)	(ITIL® Service Transition) A subgroup of the change advisory board that makes decisions about emergency changes. Membership may be decided at the time a meeting is called and depends on the nature of the emergency change.

Term	Definition
escalation	(ITIL® Service Operation) An activity that obtains additional resources when these are needed to meet service level targets or customer expectations. Escalation may be needed within any IT service management process but is most commonly associated with incident management, problem management, and the management of customer complaints. There are two types of escalation: functional escalation and hierarchic escalation.
event	(ITIL® Service Operation) A change of state that has significance for the management of an IT service or other configuration item. The term is also used to mean an alert or notification created by any IT service, configuration item, or monitoring tool. Events typically require IT operations personnel to take actions and often lead to incidents being logged.
external customer	A customer who works for a different business from the IT service provider. See also external service provider; internal customer.
external service provider	(ITIL® Service Strategy) An IT service provider that is part of a different organization from its customer. An IT service provider may have both internal and external customers. See also Type III service provider.
facilities management	(ITIL® Service Operation) The function responsible for managing the physical environment where the IT infrastructure is located. Facilities management includes all aspects of managing the physical environment—for example, power and cooling, building access management, and environmental monitoring.
failure	(ITIL® Service Operation) Loss of ability to operate to specification or to deliver the required output. The term may be used when referring to IT services, processes, activities, configuration items, etc. A failure often causes an incident.
fast recovery	(ITIL® Service Design) A recovery option that is also known as hot standby. Fast recovery normally uses a dedicated fixed facility with computer systems and software configured ready to run the IT services. Fast recovery typically takes up to 24 hours but may be quicker if there is no need to restore data from backups.
fit for purpose	(ITIL® Service Strategy) The ability to meet an agreed level of utility. Fit for purpose is also used informally to describe a process, configuration item, IT service, etc. that is capable of meeting its objectives or service levels. Being fit for purpose requires suitable design, implementation, control, and maintenance.

Term	Definition
fit for use	(ITIL® Service Strategy) The ability to meet an agreed level of warranty. Being fit for use requires suitable design, implementation, control, and maintenance.
follow the sun	(ITIL® Service Operation) A methodology for using service desks and support groups around the world to provide seamless 24/7 service. Calls, incidents, problems, and service requests are passed between groups in different time zones.
function	A team or group of people and the tools or other resources they use to carry out one or more processes or activities—for example, the service desk. The term also has two other meanings: An intended purpose of a configuration item, person, team, process, or IT service. For example, one function of an email service may be to store and forward outgoing mails, while the function of a business process may be to dispatch goods to customers. To perform the intended purpose correctly, as in 'The computer is functioning.'
functional escalation	(ITIL® Service Operation) Transferring an incident, problem, or change to a technical team with a higher level of expertise to assist in an escalation.
governance	Ensures that policies and strategy are actually implemented and that required processes are correctly followed. Governance includes defining roles and responsibilities, measuring and reporting, and taking actions to resolve any issues identified.
gradual recovery	(ITIL® Service Design) A recovery option that is also known as cold standby. Gradual recovery typically uses a portable or fixed facility that has environmental support and network cabling but no computer systems. The hardware and software are installed as part of the IT service continuity plan. Gradual recovery typically takes more than three days and may take significantly longer.
hierarchic escalation	(ITIL® Service Operation) Informing or involving more senior levels of management to assist in an escalation.
hot standby	See fast recovery; immediate recovery.
immediate recovery	(ITIL® Service Design) A recovery option that is also known as hot standby. Provision is made to recover the IT service with no significant loss of service to the customer. Immediate recovery typically uses mirroring, load balancing, and split-site technologies.
impact	(ITIL® Service Operation) (ITIL® Service Transition) A measure of the effect of an incident, problem, or change on business processes. Impact is often based on how service levels will be affected. Impact and urgency are used to assign priority.

Term	Definition
incident	(ITIL® Service Operation) An unplanned interruption to an IT service or reduction in the quality of an IT service. Failure of a configuration item that has not yet affected service is also an incident—for example, failure of one disk from a mirror set.
incident record	(ITIL® Service Operation) A record containing the details of an incident. Each incident record documents the lifecycle of a single incident.
information security management (ISM)	(ITIL® Service Design) The process responsible for ensuring that the confidentiality, integrity, and availability of an organization's assets, information, data, and IT services match the agreed needs of the business. Information security management supports business security, has a wider scope than that of the IT service provider, and includes handling of paper, building access, phone calls, etc. for the entire organization. See also security management information system.
information security policy	(ITIL® Service Design) The policy that governs the organization's approach to information security management.
information technology (IT)	The use of technology for the storage, communication, or processing of information. The technology typically includes computers, telecommunications, applications, and other software. The information may include business data, voice, images, video, etc. Information technology is often used to support business processes through IT services.
intermediate recovery	(ITIL® Service Design) A recovery option that is also known as warm standby. Intermediate recovery usually uses a shared portable or fixed facility that has computer systems and network components. The hardware and software will need to be configured and data will need to be restored as part of the IT service continuity plan. Typical recovery times for intermediate recovery are one to three days.
internal customer	A customer who works for the same business as the IT service provider. See also external customer; internal service provider.
internal service provider	(ITIL® Service Strategy) An IT service provider that is part of the same organization as its customer. An IT service provider may have both internal and external customers. See also Type I service provider; Type II service provider.
internet service provider (ISP)	An external service provider that provides access to the internet. Most ISPs also provide other IT services, such as web hosting.

Term	Definition
ISO 9000	A generic term that refers to a number of international standards and guidelines for quality management systems. See www.iso.org for more information.
ISO 9001	An international standard for quality management systems. See also ISO 9000.
ISO/IEC 20000	An international standard for IT service management.
ISO/IEC 27001	(ITIL® Continual Service Improvement) (ITIL® Service Design) An international specification for information security management. The corresponding code of practice is ISO/IEC 27002.
ISO/IEC 27002	(ITIL® Continual Service Improvement) An international code of practice for information security management. The corresponding specification is ISO/IEC 27001.
IT accounting	See accounting.
IT infrastructure	All of the hardware, software, networks, facilities, etc. that are required to develop, test, deliver, monitor, control, or support applications and IT services. The term includes all of the information technology but not the associated people, processes, and documentation.
IT operations	(ITIL® Service Operation) Activities carried out by IT operations control, including console management/operations bridge, job scheduling, backup and restore, and print and output management. IT operations is also used as a synonym for service operation.
IT operations control	(ITIL® Service Operation) The function responsible for monitoring and control of the IT services and IT infrastructure. See also operations bridge.
IT service	A service provided by an IT service provider. An IT service is made up of a combination of information technology, people, and processes. A customer-facing IT service directly supports the business processes of one or more customers, and its service level targets should be defined in a service level agreement. Other IT services, called supporting services, are not directly used by the business but are required by the service provider to deliver customer-facing services. See also service; service package.
IT service continuity plan	(ITIL® Service Design) A plan defining the steps required to recover one or more IT services. The plan also identifies the triggers for invocation, people to be involved, communications, etc. The IT service continuity plan should be part of a business continuity plan.

Term	Definition
IT service management (ITSM)	The implementation and management of quality IT services that meet the needs of the business. IT service management is performed by IT service providers through an appropriate mix of people, process, and information technology. See also service management.
IT Service Management Forum (itSMF)	The IT Service Management Forum is an independent organization dedicated to promoting a professional approach to IT service management. The itSMF is a not-for-profit membership organization with representation in many countries around the world (itSMF chapters). The itSMF and its membership contribute to the development of ITIL® and associated IT service management standards. See www.itsmf.com for more information.
IT service provider	(ITIL® Service Strategy) A service provider that provides IT services to internal or external customers.
ITIL®	A set of best-practice publications for IT service management. Owned by the Cabinet Office (part of HM Government), ITIL® gives guidance on the provision of quality IT services and the processes, functions, and other capabilities needed to support them. The ITIL® framework is based on a service lifecycle and consists of five lifecycle stages (service strategy, service design, service transition, service operation, and continual service improvement), each of which has its own supporting publication. There is also a set of complementary ITIL® publications providing guidance specific to industry sectors, organization types, operating models, and technology architectures. See www.itilofficialsite.com for more information.
key performance indicator (KPI)	(ITIL® Continual Service Improvement) (ITIL® Service Design) A metric that is used to help manage an IT service, process, plan, project, or other activity. Key performance indicators are used to measure the achievement of critical success factors. Many metrics may be measured, but only the most important of these are defined as key performance indicators and used to actively manage and report on the process, IT service, or activity. They should be selected to ensure that efficiency, effectiveness, and cost effectiveness are all managed.

Term	Definition
known error	(ITIL® Service Operation) A problem that has a documented root cause and a workaround. Known errors are created and managed throughout their lifecycle by problem management. Known errors may also be identified by development or suppliers.
known error database (KEDB)	(ITIL® Service Operation) A database containing all known error records. This database is created by problem management and used by incident and problem management. The known error database may be part of the configuration management system or may be stored elsewhere in the service knowledge management system.
known error record	(ITIL® Service Operation) A record containing the details of a known error. Each known error record documents the lifecycle of a known error, including the status, root cause, and workaround. In some implementations, a known error is documented using additional fields in a problem record.
lifecycle	The various stages in the life of an IT service, configuration item, incident, problem, change, etc. The lifecycle defines the categories for status and the status transitions that are permitted. For example: The lifecycle of an application includes requirements, design, build, deploy, operate, optimize The expanded incident lifecycle includes detection, diagnosis, repair, recovery, and restoration The lifecycle of a server may include ordered, received, in test, live, disposed etc.
maintainability	(ITIL® Service Design) A measure of how quickly and effectively an IT service or other configuration item can be restored to normal working after a failure. Maintainability is often measured and reported as MTRS. Maintainability is also used in the context of software or IT service development to mean ability to be changed or repaired easily.
major incident	(ITIL® Service Operation) The highest category of impact for an incident. A major incident results in significant disruption to the business.
manual workaround	(ITIL® Continual Service Improvement) A workaround that requires manual intervention. Manual workaround is also used as the name of a recovery option in which the business process operates without the use of IT services. This is a temporary measure and is usually combined with another recovery option.
modeling	A technique that is used to predict the future behavior of a system, process, IT service, configuration item, etc. Modeling is commonly used in financial management, capacity management, and availability management.

Term	Definition
normal change	(ITIL® Service Transition) A change that is not an emergency change or a standard change. Normal changes follow the defined steps of the change management process.
operational level agreement (OLA)	(ITIL® Continual Service Improvement) (ITIL® Service Design) An agreement between an IT service provider and another part of the same organization. It supports the IT service provider's delivery of IT services to customers and defines the goods or services to be provided and the responsibilities of both parties. For example, there could be an operational level agreement: Between the IT service provider and a procurement department to obtain hardware in agreed times Between the service desk and a support group to provide incident resolution in agreed times. See also service level agreement.
operations bridge	(ITIL® Service Operation) A physical location where IT services and IT infrastructure are monitored and managed.
operations control	See IT operations control.
outcome	The result of carrying out an activity, following a process, or delivering an IT service, etc. The term is used to refer to intended results as well as to actual results.
pattern of business activity (PBA)	(ITIL® Service Strategy) A workload profile of one or more business activities. Patterns of business activity are used to help the IT service provider understand and plan for different levels of business activity.
Plan-Do-Check-Act (PDCA)	(ITIL® Continual Service Improvement) A four-stage cycle for process management, attributed to Edward Deming. Plan-Do-Check-Act is also called the Deming Cycle. Plan—design or revise processes that support the IT services; Do—implement the plan and manage the processes; Check—measure the processes and IT services, compare with objectives and produce reports; Act—plan and implement changes to improve the processes.
post-implementation review (PIR)	A review that takes place after a change or a project has been implemented. It determines if the change or project was successful and identifies opportunities for improvement.
PRINCE2®	See PRojects IN Controlled Environments.
proactive problem management	(ITIL® Service Operation) Part of the problem management process. The objective of proactive problem management is to identify problems that might otherwise be missed. Proactive problem management analyzes incident records and uses data collected by other IT service management processes to identify trends or significant problems.

Term	Definition
problem	(ITIL® Service Operation) A cause of one or more incidents. The cause is not usually known at the time a problem record is created, and the problem management process is responsible for further investigation.
problem record	(ITIL® Service Operation) A record containing the details of a problem. Each problem record documents the lifecycle of a single problem.
process	A structured set of activities designed to accomplish a specific objective. A process takes one or more defined inputs and turns them into defined outputs. It may include any of the roles, responsibilities, tools, and management controls required to reliably deliver the outputs. A process may define policies, standards, guidelines, activities, and work instructions if they are needed.
process control	The activity of planning and regulating a process with the objective of performing the process in an effective, efficient, and consistent manner.
process manager	A role responsible for the operational management of a process. The process manager's responsibilities include planning and coordination of all activities required to carry out, monitor, and report on the process. There may be several process managers for one process—for example, regional change managers or IT service continuity managers for each data centre. The process manager role is often assigned to the person who carries out the process owner role, but the two roles may be separate in larger organizations.
process owner	The person who is held accountable for ensuring that a process is fit for purpose. The process owner's responsibilities include sponsorship, design, change management, and continual improvement of the process and its metrics. This role can be assigned to the same person who carries out the process manager role, but the two roles may be separate in larger organizations.
project	A temporary organization, with people and other assets, that is required to achieve an objective or other outcome. Each project has a lifecycle that typically includes initiation, planning, execution, and closure. Projects are usually managed using a formal methodology, such as PRojects IN Controlled Environments (PRINCE2) or the Project Management Body of Knowledge (PMBOK).
PRojects IN Controlled Environments (PRINCE2)	The standard UK government methodology for project management. See www.princeofficialsite.com for more information. See also Project Management Body of Knowledge (PMBOK).

Term	Definition
Project Management Body of Knowledge (PMBOK)	A project management standard maintained and published by the Project Management Institute. See www.pmi.org for more information. See also PRojects IN Controlled Environments (PRINCE2).
Project Management Institute (PMI)	A membership association that advances the project management profession through globally recognized standards and certifications, collaborative communities, an extensive research program, and professional development opportunities. PMI is a not-for-profit membership organization with representation in many countries around the world. PMI maintains and publishes the Project Management Body of Knowledge (PMBOK). See www.pmi.org for more information. See also PRojects IN Controlled Environments (PRINCE2).
quality	The ability of a product, service, or process to provide the intended value. For example, a hardware component can be considered to be of high quality if it performs as expected and delivers the required reliability. Process quality also requires an ability to monitor effectiveness and efficiency and to improve them if necessary. See also quality management system.
quality assurance (QA)	(ITIL® Service Transition) The process responsible for ensuring that the quality of a service, process, or other service asset will provide its intended value. Quality assurance is also used to refer to a function or team that performs quality assurance. This process is not described in detail within the core ITIL® publications.
quality management system (QMS)	(ITIL® Continual Service Improvement) The framework of policy, processes, functions, standards, guidelines, and tools that ensures an organization is of a suitable quality to reliably meet business objectives or service levels. See also ISO 9000.
RACI	(ITIL® Service Design) A model used to help define roles and responsibilities. RACI stands for responsible, accountable, consulted and informed.
reciprocal arrangement	(ITIL® Service Design) A recovery option. An agreement between two organizations to share resources in an emergency—for example, high-speed printing facilities or computer room space.

Term	Definition
record	A document containing the results or other output from a process or activity. Records are evidence of the fact that an activity took place and may be paper or electronic—for example, an audit report, an incident record, or the minutes of a meeting.
recovery	(ITIL® Service Design) (ITIL® Service Operation) Returning a configuration item or an IT service to a working state. Recovery of an IT service often includes recovering data to a known consistent state. After recovery, further steps may be needed before the IT service can be made available to the users (restoration).
recovery option	(ITIL® Service Design) A strategy for responding to an interruption to service. Commonly used strategies are manual workaround, reciprocal arrangement, gradual recovery, intermediate recovery, fast recovery, and immediate recovery. Recovery options may make use of dedicated facilities or third-party facilities shared by multiple businesses.
relationship	A connection or interaction between two people or things. In business relationship management, it is the interaction between the IT service provider and the business. In service asset and configuration management, it is a link between two configuration items that identifies a dependency or connection between them. For example, applications may be linked to the servers they run on, and IT services have many links to all the configuration items that contribute to that IT service.
release	(ITIL® Service Transition) One or more changes to an IT service that are built, tested, and deployed together. A single release may include changes to hardware, software, documentation, processes, and other components.
release package	(ITIL® Service Transition) A set of configuration items that will be built, tested, and deployed together as a single release. Each release package will usually include one or more release units.
release record	(ITIL® Service Transition) A record that defines the content of a release. A release record has relationships with all configuration items that are affected by the release. Release records may be in the configuration management system or elsewhere in the service knowledge management system.
release unit	(ITIL® Service Transition) Components of an IT service that are normally released together. A release unit typically includes sufficient components to perform a useful function. For example, one release unit could be a desktop PC, including hardware, software, licenses, documentation, etc. A different release unit may be the complete payroll application, including IT operations procedures and user training.
release window	See change window.

Term	Definition
reliability	(ITIL® Continual Service Improvement) (ITIL® Service Design) A measure of how long an IT service or other configuration item can perform its agreed function without interruption. Usually measured as MTBF or MTBSI. The term can also be used to state how likely it is that a process, function, etc. will deliver its required outputs. See also availability.
remediation	(ITIL® Service Transition) Actions taken to recover after a failed change or release. Remediation may include back-out, invocation of service continuity plans, or other actions designed to enable the business process to continue.
request for change (RFC)	(ITIL® Service Transition) A formal proposal for a change to be made. It includes details of the proposed change and may be recorded on paper or electronically. The term is often misused to mean a change record or the change itself.
request fulfillment	(ITIL® Service Operation) The process responsible for managing the lifecycle of all service requests.
request model	(ITIL® Service Operation) A repeatable way of dealing with a particular category of service request. A request model defines specific agreed steps that will be followed for a service request of this category. Request models may be very simple with no requirement for authorization (e.g., password reset) or may be more complex with many steps that require authorization (e.g., provision of an existing IT service). See also request fulfillment.
resilience	(ITIL® Service Design) The ability of an IT service or other configuration item to resist failure or to recover in a timely manner following a failure. For example, an armored cable will resist failure when put under stress.
resolution	(ITIL® Service Operation) Action taken to repair the root cause of an incident or problem or to implement a workaround. In ISO/IEC 20000, resolution processes is the process group that includes incident and problem management.
resource	(ITIL® Service Strategy) A generic term that includes IT infrastructure, people, money, or anything else that might help to deliver an IT service. Resources are considered to be assets of an organization. See also capability; service asset.

Term	Definition
response time	A measure of the time taken to complete an operation or transaction. Used in capacity management as a measure of IT infrastructure performance and in incident management as a measure of the time taken to answer the phone or to start diagnosis.
restoration of service	See restore.
restore	(ITIL® Service Operation) Taking action to return an IT service to the users after repair and recovery from an incident. This is the primary objective of incident management.
retire	(ITIL® Service Transition) Permanent removal of an IT service or other configuration item from the live environment. Being retired is a stage in the lifecycle of many configuration items.
return on investment (ROI)	(ITIL® Continual Service Improvement) (ITIL® Service Strategy) A measurement of the expected benefit of an investment. In the simplest sense, it is the net profit of an investment divided by the net worth of the assets invested.
rights	(ITIL® Service Operation) Entitlements or permissions granted to a user or role—for example, the right to modify particular data or to authorize a change.
risk	A possible event that could cause harm or loss or affect the ability to achieve objectives. A risk is measured by the probability of a threat, the vulnerability of the asset to that threat, and the impact it would have if it occurred. Risk can also be defined as uncertainty of outcome and can be used in the context of measuring the probability of positive outcomes as well as negative outcomes.
risk assessment	The initial steps of risk management: analyzing the value of assets to the business, identifying threats to those assets, and evaluating how vulnerable each asset is to those threats. Risk assessment can be quantitative (based on numerical data) or qualitative.
risk management	The process responsible for identifying, assessing, and controlling risks. Risk management is also sometimes used to refer to the second part of the overall process after risks have been identified and assessed, as in 'risk assessment and management'. This process is not described in detail within the core ITIL® publications. See also risk assessment.

Term	Definition
role	A set of responsibilities, activities, and authorities assigned to a person or team. A role is defined in a process or function. One person or team may have multiple roles—for example, the roles of configuration manager and change manager may be carried out by a single person. Role is also used to describe the purpose of something or what it is used for.
root cause	(ITIL® Service Operation) The underlying or original cause of an incident or problem.
scope	The boundary or extent to which a process, procedure, certification, contract, etc. applies. For example, the scope of change management may include all live IT services and related configuration items; the scope of an ISO/IEC 20000 certificate may include all IT services delivered out of a named data centre.
security	See information security management.
security management information system (SMIS)	(ITIL® Service Design) A set of tools, data, and information that is used to support information security management. The security management information system is part of the information security management system. See also service knowledge management system.
security policy	See information security policy.
service	A means of delivering value to customers by facilitating outcomes customers want to achieve without the ownership of specific costs and risks. The term 'service' is sometimes used as a synonym for core service, IT service, or service package. See also utility; warranty.
service asset	Any resource or capability of a service provider. See also asset.
service capacity management (SCM)	(ITIL® Continual Service Improvement) (ITIL® Service Design) The sub-process of capacity management responsible for understanding the performance and capacity of IT services. Information on the resources used by each IT service and the pattern of usage over time are collected, recorded, and analyzed for use in the capacity plan.
service catalog	(ITIL® Service Design) (ITIL® Service Strategy) A database or structured document with information about all live IT services, including those available for deployment. The service catalog is part of the service portfolio and contains information about two types of IT service: customer-facing services that are visible to the business and supporting services required by the service provider to deliver customer-facing services.

Term	Definition
service contract	(ITIL® Service Strategy) A contract to deliver one or more IT services. The term is also used to mean any agreement to deliver IT services, whether this is a legal contract or a service level agreement.
service design package (SDP)	(ITIL® Service Design) Document(s) defining all aspects of an IT service and its requirements through each stage of its lifecycle. A service design package is produced for each new IT service, major change, or IT service retirement.
service desk	(ITIL® Service Operation) The single point of contact between the service provider and the users. A typical service desk manages incidents and service requests and also handles communication with the users.
service improvement plan (SIP)	(ITIL® Continual Service Improvement) A formal plan to implement improvements to a process or IT service.
service knowledge management system (SKMS)	(ITIL® Service Transition) A set of tools and databases that is used to manage knowledge, information, and data. The service knowledge management system includes the configuration management system, as well as other databases and information systems. The service knowledge management system includes tools for collecting, storing, managing, updating, analyzing, and presenting all the knowledge, information, and data that an IT service provider will need to manage the full lifecycle of IT services.
service level	Measured and reported achievement against one or more service level targets. The term is sometimes used informally to mean service level target.
service level agreement (SLA)	(ITIL® Continual Service Improvement) (ITIL® Service Design) An agreement between an IT service provider and a customer. A service level agreement describes the IT service, documents service level targets, and specifies the responsibilities of the IT service provider and the customer. A single agreement may cover multiple IT services or multiple customers. See also operational level agreement.
service level package (SLP)	See service option.
service level requirement (SLR)	(ITIL® Continual Service Improvement) (ITIL® Service Design) A customer requirement for an aspect of an IT service. Service level requirements are based on business objectives and used to negotiate agreed service level targets.
service management	(ITIL® Service Operation) The expected time that a configuration item will be unavailable due to planned maintenance activity.

Term	Definition
service manager	A generic term for any manager within the service provider. Most commonly used to refer to a business relationship manager, a process manager, or a senior manager with responsibility for IT services overall.
service model	(ITIL® Service Strategy) A model that shows how service assets interact with customer assets to create value. Service models describe the structure of a service (how the configuration items fit together) and the dynamics of the service (activities, flow of resources, and interactions). A service model can be used as a template or blueprint for multiple services.
service option	(ITIL® Service Design) (ITIL® Service Strategy) A choice of utility and warranty offered to customers by a core service or service package. Service options are sometimes referred to as service level packages.
service owner	(ITIL® Service Strategy) A role responsible for managing one or more services throughout their entire lifecycle. Service owners are instrumental in the development of service strategy and are responsible for the content of the service portfolio.
service package	(ITIL® Service Strategy) Two or more services that have been combined to offer a solution to a specific type of customer need or to underpin specific business outcomes. A service package can consist of a combination of core services, enabling services and enhancing services. A service package provides a specific level of utility and warranty. Customers may be offered a choice of utility and warranty through one or more service options. See also IT service.
service pipeline	(ITIL® Service Strategy) A database or structured document listing all IT services that are under consideration or development but are not yet available to customers. The service pipeline provides a business view of possible future IT services and is part of the service portfolio that is not normally published to customers.
service portfolio	(ITIL® Service Strategy) The complete set of services that is managed by a service provider. The service portfolio is used to manage the entire lifecycle of all services and includes three categories: service pipeline (proposed or in development), service catalog (live or available for deployment), and retired services.
service provider	(ITIL® Service Strategy) An organization supplying services to one or more internal customers or external customers. Service provider is often used as an abbreviation for IT service provider. See also Type I service provider; Type II service provider; Type III service provider.

Term	Definition
service reporting	(ITIL® Continual Service Improvement) Activities that produce and deliver reports of achievement and trends against service levels. The format, content, and frequency of reports should be agreed with customers.
service request	(ITIL® Service Operation) A formal request from a user for something to be provided—for example, a request for information or advice, to reset a password, or to install a workstation for a new user. Service requests are managed by the request fulfillment process, usually in conjunction with the service desk. Service requests may be linked to a request for change as part of fulfilling the request.
serviceability	(ITIL® Continual Service Improvement) (ITIL® Service Design) The ability of a third-party supplier to meet the terms of its contract. This contract will include agreed levels of reliability, maintainability, and availability for a configuration item.
seven-step improvement process	(ITIL® Continual Service Improvement) The process responsible for defining and managing the steps needed to identify, define, gather, process, analyze, present, and implement improvements. The performance of the IT service provider is continually measured by this process and improvements are made to processes, IT services, and IT infrastructure in order to increase efficiency, effectiveness, and cost effectiveness. Opportunities for improvement are recorded and managed in the CSI register.
shared service unit	See Type II service provider.
single point of contact	(ITIL® Service Operation) Providing a single consistent way to communicate with an organization or business unit. For example, a single point of contact for an IT service provider is usually called a service desk.
SLAM chart	(ITIL® Continual Service Improvement) A service level agreement monitoring chart is used to help monitor and report achievements against service level targets. A SLAM chart is typically color-coded to show whether each agreed service level target has been met, missed, or nearly missed during each of the previous 12 months.
stakeholder	A person who has an interest in an organization, project, IT service, etc. Stakeholders may be interested in the activities, targets, resources, or deliverables. Stakeholders may include customers, partners, employees, shareholders, owners, etc. See also RACI.

Term	Definition
standard change	(ITIL® Service Transition) A pre-authorized change that is low risk, relatively common, and follows a procedure or work instruction—for example, a password reset or provision of standard equipment to a new employee. Requests for change are not required to implement a standard change, and they are logged and tracked using a different mechanism, such as a service request. See also change model.
status accounting	(ITIL® Service Transition) The activity responsible for recording and reporting the lifecycle of each configuration item.
strategic asset	(ITIL® Service Strategy) Any asset that provides the basis for core competence, distinctive performance, or sustainable competitive advantage or that allows a business unit to participate in business opportunities. Part of service strategy is to identify how IT can be viewed as a strategic asset rather than an internal administrative function.
super user	(ITIL® Service Operation) A user who helps other users and assists in communication with the service desk or other parts of the IT service provider. Super users are often experts in the business processes supported by an IT service and will provide support for minor incidents and training.
supplier	(ITIL® Service Design) (ITIL® Service Strategy) A third party responsible for supplying goods or services that are required to deliver IT services. Examples of suppliers include commodity hardware and software vendors, network and telecom providers, and outsourcing organizations. See also underpinning contract.
supplier and contract management information system (SCMIS)	(ITIL® Service Design) A set of tools, data, and information that is used to support supplier management. See also service knowledge management system.
technical management	(ITIL® Service Operation) The function responsible for providing technical skills in support of IT services and management of the IT infrastructure. Technical management defines the roles of support groups, as well as the tools, processes, and procedures required.
test	(ITIL® Service Transition) An activity that verifies that a configuration item, IT service, process, etc. meets its specification or agreed requirements.

Term	Definition
third party	A person, organization, or other entity that is not part of the service provider's own organization and is not a customer—for example, a software supplier or a hardware maintenance company. Requirements for third parties are typically specified in contracts that underpin service level agreements. See also underpinning contract.
third-line support	(ITIL® Service Operation) The third level in a hierarchy of support groups involved in the resolution of incidents and investigation of problems. Each level contains more specialist skills, or has more time or other resources.
threat	A threat is anything that might exploit a vulnerability. Any potential cause of an incident can be considered a threat. For example, a fire is a threat that could exploit the vulnerability of flammable floor coverings. This term is commonly used in information security management and IT service continuity management but also applies to other areas, such as problem and availability management.
transition	(ITIL® Service Transition) A change in state, corresponding to a movement of an IT service or other configuration item from one lifecycle status to the next.
trend analysis	(ITIL® Continual Service Improvement) Analysis of data to identify time-related patterns. Trend analysis is used in problem management to identify common failures or fragile configuration items and in capacity management as a modeling tool to predict future behavior. It is also used as a management tool for identifying deficiencies in IT service management processes.
tuning	The activity responsible for planning changes to make the most efficient use of resources. Tuning is most commonly used in the context of IT services and components. Tuning is part of capacity management, which also includes performance monitoring and implementation of the required changes. Tuning is also called optimization, particularly in the context of processes and other nontechnical resources.
Type I service provider	(ITIL® Service Strategy) An internal service provider that is embedded within a business unit. There may be several Type I service providers within an organization.
Type II service provider	(ITIL® Service Strategy) An internal service provider that provides shared IT services to more than one business unit. Type II service providers are also known as shared service units.
Type III service provider	(ITIL® Service Strategy) A service provider that provides IT services to external customers.

Term	Definition
underpinning contract (UC)	(ITIL® Service Design) A contract between an IT service provider and a third party. The third party provides goods or services that support delivery of an IT service to a customer. The underpinning contract defines targets and responsibilities that are required to meet agreed service level targets in one or more service level agreements.
urgency	(ITIL® Service Design) (ITIL® Service Transition) A measure of how long it will be until an incident, problem, or change has a significant impact on the business. For example, a high-impact incident may have low urgency if the impact will not affect the business until the end of the financial year. Impact and urgency are used to assign priority.
user	A person who uses the IT service on a day-to-day basis. Users are distinct from customers, as some customers do not use the IT service directly.
utility	(ITIL® Service Strategy) The functionality offered by a product or service to meet a particular need. Utility can be summarized as 'what the service does' and can be used to determine whether a service is able to meet its required outcomes or is fit for purpose. The business value of an IT service is created by the combination of utility and warranty.
validation	(ITIL® Service Transition) An activity that ensures a new or changed IT service, process, plan, or other deliverable meets the needs of the business. Validation ensures that business requirements are met even though these may have changed since the original design.
verification and audit	(ITIL® Service Transition) The activities responsible for ensuring that information in the configuration management system is accurate and that all configuration items have been identified and recorded. Verification includes routine checks that are part of other processes—for example, verifying the serial number of a desktop PC when a user logs an incident. Audit is a periodic, formal check.
vision	A description of what the organization intends to become in the future. A vision is created by senior management and is used to help influence culture and strategic planning.
vital business function (VBF)	(ITIL® Service Design) Part of a business process that is critical to the success of the business. Vital business functions are an important consideration of business continuity management, IT service continuity management, and availability management.
vulnerability	A weakness that could be exploited by a threat—for example, an open firewall port, a password that is never changed, or a flammable carpet. A missing control is also considered to be a vulnerability.

Term	Definition
warm standby	See intermediate recovery.
warranty	(ITIL® Service Strategy) Assurance that a product or service will meet agreed requirements. This may be a formal agreement, such as a service level agreement or contract, or it may be a marketing message or brand image. Warranty refers to the ability of a service to be available when needed, to provide the required capacity, and to provide the required reliability in terms of continuity and security. Warranty can be summarized as 'how the service is delivered' and can be used to determine whether a service is fit for use. The business value of an IT service is created by the combination of utility and warranty.
work instruction	A document containing detailed instructions that specify exactly what steps to follow to carry out an activity. A work instruction contains much more detail than a procedure and is only created if very detailed instructions are needed.
work order	A formal request to carry out a defined activity. Work orders are often used by change management and by release and deployment management to pass requests to technical management and application management functions.
workaround	(ITIL® Service Operation) Reducing or eliminating the impact of an incident or problem for which a full resolution is not yet available—for example, by restarting a failed configuration item. Workarounds for problems are documented in known error records. Workarounds for incidents that do not have associated problem records are documented in the incident record.

ABBREVIATIONS

Abbreviation	Term
AMIS	Availability management information system
BCM	Business continuity management
BCP	Business continuity plan
BIA	Business impact analysis
BRM	Business relationship manager
CAB	Change advisory board
CI	Configuration item
CMDB	Configuration management database
CMIS	Capacity management information system
CMS	Configuration management system
CSF	Critical success factor
CSI	Continual service improvement
DIKW	Data-to-Information-Knowledge-to-Wisdom
DML	Definitive media library
ECAB	Emergency change advisory board
ISM	Information security management
ISMS	Information security management system
ISP	Internet service provider
IT	Information technology
ITSCM	IT service continuity management
ITSM	IT service management
ITSMF	IT service management forum
KEDB	Known error database
KPI	Key performance indicator
OLA	Operational level agreement
PBA	Pattern of business activity
PDCA	Plan-do-check-act
PIR	Post-implementation review
PMBOK	Project management body of knowledge

Abbreviation	Term
PMI	Project management institute
PRINCE2	Projects in controlled environments
PSO	Projected service outage
QMS	Quality management system
RACI	Responsible, accountable, consulted, and informed
RFC	Request for change
ROI	Return on investment
SACM	Service asset and configuration management
SCMIS	Supplier and contract management information system
SDP	Service design package
SIP	Service improvement plan
SKMS	Service knowledge management system
SLA	Service level agreement
SLM	Service level management
SLP	Service level package
SLR	Service level requirement
SMART	Specific, measurable, achievable, relevant, and time-bound
SMIS	Security management information system
UC	Underpinning contract
VBF	Vital business function
VOI	Value on investment

CERTIFICATION

ITIL® Certification Pathways

There are many pathway options that are available once you have acquired your ITIL® Foundation Certification. Below illustrates the possible pathways that are available to you. Currently it is intended that the highest certification is the ITIL® V3 Expert, considered to be equal to that of Diploma Status.

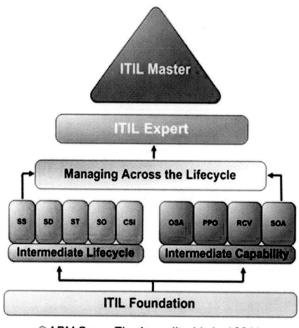

©APM Group-The Accreditor Limited 2011

Figure 12.A—ITIL® Certification Pathway

For more information on certification and available programs, please visit our **website:** http://theartofservice.com

ISO/IEC 20000 Pathways

ISO/IEC 20000 STANDARD IS BECOMING a basic requirement for IT service providers and is fast becoming the most recognized symbol of quality regarding IT Service Management processes. Once you have acquired your ITIL® Foundation Certification, you are eligible to pursue the ISO/IEC 20000 certification pathways. ISO/IEC 20000 programs aim to assist IT professionals master and understand the standard and issues relating to earning standards compliance.

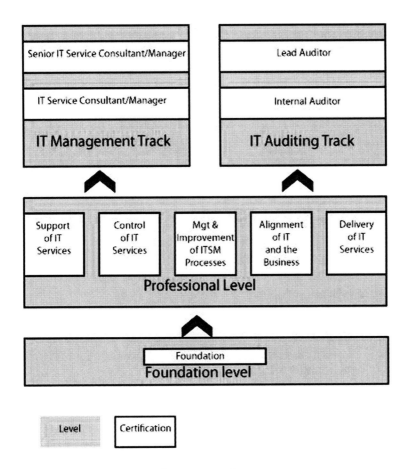

Figure 12.B—ISO/IEC 20000 Certification Pathway

For more information on certification and available programs, please visit our **website:** http://theartofservice.com

INDEX

D